汉语国际中医药文化推广及特色专业建设项目·**双语教材**

Chinese International Chinese Medical Culture Promotion and
Characteristic Major Construction Project · Bilingual Textbooks

常用保健中药及膳食配方

Common Chinese Medicine for Health Care and Medicated Recipes

主　编｜许东升　左　艇

Chief Editors｜XuDongsheng　Zuo Ting

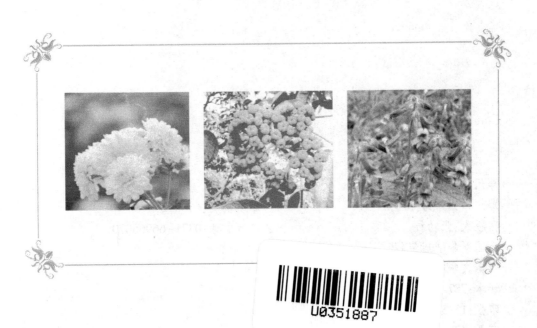

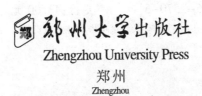

郑州大学出版社

Zhengzhou University Press

郑　州

Zhengzhou

图书在版编目(CIP)数据

常用保健中药及膳食配方/许东升,左艇主编. —郑州:郑州
大学出版社,2017.10

ISBN 978-7-5645-2570-5

Ⅰ.①常… Ⅱ.①许…②左… Ⅲ.①中药材-养生(中医)
Ⅳ.①R212②R282

中国版本图书馆 CIP 数据核字(2015)第 231452 号

郑州大学出版社出版发行
郑州市大学路 40 号　　　　　　　　　邮政编码:450052
出版人:张功员　　　　　　　　　　　发行电话:0371-66966070
全国新华书店经销
河南文华有限公司印制
开本:787 mm×1 092 mm　1/16
印张:15.5
字数:478 千字
版次:2017 年 10 月第 1 版　　　　　　印次:2017 年 10 月第 1 次印刷

书号:ISBN 978-7-5645-2570-5　　　　定价:43.00 元

汉语国际中医药文化推广及特色专业建设项目/《常用保健中药及膳食配方》编委会

Chinese International Chinese Medical Culture Promotion and Characteristic Major Construction Project *Common Chinese Medicine for Health Care and Medicated Recipes* Editorial Board

序

　　孙思邈是我国唐代著名的医学家、养生家,由于养生得法享年百余岁。对于饮食,道家较早提出统治者应当满足人们的温饱同时提倡人们注意节俭少食,老子把能否以人们的甘其食作为统治者治理一方的政绩作为考察标准之一并做到甘其食;庄子倡导食不知所味与老子的甘其食在内涵上是一致的,基本上是以人们的温饱问题为前提而不特别讲究美味佳肴。到了夏商周时代,祖国医学和烹饪学已经发展日趋成熟,人们已经熟知饮食营养和中药治疗对于人体健康来讲同样重要,从整体观出发通过自身的调摄(尤其是某些药物与食物的搭配)以达到强身健体、防病治病、延年益寿的目的。以周朝的医事制度为例,食医居所有医师之首,充分体现了人们当时对食疗的重视。中医养生由整体观出发,讲求人体与环境的和谐与宝命全形,重视身心的交互影响,强调对时令地域的顺应,而且特别注意生活调理和体质锻炼,以扶助自身正气。

　　养生因人而异:健康人群——防患未然;亚健康者——防微杜渐;患病之人——祛病康复;不治之症——带病延年。故言"五谷为养""民以食为天""药补不如食补"。中国民间的养生与修炼之道蕴含着民族文化的哲理,讲究人与自然的协调统一。《素问·五常政大论》提及:"病有久新,方有大小,有毒无毒,固宜常制矣。大毒治病,十去其六;常毒治病,十去其七;小毒治病,十去其八;无毒治病,十去其九。谷肉果菜,食养尽之,无使过之,伤其正也。不尽,行复如法。"于是,遵循自然规律,调节人的日常活动,成为中国养生的基础。

Preface

Sun Simiaowho lived in Tangdynastywas a famous medical scientist and an expert in health preservation. Due to proper health preserving methods, He lived for more than one hundred years. In ancient times, Daoists put forward that governors should meet people's basic demands of food and clothing. Meanwhile, they advocated the thrifty in diet. Laozi tooke the ability of meeting people's eating demands as a standard to evaluate the governors' political achievements. Zhuangzi advocated the concept of eating without tasting the flavor, which means the basic life necessities are people's main concern. In the dynasties of Xia, Shang and Zhou, the traditional medicine and gastronomy became more and more mature. People then were familiar with the equal importance of food nuitrion and Chinese medicinal treatment. Based on the wholism, they took care of themselves through the proper combination of some drugs and food to strengthen the body, prevent and treat diseases and lengthen their life. Take the medical system in Zhou dynasty as an example, dieticians rank at the top of all kinds of doctors, which fully presented people's emphasis on diet therapy. According to the Traditional Chinese Medicine (TCM), to keep themselves healthy and support their vital qi, people should keep their bodies and the environment in harmony to keep healthy, valuing the interaction between the body and mind, emphasizing the adaptation to seasons and regions, especially paying attention to life regulation and physical exercises.

Health preservation methods vary from person to person; healthy people should take preventive measures; subhealthy people should take every precaution at beginning; diseased people should get rid of illnesses and rehabilitate; people with incurable diseases shuld extend the longevity with diseases. There are some sayings about that: "Nourish with grains"; "People take the food as their god. "; "Medicinal nourishment is inferior to food nourishment". The popular methods of health preservation and cultivation contain the philosophy of the national culture and stress on the harmony and unity of human and the nature. According to the Wuchangzheng Dalunpian (Major discussion on the administration of five-motions) in Suwen (Essential questions from Huangdi's canon of medicine), "Diseases are either chronic or new; prescriptions are either large or small; drugs are either toxic or nontoxic. There are certainly rules for taking them. To use drugs with great toxicity to treat a disease, the rule is to stop the use of it when 60% of the disease is cured; to use drugs with moderate toxicity to treat a disease, the rule is to stop the use of it when 70% of disease is cured; to use drugs with mild toxicity to treat disease, the rule is to stop the use of it when 80% of the disease is cured; to use drugs with no toxicity to treat disease, the rule is to stop the use of it when 90% of the disease is cured. Then the patient should take food, meat, fruit and vegetables to build up the health. Care should be taken to prevent excessive use of drugs lest Zhengqi (Healthy qi) be damaged. If Xie (Evil) is not fully eliminated, drugs can be used with the methods mentioned above. " Therefore, corforming to the natural law and regulating people's daily activities have become the foundation of Chinese health preservation.

前言

随着经济和社会的快速发展、工作生活环境及饮食习惯的改变，同时也伴随着日益增长的压力给人们带来了无尽的隐形疾病或者说为各种疾病的发生埋下了伏笔，而这个伏笔就是"亚健康"。据世界卫生组织一项全球性调查结果表明，全世界真正健康的人仅占5%，经医生检查、诊断有病的人也只占20%，75%的人处于亚健康状态。我国约有60%人处于亚健康状态。这样的形势，使得亚健康状态越来越引起广大医学工作者的关注。对这类疾病的认知和治疗缺乏深入了解，不仅延误患者病情还造成医疗资源的过度浪费。

针对上述情况，为适应需求，编者本着中医养生学是一种健康的身体管理学的观念，全面系统总结了各个常见系统的常见病的养生方剂及药膳。全书共分为三大部分：首先是第一部分——常用百种天然药物，着重介绍了常见常用的养生保健单味中药，日常可药食两用。其次是第二部分——各系统常见病的治疗及其预防，主要内容为养生药膳部分，内容丰富，条理清晰，体例规范。最后列举了一部分历代的医家功效显著的养生方剂，以供老年人和慢性病患者使用，但是在运用过程中有任何疑问需要咨询相关专业人士，切记不可随意乱用，要结合自己的体质和病情情况，辨证施治，以避免任何意外发生。

编　者

Foreword

With the rapid development of economy and society, accompanied by the change of working and living environments and eating habits, the increasing pressure has paved the way for the " sub-health " , which means endless hidden diseases. According to a global investigation result of the World Health Organization, the truly healthy people account for only 5% of the world population, people with diagnosed diseases account for only 20% , and 75% of people are in the sub-health state. In China, about 60% of people are in the sub-health state. Such a situation, the sub-health state has drawn increasing concern of more and more medical workers. Lacking deep understanding of the cognition and treatment of these diseases not only delay the patient's condition but also caused the excessive waste of medical resources.

Under such circumstances, in order to meet the demand, based on the concept of taking TCM nurturing as a healthy body management discipline, editors of this book completely and systematically summarizes the nurturing formula and medicated food for common diseases of every system. The book is divided into three parts: first, one hundred common natural drugs are introduced from their functions in drugs and food. Second, the treatment and prevention of common diseases in every system are introduced. At last, some nurturing formula of famous doctors in the history are introduced for elderly people and patients with chronic diseases. During the application process, if you have any doubts, please inquire professionals. Remember not to use it causully. Please make treatments according to different syndromes, constitutions and states of illness so as to avoid any accidents.

Editors

目录

方剂及药膳篇 Prescriptions

常用保健中药篇
Common Health Care Chinese Medicine

1. 枸杞子 Barbary Wolf Berry

Gouqi Zi (Fructus Lycii)

形态特征：为茄科植物宁夏枸杞的干燥成熟果实，呈类纺锤形或椭圆形，表面红色或暗红色，顶端有小突起状的花柱痕，基部有白色的果梗痕。果皮柔韧，皱缩；果肉肉质，柔润。

Morphology：The dry ripe fruit of Ningxia Gouqi (Fructus Lycii) (Fam. Solanaceae). It has a spindle or oval-like shape with red or dark red surface, the apex with small bumps style mark on the top and white stem scar on the base. The fruit skin is flexible, tough and wrinkled; the fruit is fleshy and soft.

别称：又称甜菜子、红青椒、枸蹄子、枸杞果、地骨子、枸茄茄、红耳坠、血枸子、枸地芽子、枸杞豆、血杞子、津枸杞。

Byname：Also called Tian Caizi, Hong Qingjiao, Gou Tizi, Gouqi Guo, Digu Zi, Gou Qieqie, Hong Er'zhui, Xue Gouzi, Gou Diyazi, Gouqi Dou, Xue Qizi, Jin Gouqi.

功效：养肝，滋肾，润肺。

Efficacy：Nourishing the liver and kidney and moistening the lung.

主治病症：肝肾亏虚；头晕目眩；目视不清；腰膝酸软；阳痿遗精；虚劳咳嗽；消渴引饮。

Indications：Liver-kidney deficiency, dizziness, weak eyesight, sore and weak waist and knees, impotence and seminal emission, cough due to consumptive disease, dispersion thirst with intake of fluid.

性味归经：入肺、肾经。

Medicinal properties：Enters lung and kidney meridians.

用量用法：内服煎汤，5~15 g；或入丸、散、膏、酒剂。

Usage and dosage：5 ~ 15 g is used in decoction, pill, powder, paste preparations or medicated wine.

注意事项：能治肝虚、迎风流泪、目暗视弱，并可长肌肉、益面色。枸杞子有滋补肝肾、益精明目作用。

Notes：It is applied for people with liver deficiency, lacrimation due to wind irritation, weak eyesight and is also beneficial for muscle and complexion, with the functions of nourishing the liver and kidney nourishment, vital essence replenishment and eyesight improvement.

2. 黄精 Solomonseal Rhizome

Huang Jing(Polygonatum Sibiricum)

形态特征：为百合科植物滇黄精、黄精或多花黄精的干燥根茎。呈肉质的结节块状。表面淡黄色至黄棕色，具环节，有皱纹及须根痕，结节上侧茎痕呈圆盘状。质硬而韧，不易折断，断面角质，淡黄色至黄棕色。

Morphology：The dry rhizome of, Dian huang Jing(Polygonatum kingianum Coll. et Hemsl.), Huang Jing(Polygonatum Sibiricum) or Duohua Huang Jing(Polygonatum cyrtonema)(Fam. Lilaceae). It has a fleshy nodules block-like shape, faint yellow to yellowish brown surface, with segment, wrinkles, and fibrous root scar on it. There are disc-like marks on nodules. The texture is solid and tough, hard to break; section is cutin, pale yellow to yellowish brown color.

别称：又称老虎姜、鸡头参。

Byname：Also called Laohu Jiang, Jitou Shen.

功效：补气养阴，健脾，润肺，益肾

Efficacy：Reinforcing qi and nourishing yin; strengthening spleen; moisturizing lung; tonifying kidney.

主治病症：阴虚劳嗽；肺燥咳嗽；脾虚乏力；食少口干；消渴；肾亏腰膝酸软；阳痿遗精；耳鸣目暗；须发早白；体虚羸瘦。

Indication：Over-strained cough due to yin deficiency; xeropulmonary cough; acratia due to spleen deficiency; poor eating and dry mouth; wasting-thirst; sour-weak waist and knee due to kidney deficiency; impotence and seminal emission; tinnitus and poor eye-sight; early white beard and hair; weakness and thinness.

性味归经：甘，平。入脾、肺、肾经。

Medicinal properties：Sweet and bland in flavor; enters the spleen, lung and kidney meridians.

用量用法：煎服，10～30 g。

Usage and dosage：10～30 g is used in decoction.

注意事项：凡脾虚有湿，咳嗽痰多及中寒泄泻者均忌用黄精。

Notes：It is contraindicated for spleen deficiency with dampness, cough with excessive phlegm and middle cold with diahhrea.

3. 地黄 Rehmannia Root

Di Huang(Radix Rehmanniae)

形态特征：为玄参科植物地黄的新鲜或干燥块根。多呈不规则的团块状,中间膨大,两端细小。表面棕黑色,极皱缩,具不规则的横曲纹。体重,质较软而韧,不易折断,断面棕黑色或乌黑色,有光泽,具黏性。

Morphology：The fresh or dry root of Di Huang (Radix Rehmanniae) (Fam. Scrophulariaceae). Usually it is an irregular block, the center enlarged and small on both ends. The surface is dark brown, easy to shrink, with irregular transversal twist lines. It is heavy in weight, soft and tough, hard to break, section dark brown or black, shiny and sticky.

别称：酒壶花、山烟根。

Byname：Jiuhu Hua, Shanyan Gen

功效：生地黄：清热凉血,养阴,生津。

Efficacy：Shengdihuang(Rehmannia Root)：removing heat to cool blood, nourishing yin, regenerating body fluid.

主治病症：用于热病伤阴,舌绛烦渴,发斑发疹,吐血,衄血,咽喉肿痛。

Indication：Consumption of yin caused by febrile disease, dark red tongue and polydipsia, macula and exanthesis; hematemesis, non-traumatic hemorrhage, swelling and sour throat.

性味归经：熟地味甘,微温;生地黄甘,寒。入心、肝、肾经。

Medicinal properties：The cooked rehmannia root(Radix Rehmanniae Preparata)is sweet in flavor and slightly warm in property; the dried/fresh rehmannia root (Radix Rehmaniae Recens)sweet in flavor and cold in property; enters the heart, liver and kidney meridians.

用量用法：煎服,10 ~ 30 g。

Usage and dosage：10 ~ 30 g is used in decoction.

4. 韭菜 Chinese Leek

Jiu Cai(Allium Tuberosum Rottl.)

形态特征：为百合科植物韭的叶。

Morphology：The leave of Chinese leek(Allium tuberosum Rottl.)(Fam. Lilaceae)

别称：又名草钟乳、起阳草或壮阳草等。

Byname：Cao Zhongru, Qiyang Cao, Zhuangyang Cao

功效：补肾壮阳,健脾暖胃。

Efficacy：Reinforcing kidney to strengthen yang, strengthening spleen and warming stomach.

主治病症：肾阳虚弱,腰膝酸冷,阳痿早泄,小便频数等;脾胃虚寒,噎嗝反胃,腹中冷痛,泄泻或便秘等。

Indication：Kidney yang deficiency, sour – cold lumbus and knees; impotence and premature ejaculation, frequent urination; spleen–stomach insufficiency–cold, dysphagia and regurgitation, abdominal crymodynia, diarrhea or constipation.

性味归经：性温,味辛。入脾、胃、肾经。

Medicinal properties：Warm in property, pungent in flavor; spleen, enters the stomach and kidney meridians.

用量用法：内服捣汁饮,每日 50～100 g,或炒熟做菜食。外用:取汁滴注,炒热煨或煎水熏洗。

Usage and dosage：50～100 g is taken after being smashed into juice or fried to make a dish daily; or dripped with smashed juice, stewed after being fried hot or steam bathed with its decoction externally.

注意事项：韭菜性偏温热,凡阴虚内热或眼疾、疮疡毒不宜食用。

Notes：It is contraindicated for yin deficiency with internal heat, eye diseases, swelling and toxin of sores because of its slightly warm and hot property.

5. 核桃仁 Walnut Kernel

Hetao Ren(Semen Juglandis)

形态特征：为胡桃科植物胡桃的干燥成熟种子。本品多破碎,为不规则的块状,有皱曲的沟槽,大小不一;完整者类球形。种皮淡黄色或黄褐色,膜状,维管束脉纹深棕色。

Morphology：The dry ripe seed of walnut (Juglans regia L. var. sinensis DC.) (Fam. Juglandaceae). It is mostly broken, irregular clumps, have wrinkling grooves, and variable in size . The integrate seed is a kind of spherical. The seed coat is light yellow or yellow–brown in color, membranous, vascular bundles veins are dark brown.

别称：又名胡桃肉。

Byname：Hutao Rou

功效：补肾固精,温肺定喘,乌发润肌,润肠通便。

Efficacy：Tonifying kidney to arrest spontaneous emission, warming lung and relieving asthma, darkening hair and moistening skin, loosening bowel to relieve constipation.

主治病症：肺肾亏虚,久咳气短而喘,遇寒及活动加剧,甚则张口抬肩;或肾气虚衰,腰痛膝软,耳鸣乏力,阳痿早泄,梦遗滑精以及须发早白、大便燥结等。

Indication：Deficiency of lung and kidney, short breath and wheezing due to long–term cough(more serious in cold weather); deficiency of kidney qi, aching waist and weak knee, strepitus aurium and weak, impotence and premature ejaculation, spermatorrhea, early white beard and hair whiten and dry feces.

性味归经：性温，味甘。入肺、肾经。

Medicinal properties：Warm in property，sweet in flavor；enters the lung and kidney meridians.

用量用法：内服，每日 10～30 g，水煎服或研末服。

Usage and dosage：10～30 g is used in decoction or powder preparations daily.

注意事项：核桃仁性温，含多量油脂，不宜多食，否则易生热聚痰。凡痰内盛引起的痰黄、发热气喘、烦躁呕恶和阴虚火旺的吐血、鼻出血等均忌用。大便稀薄者也不宜用。

Notes：Since the kernel is warm in property and is abundant in oil，large intake of it generates heat and accumulates the phlegm. It is contraindicated for yellow phlegm due to excessive internal phlegm，fever with asthma，irritation with nausea and retching，blood ejection and nasal hemorrhage，etc. It's also unsuitable for people with thin sloppy stool.

6. 百合 Lily Bulb

Bai He（Bulbus Lilii）

形态特征：为百合科植物卷丹、百合或细叶百合的干燥肉质鳞叶。呈长椭圆形。表面黄白色至淡棕黄色，有的微带紫色，有数条纵直平行的白色维管束。顶端稍尖，基部较宽，边缘薄，微波状，略向内弯曲。质硬而脆，断面较平坦，角质样。

Morphology：The dry fleshy scale leaf of Juandan（Lilium tigrinum Ker Gawl.）Baihe（Bulbus Lilii），Xiye Baihe（Lilium tenifolium Fisch.）. It is long oval in shape. The surface is yellow–white to light tan，and some slightly purple，with several longitudinal parallel vascular bundles on it. The leaf is slightly pointed at the top，base broad，margin thin，wavy，and slightly bent inwards，with a hard and brittle quality and flat cutin section.

别称：又名百合蒜、夜合花、白花百合、蒜脑薯等。

Byname：Also called Baihe Suan，Yehe Hua，Baihua Baihe，Suannao Shu

功效：养阴润肺，清心安神。

Efficacy：Nourishing yin and moisturizing lung，easing mental anxiety.

主治病症：主治心阴亏虚，虚烦口渴，心悸怔忡，失眠多梦，神志恍惚；肺阴亏虚，干咳少痰，痰中带血，潮热盗汗等。

Indication：Heart yin deficiency，deficient dysphoria and dipsia，severe palpitation，insomnia and dreaminess，staring spells；lung yin deficiency，dry cough with little phlegm，blood phlegm，hectic fever and night sweat.

性味归经：性微寒，味甘、微苦。入心、肺经。

Medicinal properties：Slightly cold in property，sweet and slightly bitter in flavor；enters heart and lung meridians.

用量用法：内服煎汤，每日 9～30 g；蒸食或煮粥食。外用：捣敷。

Usage and dosage: 9 ~ 30 g is used in decoction daily or taken after being steamed or cooked in porridge; or smashed and applied externally.

注意事项:百合性偏寒凉,脾胃虚寒所致的脘腹冷痛、泄泻和外感风寒所致的咳嗽均忌用。

Notes: Since the lily bulb is slightly cold and cool in property, it is contraindicated for cold pain in the stomach duct and abdomen due to the deficiency and coldness of spleen and stomach, diarrhea and cough due to external wind cold.

7. 松子仁 Pinenut Kernel

Songzi Ren(Pinus Pinea)

形态特征:本品为松科植物红松的种子。

Morphology: The seed of the Korean pine(Pinus Koraiensis)(Fam. Pinaceae)

功效:滋阴润肺,润肠通便,养肝息风。

Efficacy: Nourishing yin and moisturizing lung, loosening bowel to relieve constipation, nourishing liver and extinguishing wind.

主治病症:肺阴亏虚,干咳少痰,时有咯血,皮肤干燥等;大肠阴亏,大便秘结,排便困难等;肝血亏虚,头晕目眩,耳鸣咽干,视物模糊等。

Indication: Lung yin deficiency, dry cough with little phlegm, hemoptysis, xerosis cutis; large intestine yin – deficiency, constipation, difficult defecation; hepatic blood deficiency, dizziness, tinnitus and dry pharynx, poor eyesight.

性味归经:性微温,味甘。入肺、大肠、肝经。

Medicinal properties: Slightly warm in property and sweet in flavor; enters lung and kidney meridians.

用量用法:内服煎汤,每日 5 ~ 45 g,或入膏丸。也可炒熟食用。

Usage and dosage: 5 ~ 15 g is used in the decoction daily; or used in paste and pills or fried to be taken.

注意事项:海松子滋腻滑肠,脾胃虚弱,大便溏泄和脾湿内盛,胸闷食少,脘胀呕吐均忌用。霉变的海松子不能食用。

Notes: Rich and slimy korean pine seeds lubricate the intestines, which are contraindicated for people suffering from the deficiency of spleen and stomach with loose stool and exuberant spleen dampness with thoracic oppression, decreased food intake and abdominal distention with vomiting. Moldy Korean pine seeds are inedible.

8. 黑大豆 Black Bean

Hei Dadou(Glycinemax(L.)Merr)

形态特征：本品为豆科植物大豆的干燥成熟种子。

Morphology：The dry ripe seed of the soy bean (Glycinemax(L.)merr.) (Fam. Leguminosae).

别称：又名乌豆、黑豆、冬豆子。

Byname：Wudou, Heidou, Dongdou Zi

功效：滋养肝肾，补虚止汗，健脾利水，活血解毒。

Efficacy：Nourishing liver and kidney, improving deficiency to stoping excessive sweating, strengthening spleen to alleviate water retention, activating blood circulation for detoxication.

主治病症：肝肾阴虚，腰腿酸痛，头目眩晕，耳鸣耳聋，皮肤干燥等；脾虚水泛，周身水肿，小便短少等。

Indication：Liver kidney yin deficiency, sour-aching waist and leg, dizziness, tinnitus and deaf, xerosis cutis; severe water retention due to spleen deficiency, dropsy all over the body and oliguresis.

性味归经：性平，味甘。入肝、脾、肾经。

Medicinal properties：Neutral in property and sweet in flavor; enters the lung and kidney meridians.

用量用法：内服，煎汤，10~30 g，入丸、散。外用：研末掺或煮汁涂。

Usage and dosage：10 ~ 30 g is used in decoction, pills and powder; or ground into powder and mixed with water or boiled to make juice for external application.

注意事项：黑大豆炒食易壅热，伤脾腹胀，老年体虚者不宜炒食。

Notes：Fried black beans often cause heat stagnation, spleen damage and abdominal distention. Elderly people with deficiency are not suitable to take the fried beans.

9. 龙眼肉 Longan Aril

Longyan Rou(Arillus Longan)

形态特征：为无患子科植物龙眼的假种皮。为纵向破裂的不规则薄片，或呈囊状。棕黄色至棕褐色，半透明。外表面皱缩不平，内表面光亮而有细纵皱纹。薄片者质柔润，囊状者质稍硬。

Morphology：The aril of longan (Dimocarpus longgana Lour) (Fam. Sapindaceae). Shown as longitudinal broken irregular flakes or cystic in shape, with tan to brown color, translucent. The surface is shrinking and the inner surface is bright, with fine longitudinal wrinkles. The wafer is soft and moist, and the cystic form is a bit hard.

别称：俗称桂圆肉。

Byname：It is commonly called Guiyuan Rou.

功效：益心脾,补气血,安神。

Efficacy：Benefiting heart and spleen, reinforcing qi and blood, calming nerves.

主治病症：气血不足,虚劳羸瘦,面色无华,神疲乏力,浮肿等;心血亏虚,心悸失眠、眼花,健忘易惊等。

Indication：Insufficiency of vital energy and blood, thinness due to consumption, dark complexion, spiritlessness and powerlessness, edema; heart blood deficiency, palpitation and insomnia, dim eyesight, amnesia and hyperarousal.

性味归经：性温,味甘。入心、脾经。

Medicinal properties：Warm in property and sweet in flavor; enters the heart and spleen meridians.

用量用法：内服,煎汤,6~15 g;熬膏、浸酒或入丸剂。

Usage and dosage：6~15 g is used in decoction, paste, wine or pill preparations.

注意事项：凡内有痰火及湿滞停饮者禁服。

Notes：Contraindicated for people with internal phlegm-fire and damp stagnation and fluid retention.

10. 山药 Common Yam Rhizome

Shan Yao (Rhizoma Dioscoreae)

形态特征：为薯蓣科植物薯蓣的干燥根茎。为不规则的厚片,皱缩不平,切面白色或黄白色,质坚脆,粉性。

Morphology：The dry rhizome of Dioscoreaceae (Dioscorea opposite) (Fam. Dioscoreaceae). It is irregular slabs, wrinkled. The cut section is white or yellowish-white, hard, brittle and powdery in quality.

别称：又名薯蓣、山芋、山薯、蛇芋、怀山药、野白薯等。

Byname：Shuyu, Shanyu, Shanshu, Sheyu, Huai Shanyao, Ye Baishu

功效：补益脾肺,固肾益精,滋养气阴。

Efficacy：Benefiting spleen and lung, strengthening kidney to increase essence, nourishing qi and yin.

主治病症：脾胃气虚,食少,泄泻,神疲,体倦等;肺阴虚,干咳,口燥咽干,男子遗精,女子月经不调等;气阴不足,消渴,口渴思饮,尿多乏力等。

Indication：Deficiency of spleen-qi and stomach-qi, poor eating, diarrhea, spiritlessness and powerlessness; lung yin deficiency, dry cough, dry mouth and pharynx, spermatorrhea and menoxenia; deficiency of qi and yin, wasting thirst, dipsia, frequent urination and acratia.

性味归经：性平，味甘。入脾、肺、肾经。

Medicinal properties：Neutral in property and sweet in flavor; enters the lung and kidney meridians.

用量用法：内服煎汤，每日用量 30 ~ 60 g；或入丸、散。外用：捣敷。

Usage and dosage：30 ~ 60 g is used in decoction daily; or used in pill and powder preparations; or is smashed and applied externally.

注意事项：有实邪者忌服。不宜与甘遂同用。

Notes：Contraindicated for people with excessive syndrome. It is incompatible with Gansui root(Radix Euphorbiae Kansui).

11. 莲子 Lotus Seed

Lianzi(Stamen Nelumbinis)

形态特征：为睡莲科植物莲的干燥成熟种子。略呈椭圆形或类球形。表面红棕色，有细纵纹和较宽的脉纹。一端中心呈乳头状突起，棕褐色，多有裂口，其周边略下陷。质硬，种皮薄，不易剥离。

Morphology：The dry ripe seed of Lotus (Nelumbonucifera) (Fam. Nymphaeaceae). It is slightly oval or spherical-like in shape. The surface is reddish brown, with thin vertical lines and wide veins on it. The center is brown papillae on one end, having many cracks and slightly sinks around the edge. It is hard , with thin seed skin, not easy to peel.

别称：又名藕实、莲实、莲蓬子。

Byname：Oushi, Lianshi, Lianpeng Zi

功效：补益心气，健脾止泻，补肾固精。

Efficacy：Benefiting heart qi, strengthening spleen to check diarrhea, tonifying kidney to arrest spontaneous emission.

主治病症：脾虚，便溏，痢疾，食欲不振；或心肾不交，失眠多梦，心悸，五心烦热；或肾虚失摄，精关不固，遗精，滑泄，带下量多，尿频，遗尿，尿失禁等症。

Indication：Kidney asthenia, loose stool, dysentery, poor appetite; or heart yang kidney yin incoordination, insomnia and dreaminess, palpitation, burning sensation of five centres; or kidney's failure to absorb qi and arrest spontaneous emission due to kidney asthenia, spermatorrhea, slipping diarrhea, more morbid leucorrhea, frequent micturition, enuresis and uroclepsia.

性味归经：性平，味甘、涩。入心、脾、肾经。

Medicinal properties：Neutral in property and sweet and astringent in flavor; enters the heart, spleen and kidney meridians.

用量用法：内服煎汤，每日 10 ~ 50 g；或入丸、散。

Usage and dosage:10 ~ 50 g is used in decoction daily,or used in pill and powder preparations.

注意事项:本品收涩,易于恋邪,凡腹胀痞满,大便燥结及感冒、疟疾、痔疮、疳积等不宜食用。

Notes:The lotus seed induces astringency and is apt to keep the pathogens. Therefore it's unsuitable for people with abdominal fullness and distention with dry stool,or common cold,malaria,hemorrhoid or infantile malnutrition.

12. 益智仁 Bitter Cardamon

Yizhi Ren(Fructus Alpiniae Oxyphyllae)

形态特征:为姜科植物益智的干燥成熟果实。呈椭圆形,两端略尖。表面棕色或灰棕色,有纵向凹凸不平的突起棱线 13 ~ 20 条,顶端有花被残基,基部常残存果梗。果皮薄而稍韧,与种子紧贴,种子集结成团,中有隔膜将种子团分为 3 瓣。

Morphology:The dry ripe fruit of Yizhi(Fructus Alpinae Oxyphyllae)(Fam. Zingiberaceae). It is oval and slightly pointed on both ends. The surface is brown or gray brown,with 13 ~ 20 longitudinal uneven ridge lines. It has perianth residues on the top and often has remaining fruit stem on the base. The fruit skin is thin and a bit tough,clung and gathered together with seed. The seed mass is divided into 3 sections by diaphragm.

功效:温补固摄,暖脾止泻摄唾,温肾固精缩尿。

Efficacy:Warming and tonifying kidney to promote absorption of qi,warming spleen to check diarrhea,warming kidney to arrest spontaneous emission and polyuria.

主治病症:脾肾虚寒,腹痛腹泻;或肾气虚寒,小便频数,遗尿,遗精,白浊;或脾胃虚寒所致的慢性泄泻及口中唾液外流而不能控制者。

Indication:Asthenia cold spleen and kidney,abdominal pain and diarrhea;asthenia cold spleen qi,frequent urination,enuresis,spermatorrhea and gonoblennorrhea;or chronic diarrhea and uncontrolled saliva outflow due to spleen-stomach insufficiency-cold.

性味归经:性温,味辛。归脾、肾经。

Medicinal properties:Warm in property and pungent in flavor,enters the spleen and kidney meridians.

用量用法:内服煎汤,3 ~ 9 g;或入丸、散。

Usage and dosage:3 ~ 9 g is used in decoction,pill or powder preparations.

注意事项:本品燥热,能伤阴动火,故阴虚火旺或热证尿频、遗精、多涎者忌用。

Notes:With dry and hot properties,the bitter cardamon damages yin and flares up,therefore is contraindicated for people with yin deficiency and excessive fire,or heat syndrome,polyuria,spermatorrhea and hypersalivation,etc.

13. 墨旱莲 Eclipta

Hanlian Cao(Eclipta Alba)

形态特征:为菊科植物鳢肠的干燥地上部分。全体被白色茸毛。茎呈圆柱形,有纵棱;表面绿褐色或墨绿色。叶对生,近无柄,叶片皱缩卷曲或破碎,完整者展平后呈长披针形,全缘或具浅齿,墨绿色。头状花序。瘦果椭圆形而扁。

Morphology:The dry ground part of lichang(Eclipta prostrate)(Fam. Asteraceae). It is covered with white fuzz. The stems is cylindrical, with longitudinal ribs, and its surface is greenish brown or blackish green. The leaves are opposite, nearly sessile, curly wrinkled or broken. A complete leaf is long lanceolate after flattened, with entire or slightly jagged margin, blackish green in color. It is capitulum. Its achene is flat oval.

别称:如搓揉鲜草茎叶,则有墨汁样液体流出,所以又名"墨旱莲"。

Byname:It is also called"Mo Hanlian"(Inky Herba Ecliptae)since inky fluids flow from the stems and leaves after being rubbed. It is the whole herb of Lichang(Eclipta prostrata)(also called Jinling Cao). (Fam. Composite)

功效:本品是补益肝肾阴液,凉血止血的佳品。

Efficacy:Reinforcing liver benefiting kidney,cooling blood to stop bleeding.

主治病症:肝肾阴虚,头晕目眩,须发早白和各种热性出血等病证。

Indication:Liver kidney yin insufficiency,dizziness,early-whitening beard and hair and all kinds of febrile bleeding symptoms.

性味归经:性寒,味甘、酸。归肝、肾经。

Medicinal properties:Cold in property,sweet and sour in flavor;enters the liver and kidney meridians.

用量用法:常用 10 ~ 15 g,鲜品加倍。亦可人丸、散,或捣计服。

Usage and dosage:The usual dose is 10 ~ 15 g and double when used raw. It can also be used in pill and powder preparations or smashed into juice to be taken.

注意事项:本品性寒,故一般脾胃虚寒,大便泄泻及虚寒性出血者不宜服用。

Notes:The drug is cold-natured,thus it is unsuitable for people with deficient and cold spleen and stomach,diarrhea and hemorrhage due to cold deficiency.

14. 玉竹 Fragrant Solomonseal Rhizome

Yuzhu(Rhizoma Polygonati Odorati)

形态特征:为百合科植物玉竹的干燥根茎。本品呈长圆柱形,略扁,少有分枝。表面黄白色或淡黄棕色,半透明,具纵皱纹和微隆起的环节,有白色圆点状的须根痕和圆盘状茎痕。质硬而脆或稍软,易折断,断面角质样或显颗粒性。气微,味甘,嚼之发黏。

Morphology:The rhizome of Yuzhu (Rhizoma Polygonati Odorati) (Fam. Liliaceae). The product is long cylindrical, a little flat, with few branches. The surface is yellowish-white or yellowish brown, translucent, having longitudinal wrinkles, slightly raised links, white round dot of fibrous scar and disc-like stem scars. It is hard, brittle or slightly soft, easy to broken. The section is cutin or granular,faint smell , sweet taste, and sticky after chewing.

功效:养阴润肺,生津养胃。

Efficacy:Nourishing yin and moisturizing lung, regenerating body fluid and nourishing stomach.

主治病症:肺阴不足之干咳少痰,甚至痰中带血,或胃阴不足,津液缺乏,口渴舌红,饥不欲食等。有补阴而不滋腻、滋养而不恋邪的优点,因此,还可用于治疗素体阴虚、感冒风热而致的发热,微恶风寒,干咳少痰,咽痛口渴,舌红少苔等症。

Indication:Dry cough with less phlegm or blood phlegm due to lung yin deficiency, or lack of body fluid,dipsia and red tongue and poor eating due to stomach yin deficiency. It can be used to treat fever,little aversion to wind cold,dry cough with little phlegm,sour throat and dipsia and red tongue due to yin deficiency and wind heat cold.

性味归经:性平偏寒,味甘。归肺、胃经。

Medicinal properties:Neutral in property and sweet in flavor; enters the lung and stomach meridians.

用量用法:常用 10 ~ 15 g。可熬膏,亦可入丸、散剂。

Usage and dosage:The usual dose is 5 ~ 15 g. It can be used to make paste,pill and powder preparations.

注意事项:本品虽性质平和,但毕竟是滋阴润燥之品,故脾虚有湿疾者不宜服用。

Notes:Though mild in nature,the drug could nourish yin and moisten dryness,thus is unsuitable for people with spleen deficiency and damp diseases.

15. 阿胶 Ass Hide Glue

E Jiao(Colla Corii Asini)

形态特征:为马科动物驴的干燥皮或鲜皮经煎煮、浓缩制成的固体胶。呈长方形块、方形块或丁状。棕色至黑褐色,有光泽。质硬而脆,断面光亮,碎片对光照视呈棕色半透明状。

Morphology:The concentration of colloform made by decoction of fresh or dried skin of ass(Fam. Equidae). It is rectangular block, square piece, or dice in shape, with brown to dark brown color and shiny. It is hard and brittle, and its section is bright. The fragment is light brown and translucent in the light.

功效：补血止血，滋阴润肺。

Efficacy：Tonifying blood and arresting bleeding, nourishing yin and moisturizing lung.

主治病症：血虚而见面色萎黄无华，指甲苍白，头晕眼花，心悸失眠，久咳等，以及咯血、吐血、尿血、便血、衄血等。因本品在治疗妇女各种出血及胎产病证方面尤有特长，故被誉为"妇科圣药"。

Indication：Blood deficiency – caused dark complexion, pale nails, dizziness, palpitation and insomnia, chronic cough, hemoptysis, hematemesis, hemuresis, hematochezia and non – traumatic hemorrhage.

性味归经：性平，味甘。归肺、肝、肾经。

Medicinal properties：Neutral in property and sweet in flavor; enters the lung, liver and kidney meridians.

用量用法：服用阿胶的方法很多，用于一般性调补，通常是用阿胶 5 ~ 10 g，加适量黄酒，隔水蒸炖烊化成液体后服用。为了便于粉碎，又常炒用，炒用者称阿胶珠。

Usage and dosage：The ass hide glue is used in many different ways for the general tonification. Usually 5 ~ 10 g is used with proper amount of yellow wine after being steamed or stewed into liquid. It is often stir-baked in order to be smashed, which is called E'jiao Zhu (Ass hide glue pellets).

注意事项：阿胶质地黏腻。消化能力弱的人不宜应用；素体内热较重，有口干舌燥，潮热盗汗时也不适宜服用阿胶。

Notes：Due to its sticky and rich properties, the ass hide glue is unsuitable for people with weak digestive abilities or people with excessive heat, dry mouth, tidal fever and night sweat.

16. 何首乌 Fleeceflower Root

He Shouwu (Radix Polygoni Multiflori)

形态特征：为蓼科植物何首乌的干燥块根，呈团块状或不规则纺锤形。表面红棕色或红褐色，皱缩不平。体重，断面浅黄棕色或浅红棕色，显粉性，皮部有 4 ~ 11 个类圆形云锦状花纹。

Morphology：The dry root of He Shouwu (Radix polygoni multiflori) (Fam. Polygonaceae). It is block or irregular spindle in shape. Its surface is red brown or reddish brown, wrinkled and heavy in weight. Its section is pale yellow brown or pale red to brown, powdery. There are 4–11 round cloud patterns on the skin.

功效：补益精血，润肠通便，解毒，截疟。

Efficacy：Tonifying blood and essence, loosening bowel to relieve constipation, detoxication, stopping malaria.

主治病症：精血亏虚的头晕眼花，须发早白，腰膝酸软，遗精，妇女带下，或肠燥便秘，或久疟、瘰疬等。

Indication：Dizziness and poor eye sight，early-whitening beard and hair，sour-weak waist and knee，spermatorrhea and morbid leucorrhea caused by deficiency of blood and essence；or constipation due to dryness of the intestine；or chronic malaria and scrofulid.

性味归经：性微温，味苦、甘、涩。归肝、肾经。

Medicinal properties：Slightly warm in property，bitter，sweet and astringent in flavor；enters the liver and kidney meridians.

用量用法：常用10～30 g。服用何首乌的方法，在古代主要是煎汤，或制成丸、膏、酒等内服。现在，药店已有首乌粉、首乌胶囊、首乌茶等商品出售，购服十分方便。何首乌因加工炮制方法不同而有制首乌、生首乌和鲜首乌之别，它们的作用也不一样。一般而言，补肾益精、滋阴养血主要用制首乌；通便、解毒宜用生首乌和鲜首乌。

Usage and dosage：The usual dose is 10～30 g. In ancient times，it is used in decoction or used to make pill，paste and wine preparations to be taken. Nowadays，it is convenient to buy the powder，capsule and tea made of He Shouwu in the drugstore. Different preparations such as prepared，raw or fresh drugs have different effects. Generally speaking，prepared ones are used to tonify the kidney，nourish the essence，enrich yin and the blood，while the raw and fresh ones are used to free the stools and detoxify.

注意事项：服用何首乌时不得同时食用动物血、无鳞鱼、葱蒜、萝卜等。煎制何首乌时忌用铁器。

Notes：The drug is incompatible with animal blood，alepidotes，scallions，garlics and radishes. It shouldn't be decocted in iron containers.

17. 白术 Largehead Atractylodes Rhizome

Baizhu（Rhizoma Atractylodis Macrocephalae）

形态特征：为菊科植物白术的干燥根茎，为不规则的肥厚团块。表面灰黄色，有瘤状突起，并有须根痕，顶端有残留茎基和芽痕。质坚硬不易折断，断面不平坦，黄白色至淡棕色，有棕黄色的点状油室散在；烘干者断面角质样，色较深或有裂隙。

Morphology：The dry roots of Baizhu（Rhizoma Atractylodis Macrocephalae）.（Fam. Compositae）. It is irregular fat lump in shape. The surface is gray with nodular bumps and fibrous scar on it，the stem base and bud scar remains on the top. It is hard and not easy to break. The section is uneven，yellowish-white to light brown，with tan oil-cavity dot scattered on it. The dried section is cutin-like，dark in color，or having cracks on it.

功效：补气健脾，燥湿利水，止汗安胎。

Efficacy：Reinforcing qi and strengthening spleen，eliminating dampness to alleviate water retention，hidroschesis and soothing fetus.

主治病症：脾虚食少，消化不良，慢性腹泻，或脾虚失运，水湿停聚之痰饮、水肿以及气虚多汗，胎动不安等症。

Indication: Poor eating due to spleen asthenia, dyspepsia, chronic diarrhea, or phlegm-rheum, edema, qi-asthenia hyperhidrosis and fetal irritability due to spleen's failure to function and water-damp stagnation.

性味归经:性温,味甘、苦。归脾、胃经。

Medicinal properties: Warm in property, sweet and bitter in flavor; enters the spleen and stomach meridians.

用量用法:每日常用量 5～15 g,水煎服。生用或炒用,也可熬膏服食及泡酒常饮。生用长于利水,止汗;炒用偏于补脾燥湿,安胎,可根据病情需要,选择应用。

Usage and dosage: The usual dose is 5～15 g daily, which is used in decoction, or used raw or fried, or used in paste and wine for taking. The raw use induces diuresisa and checks sweating; the use after stir-bake tonifies the spleen, dries the dampness and prevents miscarriage. It can be chosen according to different diseases.

注意事项:本品苦温而性燥,用之不当能耗阴伤津,所以热病津伤,口干舌燥,或阴虚内热的患者均不宜用。

Notes: The drug is bitter and warm in flavor and dry in property. The improper use of it exhausts yin and damages the fluid, thus it is unsuitable for patients with heat syndrome with fluid damage, dry mouth and tongue, or yin deficiency with internal heat.

18. 绞股蓝 Fiveleaf Gynostemma Herb

Jiaogu Lan (Gynostemma Pentaphylla)

形态特征:是葫芦科植物的根状茎或全草。

Morphology: The rhizome or whole herb of plants in the Curcurbitaceae family.

别称:又名小苦药、五叶参等。

Byname: Xiao Kuyao, Wuye Shen

功效:健脾益气,生津止渴,清热解毒,止咳祛痰。

Efficacy: Strengthening spleen and benefiting qi, promoting fluid production to quench thirst, clearing away the heat evil and expelling superficial evils, stopping cough and expelling phlegm.

主治病症:适用于脾胃气虚,气阴两伤所致的胃脘疼痛,形瘦乏力,口渴等;或咳嗽痰多者。现代常用于治疗肿瘤、慢性支气管炎、高脂血症、血小板减少症、冠心病、消化性溃疡、慢性胃炎等多种疾患。

Indication: Gastric cavity pain, thin and weak and dipsia caused by deficiency of spleen-qi and stomach-qi and impairment of both qi and yin; or cough with excessive phlegm. Nowadays, it is often used to treat tumor, chronic bronchitis, hyperlipidemia, thrombocytopenia, coronary artery disease, peptic ulcer and chronic gastritis.

性味归经:性寒,味苦、甘。归脾、肺经。

Medicinal properties:Cold in property, bitter and sweet in flavor; enters the spleen and lung meridians.

用量用法:常用量 15 ~ 30 g。研末吞服,3 ~ 6 g。亦可泡茶服。

Usage and dosage:15 ~ 30 g is the usual dose. 3 ~ 6 g is ground into powder or brewed to make tea for taking.

注意事项:少数人服药后,出现恶心、呕吐、腹胀、腹泻(或便秘)、头晕、眼花、耳鸣等中毒症状,应当注意。

Notes:Few people might have poisoning symptoms after taking the drug, such as nausea, vomit, abdominal distention, diarrhea(or constipation), dizziness, dim eyesight and tinnitus, etc. Thus it should be taken cautiously.

19. 黄牛肉 Cattle Meat(Huangniu Rou)

形态特征:黄牛肉为牛科动物黄牛的肉。

Morphology:The meat of cattle. (Fam. Bovidae)

功效:温补脾胃,益气养血,强壮筋骨,消肿利水。

Efficacy:Pryetic tonification of spleen and stomach, benefiting qi and nourishing blood, strengthening bone and musculature, subsiding swelling to alleviate water retention.

主治病症:脾胃阳虚,脘腹疼痛,泄泻,脱肛,水肿;精血亏虚,消瘦乏力,筋骨酸软等。

Indication:Yang deficiency of spleen and stomach, pain in gastric cavity, diarrhea, proctoptosis, edema; deficiency of blood and essence, marasmus and acratia, sour weak bones and muscles.

性味归经:性温,味甘。入脾、胃经。

Medicinal properties:Warm in property and sweet in flavor; enters the spleen and stomach meridians.

用量用法:内服煮食、煎剂或入丸剂。

Usage and dosage:It is boiled to take, or used in decoction or pill preparations.

注意事项:黄牛肉性偏温,凡火热、痰火、湿热之证均不宜食用。病牛肉不能食用。

Notes:The cattle meat is warm in property, therefore is unsuitable to eat for people with syndromes of fire-heat, phlegm-fire and dampness-heat. The meat of diseased cattle are inedible.

20. 黑芝麻 Black Sesame

Hei Zhima(Semen Sesami Nigri)

形态特征:为脂麻科植物脂麻的干燥成熟种子。呈扁卵圆形,长约 3 mm,宽约 2 mm。表面黑色,平滑或有网状皱纹。

Morphology：The dry ripe seed of the sesame (Fam. Pedaliaceae). It is flat ovoid, about 3 mm long, and 2 mm wide. The surface is black, smooth or with reticulate wrinkles.

别称：又名芝麻、脂麻、巨胜子、胡麻等。

Byname：Zhima, Zhima, Ju Shengzi, Huma

功效：补肝肾,润五脏,养血祛风,延缓衰老。

Efficacy：Tonifying liver and kidney, moisturizing viscera, nourishing blood to expel wind, delaying senility.

主治病症：肝肾不足,虚风眩晕,风痹瘫痪,大便干燥,病后虚羸,须发早白,妇人乳少等。

Indication：Deficiency of liver and kidney, hematasthenia convulsion and dizziness, migratory arthralgia paralysis, dry stool, weak and thin after recovery, early-whitening beard and hair and insufficient breast milk.

性味归经：性平,味甘。入肝、肾经。

Medicinal properties：Neutral in property and sweet in flavor; enters the liver and kidney meridians.

用量用法：内服煎汤,每次 9~15 g;或入丸、散。外用:捣敷。

Usage and dosage：9~15 g is used in decoction, pill or powder preparations; or smashed for the external application.

注意事项：黑芝麻滑肠,脾弱便溏者勿服。

Notes：The black sesame lubricates the intestines and is contraindicated for people with spleen deficiency and loose stool.

21. 鹌鹑蛋 Quail Egg

Anchun Dan

形态特征：为雉科动物鹌鹑的卵。

Morphology：The egg of Quails. (Fam. Phasianidae)

功效：补脾养血,强筋壮骨。

Efficacy：Invigorating spleen and nourishing blood, strengthening bone and musculature.

主治病症：心脾气血两虚,心悸失眠,胆怯健忘,头晕耳鸣,乏力纳少等;血虚筋痿,腰膝无力,关节酸痛,行走不利等。

Indication：Qi-blood asthenia of heart and spleen, palpitation and insomnia, timidity and morbid forgetfulness, dizziness and tinnitus, lack of power and poor eating; flaccidity due to malnutrition of tendons and blood deficiency, powerless of waist and knees, arthralgia and unsteady walk.

性味归经：性平,味甘。入心、肝、脾经。

Medicinal properties：Neutral in property and sweet in flavor; enters the heart, liver and spleen meridians.

用量用法：内服煮食。

Usage and dosage：It is cooked to be taken.

进补应用：

1. 气阴亏虚，口干舌燥，纳食不振，咳血，大便秘结。银耳鹌蛋：鹌蛋10个，银耳15 g，冰糖30 g。将银耳水发后，去杂质，洗净，放入碗内，加清水少量，放蒸笼蒸1 h，再将鹌鹑蛋放入冷水锅内煮开，捞出，放入冷水中，剥去外壳。另用小锅，加入清水和冰糖，待水烧开后，放入备好的银耳、鹌鹑蛋，再用文火煎煮10 min即成。当点心食用。

Application in nourishment：

It is applied for people withqi and yin deficiency, dry mouth and thirst, loss of appetite, hemoptysis and dry stool. Yin'er Chundan(White Fungus and Quail Eggs)：First, choose 10 quail eggs, 15 g white fungus and 30 g crystal sugar; then soften the white fungus by soaking them in water, remove the impurities, wash them clean, put them into a bowl, add some water, and put the bowl into the steamer to steam for an hour; then put quail eggs into a pot and boil them with some cold water; after the water boil, scoop them out and put them into cold water and then peel them; then put some clean water and crystal sugar into a small pot to boil with water; after the water boil, put in the prepared white fungus and quail eggs and boil it with small fire for 10 minutes; then take it as a snack.

2. 气血不足，饮食不振，面色无华，心悸失眠，大便稀薄，病后体弱。参精鹌蛋：鹌鹑蛋10个，党参15 g，黄精10 g，大枣10枚。将党参、黄精洗净，同放入纱布袋，扎紧袋口。大枣洗净，鹌鹑蛋放入冷水中煮开，捞出放入冷水中，剥去外壳。先将党参、黄精药袋及大枣放入砂锅内，加入清水适量，用武火煮沸，改用文火煎熬45 min，再放入剥去壳的鹌鹑蛋，文火煎熬15 min。喝汤，吃大枣及鹌鹑蛋。

It is also applied for people with qi and yin deficiency, loss of appetite, with lusterless facial complexion, palpitations, insomnia, thin sloppy stool, weakness after illness. Shenjing Chundan(Quail eggs with Tangshen and Solomonseal)：Choose 10 quail eggs, 15 g Dangshen (Tangshen), 10 g Huangjing(Solomonseal) and 10 jujubes first; then wash tangshen and the solomonseal rhizome clean, put them into the gauze bag, truss the bag mouth; wash the jujubes clean; put the quail eggs into cold water to boil, and then scoop them up and put them into cold water to peel them; then put the drug bag with tangshen and the solomonseal rhizome and jujubes into an earthenware pot, add some clean water, boil them with an intense fire and then stew them with a slow fire for 45 minutes; then put the peeled quail eggs into the pot and stew them with a slow fire for 15 minutes; then drink the soup, eat jujubes and quail eggs.

注意事项：变质鹌鹑蛋不宜食用。

Notes：Stale quail eggs are unsuitable to be eaten.

22. 鳝鱼 Mud Eel

Shanyu(Monopterus Albus)

形态特征：为鳝科动物黄鳝的肉或全体。
Morphology：The meat or whole body of the mud eel.
别称：又名黄鳝。
Byname：Huangshan
功效：补虚损，祛风湿，强筋骨。
Efficacy：Treating asthenia – consumption disease, dispelling rheumatism, strengthening bone and musculature.
主治病症：脾虚血亏，腹冷肠鸣，下痢脓血，或产后恶露淋漓不净，身体羸瘦，或痔瘘等。
Indication：Spleen asthenia and hemophthisis, abdominal coldness and intestines rumbling, diarrhea with pus and blood, or postnatal dripping lochia, thinness or hemorrhoids and fistula.
性味归经：性温，味甘。入肝、脾、肾经。
Medicinal properties：Warm in property and sweet in flavor; enters the liver, spleen and kidney meridians.
用量用法：内服煮食、捣肉为丸或焙研为散。外用：剖片敷贴。
Usage and dosage：It is cooked, smashed into pills or baked into powder for internal use; it is also cut into pieces for external application.
进补应用：
Application in nourishment：
1. 气血亏虚，身体虚弱，痔疮出血。烩鳝鱼丝：鳝鱼 500 g，花生油 50 毫升，精盐、酱油、醋、红糖、淀粉、葱、料酒、姜适量。将鳝鱼去内脏及骨，洗净，斜切成丝。锅烧热后放进花生油，油八成热时，鳝鱼丝下锅煸炒片刻，加适量精盐、酱油、醋、红糖、葱、料酒、姜丝，加水稍煮 3 ~ 5 min，酌加湿淀粉，略煮即成，当菜食用。

It is applied for people with qi and blood deficiency, physical weakness, hemorrhoid hemorrhage. Hui Shanyu Si (Braised shredded eel) : 500 g mud eel, 50 ml peanut oil, salt, soy sauce, vinegar, brown sugar, starch, spring onion, cooking wine, a morsel of ginger. Dislodge eels organs and bones, wash it and incline it into thin shreds. After the hot pot in peanut oil, fire the shredded eel in a pan for a short time when the oil is hot, and add properly some salt, soy sauce, vinegar, brown sugar, spring onion, cooking wine and shredded ginger. Then add some water and boil it for 3 ~ 5 minutes, after that, add some wet starch and cook for a while. Take it as a dish.

2. 气血不足，身体虚弱，消瘦食少、脱肛、子宫脱垂 参归鳝鱼羹：鳝鱼 500 g，当归身 15

g,党参 15 g,葱、姜、精盐适量。将鳝鱼去内脏及骨,洗净,切成段。将当归、党参洗净,装入纱布袋内,扎紧袋口。再将鳝鱼、药袋和生姜片一并放入砂锅内。加入清水适量,先用武火煮沸,再用文火煎煮 50 ~ 60 min,捞出药袋,加入适量葱、精盐调味,稍沸即成。当菜或点心食用。

It is also applied for people with qi and blood deficiency, physical weakness, emaciation and low food intake, archoptosis, metroptosis. Shengui Shanyu Geng (Eel soup Stewed with Angelica and Dangshen):500 g mud eel, 15 g Danggui (Chinese angelica), 15 g Dangshen (Tangshen), spring onion, ginger and salt. Dislodge eels organs and bones, wash it and coarsely chop it. Put the washed danggui and dangshen into a gauze bag and tie tightly the pocket. Next, put the eel, medical bag and sliced ginger into marmite and add some water. Boil it with intense fire and then with gentle heat for 50 ~ 60 minutes, after that, get out the medical bag and add some spring onion and salt, cook it for a few minutes. Take it as a dish.

3. 虚寒久痢,痢下暗稀薄,夹有红色黏沫,或大便混有黄白黏液,腹痛绵绵,喜按喜温·饮食减少,神疲怕冷。鳝鱼红糖散:鳝鱼 1 条,红糖 10 g。鳝鱼去内脏及骨,洗净,晾去水汽,再将鳝鱼置新瓦上,用文火焙干(存性),与红糖一同研成细末。每次 10 g,每日 3 次,用温开水送吞。

It is also applied for people with deficiency and cold syndrome, long dysentery with dark color, diarrhoea with red sticky foam, or stool with yellow and white sticky mucus, slight abdominal pain, prefer abdominal pressure and warm, eating less, mental weakness and afraid of cold. Shanyu Hongtang San(Eel and Brown Sugar Powder):a mud eel and 10 g brown sugar. Dislodge eels organs and bones, wash it and air the water on it. Then dry out the eel on the new tile, and grind the dried eel with red sugar. 3 times a day, 10 g in a dose, swallow with boiled warm water.

4. 中气下陷,脱肛,内痔出血,子宫脱垂 鳝鱼汤:鳝鱼 2 条,姜、精盐适量。将黄鳝去内脏及骨,洗净,放入锅内,加入清水和适量精盐、姜片,先用武火煮沸,再用文火炖煮 30 min 左右,以鳝鱼熟烂为度。当菜食用。

It is also applied for people with middle qi collapse syndrome, rectal prolapse, internal hemorrhoid with bleeding and metroptosis. Shanyu Tang(Eel soup):two eels, proper amount of ginger and salt. Remove the viscera and bones of eels, wash them clean, put them into the pot, add some clean water and proper amount of salt and ginger slices, boil them with an intense fire, and then stew them with a slow fire for 30 minutes, till eels are thoroughly cooked and mushy. Take it as a dish.

注意事项:鳝鱼性温助热,凡发热、阴虚内热、疟疾、胸腹胀满等症均忌用。

Notes:Eels are warm in nature, thus are contraindicated for people with fever, internal heat with yin deficiency, malaria, distention and fullness of the chest and abdomen, etc.

23. 莲藕 Lotus Root(Lian'ou)

形态特征:为睡莲科植物藕的肥大根茎。

Morphology：The hypertrophic rhizome of the lotus. (Fam. Nymphaeaceae)

功效：熟用健脾开胃,养血止泻;生用清热生津,凉血止血。

Efficacy：Cooked：strengthening spleen and promoting appetite, nourishing blood to check diarrhea; raw：removing heat to promote salivation, cooling blood to stop bleeding.

主治病症：脾虚血少,不思饮食,面色萎黄,大便泄泻,少气懒言等;阴虚血热,烦闷口渴,发热,吐血、衄血,热淋,崩漏等。

Indication：Spleen asthenia and blood insufficiency, anorexia, withering and yellow complexion, diarrhea, deficient breath with less speech; yin deficiency with blood heat, discomfort and thirsty, fever, hematemesis, non-traumatic hemorrhage, heat strangury, uterine bleeding.

性味归经：性寒,味甘。入心、脾、胃经。

Medicinal properties：Cold in property and sweet in flavor; enters the heart, spleen and stomach meridians.

用量用法：内服生食、打汁或煮食,外用捣敷。

Usage and dosage：It is eaten raw, in juice or after being cooked; or it is smashed for external application.

进补应用：

Application in nourishment：

1. 心脾不足,心悸心慌,失眠多梦,饮食减少,肢体倦怠;血热失血,吐血、咯血、衄血、便血及崩漏。藕丝羹:嫩鲜藕500 g,鸡蛋3个,京糕100 g,蜜枣100 g,青梅100 g,白糖200 g,玉米粉适量。将藕切成细丝,放入沸水中略体后捞出。京糕、蜜枣、青梅也切成细丝。鸡蛋打在碗内,加少量清水,打匀,倒入盘内,上笼蒸5 min,成为固体蛋羹,把以上四种细丝均匀摆放在蛋羹上。白糖放在炒锅内,加入适量清水,熬成糖汁,用湿玉米粉勾欠,浇在蛋羹上,当点心食用。

It is applied for people with deficiency of heart and spleen, heart palpitations scary, insomnia and dreaminess, eating less, physical tiredness, blood heat and loss of blood, spitting blood, hemoptisis, epistaxis, stool with blood, uterine bleeding. Ousi Geng (Lotus Root Slices Porridge)：500 g fresh lotus roots, 3 eggs, 100 g hawthorn cakes, 100 g candied jujubes, 100 g green plums, 200 g sugar and the corn flour. Slice the lotus, put it into the boiling water and soon take it out; cut the hawthorn cake, candied date and green plum into slices; put the scrambled eggs into a bowl, add some water, sitr it evenly, pour it into a plate and steam it for 5 minutes till it becomes solid; put the above slices evenly on the egg custard and decoct the white sugar with proper amount of clean water to get the sugar juice; pour the wet corn flour onto the egg custard to thicken it. Take it as a snack.

2. 脾胃虚弱,食欲减退,大便稀薄,身体消瘦,四肢无力;热病伤阴,咽干口渴,心烦不宁等。藕粥:鲜藕100 g,粳米100 g。粳米淘洗干净,与初加工好的藕一并放在砂锅内,加入清水,先用武火煮沸,再用文火煮熬30 min,以米熟烂为度。或酌加少量白糖,调匀,供早晚餐或点心食用。

It is also applied for people with weakness of spleen and stomach, eating less, thin stool, loosing weight, weakness in limbs, yi deficiency caused by heat disease, dry throat and thirsty, restless. Ou Zhou(Lotus Root Porridge):100 g fresh lotus root and 100 g nonglutinous rice. wash the rice and put it into an eartheren pot together with the prepared lotus root, add some water, boil it with a strong fire, and then brew it with a slow heat for 30 minutes untill the rice is well cooked and softened; or blend it with some sugar for a meal or a snack.

3. 阴虚血热出血,鼻衄、齿衄、咯血、崩漏等。热病伤阴,低热不退,咽干口渴,五心烦热等。藕汁饮:鲜藕1000 g,鲜梨500 g,生荸荠500 g,生甘蔗500 g,鲜生地250 g。将以上鲜品分别洗净,削皮,切碎,榨汁,混合均匀。分数次浸茶饮用。每日1剂。

It is also applied for people with blood heat and bleeding caused by yin deficiency, nose bleeding, gum bleeding, hemoptysis, uterine bleeding. Yin deficiency caused by heat disease, long lasting low fever, dry throat and thirsty, tiredness and upset. Ouzhi Yin(Lotus root juice): 1000 g fresh lotus roots, 500 g fresh pears, 500 g raw water chestnuts, 500 g raw sugarcane and 250 g Shengdi(dried/fresh rehmannia root). Wash the materials, peel them, cut them into pieces and squeeze the juice. Take it several times, one dose daily.

4. 脾虚肾亏,食少便溏,遗精带下;热病心烦口渴;血热咯血、尿血等。白莲酿藕:鲜藕500 g,橘红15 g,薏苡仁15 g,百合15 g,芡实15 g,莲子15 g,糯米125 g,蜜樱桃30 g,瓜片15 g,白糖50 g,猪油50 g。先将莲子刷净皮,抽去心,苡仁、百合、芡实分别择净,冲洗后装于碗中,加清水至蒸笼蒸烂待用。瓜片、橘红切丁,蜜樱桃对剖。然后取鲜藕粗壮部分,刮去外面粗皮,洗净消去一头,用竹筷透通孔眼。糯米淘洗干净,由孔眼装入藕内,压紧,把削下的一块用牙签固定,使之封闭不漏。加水煮烂后,切成厚圆片待用。再将猪油铺于碗内,相继放入蜜樱桃、瓜片、橘红丁和薏苡仁、百合、芡实、莲子,同时将藕片摆上放好后洒人白糖,放笼上蒸至极烂,翻于圆盆内即成。

It is also applied for people with deficiency of spleen and kidney, eating less, thin stool, spermatorrhea, leucorrhea, upset and thirsty caused by heat disease, heat blood, hemoptysis, hematuria. Bailian Niang'ou(Lotus Seeds Brewed with Lotus Roots):500 g fresh lotus root, 15 g Juhong(Red tangerine peel), 15 g Yiyi Ren(Coix seed), 15 g Baihe(Lily bulb), 15 g Qianshi (Gordon uryale), 15 g lotus seed, 125 g sticky rice, 30 g sweet cherries, 15 g cucumber, 50 g sugar, 50 g lard. Wash the lotus seed, dislodge the core. Clean the coix seed, lily and Gordon uryale, put them in the bowl after washing them, pull water in the bowl and steam them. Cut the cucumber and dried tangerine peel into pieces, and cut the sweet cherry into two parts. Take the thick part of the lotus, wash it, cut its head and clean the hole with chopsticks. Wash the sticky rice, put it into the holes, press it and tie the cut pieces together with the toothpick. Cook it with boiling water, and cut it into pieces. Spread the lard in the bowl and put sweet cherry, cucumber, dried tangerine peel, coix seed, lily, Gordon uryale and lotus seed one after another into the bowl, and then put lotus slices on them with sprayed sugar. Turn over the bowl to a round basin when the dish is done.

注意事项:忌用铁器煎煮。

Notes：It should not be cooked or decocted in an iron pot.

24. 菱角 Water Chestnut（Lingjiao）

形态特征：为菱科植物菱的果肉。

Morphology：The flesh of the water chestnut.（Fam. Trapaceae）

别称：又名芰实、水栗、沙角、水菱等。

Byname：Jishi，Shuili，Shajiao，Shuiling

功效：生食清暑解热，除烦止渴；熟食益气健脾，解酒毒。

Efficacy：Raw：clearing away summer heat and heat evil，eliminating uncomfort and quenching thirst；cooked：nourishing qi to invigorate spleen，relieving alcoholism.

主治病症：脾胃气虚，大便稀溏，或久泻久痢、体倦乏力等。

Indication：Deficiency of spleen－qi and stomach－qi，thin stool，chronic diarrhea or dysentery，tiredness and lack of power.

性味归经：性凉，味甘，无毒。入大肠、肝胃经。

Medicinal properties：Cold in property and sweet in flavor；non－toxic；enters the large intestine，liver and stomach meridians.

用法用量：内服生食或煮熟食用。

Usage and dosage：It is eaten raw or after being cooked.

进补应用：

Application in nourishment：

1. 脾胃气虚，慢性泄泻，营养不良等症；或防治胃病、食管癌。菱粉粥：菱粉 30 g，粳米 100 g，红糖适量。将粳米淘净放入锅内，以武火煮至半熟，调入菱粉。继用文火煮至粥成，加入红糖，拌均匀即成。供早晚餐或作点心食用。

It is applied for people with qi deficiency of spleen and stomach，chronic diarrhea，malnutrition，or prevention of stomach disease and esophageal cancer. Lingfen Zhou（Water Chestnut Porridge）：30 g tapioca flour，100 g nongglutinous rice and proper amount of brown sugar. Wash the nongglutinous rice，put it into a pot，then boil it with a strong fire till it's half cooked and put in the chestnut powder；mix them and continue to boil the porridge with a small fire；then add some brown sugar to mix it evenly. Take it as a dinner or a snack.

2. 夏日感受暑热，口渴心烦，体倦乏力，不欲饮食；或饮酒过量，口苦烦渴，咽痛。白糖煮菱角粉：菱粉 50 g，白砂糖 10 g。将菱粉放入锅内，加入适量清水，置文火上煮沸，调入白砂糖使其溶化，即成。可当点心服用。

It is also applied for people with hot in summer，thirsty and upset，physical weakness，no appetite，or overdrinking，bitter taste，intense thirsty，pharyngalgia. Baitang Zhu Lingjiaofen （Water Chestnut Stewed with Sugar）：50 g powdered water chestnut and 10 g sugar. Put the powdered water chestnut into a pot，add some water，boil it with a small fire，and then spread sugar on it. Take it as a snack.

注意事项：本品性冷，多食则令人腹胀闷满，可用暖酒和姜汁饮服 1～2 杯。

Notes：It is cold，thus overuse of it may cause abdominal fullness and distention. To relieve the discomfort，it is better to drink 1～2 cups of warm wine mixed with ginger juice.

25. 茯苓 Tuckahoe

Fuling(Poria)

形态特征：为多孔菌科真菌茯苓干燥菌核，多为去皮后切制的茯苓，呈立方块状或方块状厚片，大小不一。白色、淡红色或淡棕色。

Morphology：The dry sclerotium of Fuling (Wolfiporia cocos)(Fam. Polyporaceae). The peeled and cut Fuling is cubic blocks or block－like thick slices，variable in size and white，pink or light brown in color.

别称：俗称云苓、松苓。古人称茯苓为"四时神药"，因为它功效非常广泛，不分四季，将它与各种药物配伍，不管寒、温、风、湿诸疾，都能发挥其独特功效。

Byname：It is commonly called Yunling or Songling. In ancient times，it was named the "magic drug in all seasons"，because its widespread curative effects in all seasons. It is compatible with every kind of drug to treat all diseases with the unique efficacy.

功效：利水渗湿，健脾化痰，宁心安神。

Efficacy：Removing dampness and promoting diuresis，invigorating spleen to remove phlegm，tranquillization.

主治病症：小便不利；水肿胀满；痰饮咳逆；呕吐；脾虚食少；泄泻；心悸不安；失眠健忘；遗精白浊。

Indication：Difficulty in micturition，edema and fullness，countflow－qi cough with phlegm －rheum，vomiting，eating less due to spleen asthenia，diarrhea，palpitation，insomnia and amnesia，spermatorrhea and gonoblennorrhea.

性味归经：性甘、淡，平，入心、肺、脾、肾经。

Medicinal properties：Sweet and mild in flavor and neutral in property；enters the heart，lung，spleen and kidney meridians.

用法用量：内服：煎汤，10～15 g；或入丸散。宁心安神用朱砂拌。

Usage and dosage：10～15 g is used in decoction，pill or powder preparations for internal use；or mixed with the cinnabar to calm down the mind.

进补应用：

Application in nourishment：

1. 用于小便不利，水肿等症。茯苓功能利水渗湿，而药性平和，利水而不伤正气，为利水渗湿要药。凡小便不利、水湿停滞的症候，不论偏于寒湿，或偏于湿热，或属于脾虚湿聚，均可配合应用。如偏于寒湿者，可与桂枝、白术等配伍；偏于湿热者，可与猪苓、泽泻等配伍；属于脾气虚者，可与党参、黄芪、白术等配伍；属虚寒者，还可配附子、白术等同用。

It is applied for people with difficult urination and edema. Tuckahoe is good at inducing diuresis and diffusing dampness. Its mild character makes it possible to induce diuresis without harming the vital energy. It is used for the disease including dysuria, water stagnation, no matter the diseases pertain to cold dampness or damp heat, or damp accumulation due to spleen deficiency. People with cold dampness syndrome can take it with Guizhi (Cassia twig) and Baizhu (Largehead atractylodes rhizome). People with damp-heat syndrome can take it with Zhuling (Grifola) and Zexie (Rhizome Alismatis). People with deficient spleen qi can take it with Dangshen (Tangshen), Huangqi (Astragalus hoangtchy) and Baizhu (Largehead atractylodes rhizome). People with cold deficiency syndrome can take it with Fuzi (Monkshood) and Baizhu (Largehead atractylodes rhizome).

2.用于脾虚泄泻,带下。茯苓既能健脾,又能渗湿,对于脾虚运化失常所致泄泻、带下,应用茯苓有标本兼顾之效,常与党参、白术、山药等配伍。又可用为补肺脾,治气虚之辅佐药。

It is also applied for people with diarrhea and leucorrhea caused by spleen weakness. Tuckahoe can not only tonify spleen and clear damp but also cure interior and exterior syndrome of diarrhea and leucorrhea caused by spleen deficiency. It is often used together with Dangshen (Tangshen), Baizhu (Largehead atractylodes rhizome) and Shanyao (Chinese yam). It is also used to nourish lung and spleen, and treat qi deficiency.

3.用于痰饮咳嗽,痰湿入络,肩背酸痛。茯苓既能利水渗湿,又具健脾作用,对于脾虚不能运化水湿,停聚化生痰饮之症,具有治疗作用。可用半夏、陈皮同用,也可配桂枝、白术同用。治痰湿入络、肩酸背痛,可配半夏、枳壳同用。

It is also applied for people with phlegm retention and cough, phlegm dampness in meridian, soreness in shoulder and back. Fuling can not only clear water stagnation and dampness and nourish spleen, but also cure stagnant phlegm caused by the disorder of transportation of weak spleen. It can take with Banxia (Pinellia tuber) and Chenpi (Dried tangerine peel), or Guizhi (Cassia twig) and Baizhu (Largehead atractylodes rhizome). And it can take with Banxia (Pinellia tuber), Zhike (Orange fruit) to cure phlegm in meridian and aches in shoulder and back.

4.用于心悸,失眠等症。茯苓能养心安神,故可用于心神不安、心悸、失眠等症,常与人参、远志、酸枣仁等配伍。

It is also applied for people with palpitation and insomnia. Fuling can nourish heart nervous, so it can be used to ease upset palpitation and insomnia with Renshen (Ginseng), Yuanzhi (Polygala root) and Suanzao Ren (Core of sour jujube).

注意事项:阴虚而无湿热、虚寒滑精、气虚下陷者慎服。

Notes: It should be carefully taken by people with yin deficiency and no damp heat, people with deficient cold and spermatorrhea and people with qi deficiency and qi collapse.

26. 麦冬 Dwarf Lilyturf Tuber

Maidong(Radix Ophiopogonis)

形态特征:呈纺锤形,两端略尖。表面黄白色或淡黄色,身细纵纹。

Morphology:It is fusiform – shaped, slightly pointed at both ends. The surface is yellowish–white or yellowish, with thin longitudinal grains on it.

别称:寸麦冬、麦门冬、朱寸冬。

Byname:Cun Maidong,Maimen Dong,Zhucun Dong

功效:养阴生津,润肺清心。

Efficacy:Nourishing yin to generate body fluid,moisturizing lung and clearing away heart fire.

主治病症:虚痨咳嗽,津伤口渴,心烦失眠,内热消渴,肠燥便秘;白喉。

Indication:cough due to asthenia consumption,thirst due to running–down of body fluid, upset and insomnia, wasting – thirst due to calor internus, intestine dryness and constipation, pharyngeal diphtheria.

性味归经:甘,微苦,微寒。入心、肺、胃经。

Medicinal properties:Sweet and slightly bitter in flavor;slightly cold in the property; enters the heart,lung and stomach meridians.

用法用量:内服煎汤,10~20 g;或6~12 g入丸、散。清养肺胃之阴多去心用,滋阴清心多连心用。

Usage and dosage:10~20 g is used in decoction for internal use,or 6~12 g used in pill or powder preparations;used to enrich the lung and stomach yin without the central part,while used to nourish yin and clear the heart with the central part.

进补应用:

Application in nourishment:

1. 素体阴虚。麦冬(鲜品,去心)2500 g,捣烂,煮熟,绞取汁,加入蜂蜜500 g,放锅内(不用铝锅、铁锅)以重汤煮,不断搅拌,待液稠如饴,盛于瓷器中备用。每次用温酒调服1匙,每日2次。长服有滋补强壮、延年益寿之功。

It is applied for people with Yin deficiency:2500 g Maidong(Dwarf lilyturf tuber)(fresh, no core). Smash it,cook it and juice it. Add 500 g honey in it,and put it in any pot except the iron and aluminium ones to boil it with the soup stock. Stir the soup until it becomes sticky and put it in the china. 2 times a day,with each time a spoon of it mixed with warm wine. It is nutritious,tonic and good for longevity.

2. 慢性萎缩性胃炎。麦冬、党参、沙参、玉竹、天花粉各9 g,乌梅、知母、甘草各6 g。水煎服,每日1剂。

Chronic atrophic gastritis:9 g Maidong(Dwarf lilyturf tuber),9 g Dangshen(Tangshen),9 g Shashen (Root of straight ladybell) , 9 g Yuzhu (Dried solomonseal) , 9 g Tianhuafen (Trichosanthes root) , 6 g Wumei (Smoked plum) , 6 g Zhimu (Common anemarrhena rhizome) ,6 g Gancao(Liquorice root). Take the decoction , one dose daily.

3. 慢性胃炎。麦冬 9 g,黄芪 9 g,党参 10 g,玉竹 10 g,黄精 10 g,天花粉 12 g。水煎服,每日 1 剂。对胃阴不足者有良效。

Chronic gastritis:9 g Maidong(Dwarf lilyturf tuber) ,9 g Huangqi(Milkvetch root) ,10 g Dangshen(Tangshen) ,10 g Yuzhu(Dried solomonseal) ,10 g Huangjing(Solomonseal) and 12 g Tianhuafen(Trichosanthes root). Take the decoction, one dose daily. It is good for those with deficiency of stomach yin.

4. 糖尿病,口渴多饮。麦冬 12 g,生地 12 g,天花粉 10 g,知母 12 g,黄连 5 g。水煎服,每日 1 剂。有缓解燥渴的作用。

Diabetes , thirsty and overdrinking:12 g Maidong (Dwarf lilyturf tuber) ,12 g Shengdi (Dried/fresh rehmannia root) ,10 g Tianhuafen (Trichosanthes root) ,12 g Zhimu (Common anemarrhena rhizome) ,5 g Huanglian(Goldthread). Take the decoction, one dose daily. It is good for easing the dryness and thirst.

5. 肠燥便秘,大便干结。麦冬 15 g,生地 15 g,玄参 15 g。水煎服,每日 1 剂。有润肠通便的作用。

Intestine dryness and astriction , dry stool:15 g Maidong (Dwarf lilyturf tuber) ,15 g Shengdi(Dried/fresh rehmannia root) and 15 g Xuanshen(Figwort root). Take the decoction, one dose daily. It helps to lubricate bowels and promote defecation.

6. 暑天汗多口渴,体倦乏力。麦冬 10 g,人参 10 g,五味子 6 g。水煎服,每日 2 剂。本法对汗出虚脱,心慌心悸,血压过低之症,用之也有良效。

Sweaty and thirsty in summer , tiredness:10 g Maidong (Dwarf lilyturf tuber) ,10 g Renshen(Ginseng) and 6 g Wuwei Zi(Chinese magnoliavine fruit). Take the decoction, two doses daily. It helps those with sweat exhaustion,palpitation and low blood pressure.

注意事项:凡脾胃虚寒泄泻,胃有痰饮湿浊及暴感风寒咳嗽者均忌服。

Notes:Those with deficiency cold of spleen and stomach , diarrhea , phlegm wet cloud and cough caused by cold wind are forbidden from it.

27. 白芍 White Peony Root

Baishao(Radix Paeoniae Alba)

形态特征:为毛茛科植物芍药的干燥根。呈类圆形薄片,断面类白色或微带棕红色,可见稍隆起的筋脉纹呈放射状排列。

Morphology:The dry root of Baishao (Radix Paeoniae Alba) (Fam. Ranunculaceae). It is round-like slice; the section is white or slightly brownish-red; some raised vascular bundle texture is ranged in radical pattern.

别称：又称花子、白芍药、金芍药、杭芍、大白芍、生白芍、炒白芍、炒杭芍。

Byname：Huazi, Bai Shaoyao, Jin Shaoyao, Hangshao, Da Baishao, Sheng Baishao, Chao Baishao, Chao Hangshao

功效：养血柔肝，缓中止痛，敛阴止汗。

Efficacy：Nourishing blood and liver, relaxing the middle energizerto relieve pains, retaining yin with astringent for hidroschesis.

主治病症：胸腹胁肋疼痛，泻痢腹痛，自汗盗汗，阴虚发热，月经不调，崩漏，带下。

Indication：Pains in chest, abdomen and costa, decanta and dysentery with abdominal pain, spontaneous perspiration and night sweating, fever with yin asthenia, menoxenia, uterine bleeding, morbid leucorrhea.

性味归经：苦酸，凉。入肝、脾经。

Medicinal properties：Bitter and sour in flavor; cold in property; enters the liver and spleen meridians.

用法用量：内服煎汤，10～15 g；或入丸、散。

Usage and dosage：10～15 g is used in decoction, pill or powder preparations for internal use.

进补应用：白芍药补中焦之药，炙甘草为辅，治腹中痛。如夏月腹痛，少加黄芩；恶热而痛，加黄柏；若恶寒腹痛，加肉桂0.5 g，白芍药1 g，炙甘草0.75 g，此仲景神品药也。

Application in nourishment：

White peony root is used to consolidate the middle energizer. With the assistance of Zhi Gancao(Honey – fried licorice root), it can alleviate the pain in stomach. If stomachache happens in summer, a little dose of Huangqin(Baical skullcap root) can be added. Huangbai (Corktree bark) is added to treat aversion to heat and pain. If the stomachache is accompanied with aversion to heat, then add some Rougui(Chinese cinnamon). While if it happens with the symptom of aversion to cold, then treat it with the magic prescription of Zhang Zhongjing:0.5 g Rougui,1 g Baishao(White peony root), and 0.75 g Zhi Gancao(Honey–fried licorice root).

注意事项：白芍性寒，虚寒性腹痛泄泻者忌食；小儿出麻疹期间忌食；服用中药藜芦者忌食。

Notes：White peony root is cold in nature, thus is contraindicated for people suffering from stomachache and diarrhea with cold and deficient syndrome, children or infants in the outbreak of measles and people who are taking Lilu(Veratrum).

28. 当归 Chinese Angelica

Danggui(Radix Angelicae Sinensis)

形态特征：呈圆柱形。外皮黄棕色至棕褐色，有纵皱纹及横长皮孔样突起。质柔韧，断面黄白色，皮部有油点，木部似菊花心。香气浓郁。

Morphology：The root of Angelica sinensis（Oliv.）Diels.（Fam. Umbelliferae）. It is cylindrical. The skin is yellowish－brown to dark brown, with longitudinal wrinkles and transverse lenticel protuberance. It is flexible and the section is yellowish－white；the cortex has some oily points ；the xylem ranges in a chrysanthemum－－like pattern. It has a strong flavor.

别称：又称干归、马尾归、云归、西当归、金当归、当归身、当归尾、酒当归等。

Byname：Gangui, Mawei Gui, Yungui, Xi Danggui, Jin Danggui, Danggui Shen, Danggui Wei, Jiu Danggui

功效：补血,活血,调经止痛,润燥滑肠。

Efficacy：Enriching blood, activating blood circulation；regulating menstruation to relieve pain；moisturizing dryness－syndrome for intestines.

主治病症：血虚诸证,月经不调,经闭,痛经,症瘕结聚,崩漏,虚寒腹痛,痿痹,肌肤麻木,肠燥便难,赤痢后重,痈疽疮疡,跌扑损伤。

Indication：Blood － deficiency syndromes；menoxenia；menischesis；dysmenorrheal；obstruction in the intestine；uterine bleeding；asthenia－cold abdominalgia；wilting impediment；numbness of muscle and skin；difficulty in stool due to dryness of the intestine；serious hemato-diarrhoea in later period；carbuncle－abscess and sores ulceration；injury from falling down.

性味归经：味甘,辛,苦,性温;入肝、心、脾经。

Medicinal properties：Sweet, pungent and bitter in flavor；warm in property；enters the liver, heart and spleen meridians.

用法用量：内服煎汤,6～12 g;或入丸、散;或浸酒;或敷膏。

Usage and dosage：6～12 g is used in decoction, pill or powder preparations for internal use；or steeped in the wine or applied in the paste.

进补应用：

Application in nourishment：

1. 血虚肠燥的便秘。常与肉苁蓉火麻仁等润肠药配伍。

Constipation caused by blood deficiency and intestinal dryness. It is usuallycompatible with aperitives such as Roucongrong（Broomrape）, Huomaren（Fructus cannabis）etc.

2. 血瘀阻滞的病证,如跌打损伤,瘀肿疼痛;肢体麻木、疼痛;肩周炎;血栓闭塞性脉管炎。常与川芎、赤芍等活血药配伍。

Symptoms with blood stasis and stagnation, such as bruises and pain caused by ecchymoma, numb and pain in four extremities, scapulohumeral periarthritis and thromboangitis obliterans. It is usually compatible with blood－activating drugs such as Chuanqiong（Sichuan lovage）, Chishao（Red peony root）and so on.

3. 血虚或血瘀所致的月经不调、经闭、痛经。常与熟地黄、川芎、丹参等补血活血药配伍。

Abnormal menstruation, amenorrhea and dysmenorrhea caused by blood deficiency or blood stasis. It is usually used with the combination of medicine that can enrich blood and invigorate blood circulation such asShudihuang（Prepared rehmannia root）, Chuanqiong

(Sichuan lovage), Danshen(Red sage root) and so on.

4.痈肿疮疡者气血不足,脓成不溃或溃后不易愈合。常与黄芪配伍以扶持正气。

Welling-abscess swellings and sores caused by deficiency of both qi and blood. Usually the swellings can not ulcerate and even if they ulcerate, they can not recover by themselves. It is uaually used with Huangqi(Milkvetch root) to support and enrich healthy qi.

5.血虚证或贫血,症见眩晕、疲倦乏力、面色萎黄、舌质淡、脉细等,以及血虚腹痛、头痛。常与熟地黄、白芍,或羊肉、黄芪等补血益气之物配伍。

Blood deficiency and anemia with the symptoms of dizziness, fatigue and weakness, witheringly yellow complexion, pale tongue coating, thready pulse etc. There are other symptoms such as stomachache and headache caused by blood deficiency. It can be applied with medicines that can enrich blood and qi such as Shudihuang(Prepared rehmannia root) and Baishao(White peony root), or mutton and Huangqi(Milkvetch root) and so on.

注意事项:脾湿中满、脘腹胀闷、大便稀薄或腹泻者慎服;里热出血者忌服。

Notes: People who suffer dampness in spleen and abdominal distension, epigastric distension and depression, loose stool or diarrhea have to take it cautiously. People who suffer from hemorrhage caused by interior heat should avoid eating it.

29. 芥菜 Mustard

Jiecai(Brassica Juncea Czern. et Coss.)

形态特征:为十字花科植物芥菜的嫩茎叶。

Morphology: The tender stem and leave of Brassica juncea Czern. et Coss. (Fam. Cruciferae)

别称:又名雪里红。

Byname: Xueli Hong

功效:宣肺豁痰,温中利气。

Efficacy: Facilitating lung to clear phlegm to expel phlegm, warming spleen-stomach to guid qi downward.

主治病症:寒饮内盛,咳嗽痰滞,胸膈满闷。

Indication: Inner-abundant cold fluid-retention, cough with phlegm stagnation, septum pectorale suffocation.

性味归经:性温,味辛。入肺、胃、肾经。

Medicinal properties: Warm in property and pungent in flavor; enters the lung, stomach and kidney meridians.

用量用法:内服煎汤或捣汁。外用:研末撒或煎水洗。

Usage and dosage: It is used in decoction or smashed juice for internal use; or ground into powder to spray or decocted for washing.

进补应用：

Application in nourishment：

1. 中虚胃寒,痰饮阻滞,咳嗽胸闷。芥菜炒肉丝:猪肉丝250 g,芥菜500 g洗净。将猪肉先用油炒半熟,然后加入芥菜同炒致熟。加入葱、姜、糖、味精等调味略炒即可。当菜食用。

Deficiency in middle energizer and stomach cold,phlegm and fluid stasis and cough and chest congestion. Jiecai Chao Rousi(Mustard Fried with Shredded Pork):250 g shredded pork, 500 g mustard. Wash them and then fry the shredded porks with seed-oil to medium and then put mustard into pot fried both till they are cooked. At last,add some onion ginger,sugar and monosodium glutamate,stir-fry a little. Take it as a dish.

2. 牙龈肿烂。用芥菜杆,烧存性,研末,频敷之。

Gingival abscess and rot. Burn mustard rod into ash with its nature remained. Grind it into powder and apply frequently to the injured parts.

3. 漆疮瘤痒。芥菜煎水洗之。

Dermatitis rhus,tumor and itch. Decoct mustard with water and then wash the affected parts with the decoction.

4. 痔疮肿痛。芥菜捣烂频敷之。

Hemorrhoids and gall. Apply the affected parts with mashed mustard.

30. 刀豆 Jack Bean

Daodou(Semen Canavaliae)

形态特征:种子呈扁卵形。表面淡红色至红紫色,微皱缩,略有光泽。边缘具眉状黑色种脐,上有白色细纹3条。质硬,难破碎。种皮革质;子叶2。嚼之有豆腥味。

Morphology:The Seed is a flat oval shape. The surface is pink to red purple, slightly wrinkled and glossy. There is an eyebrow-like black hilum with 3 white lines on it. The seed is hard,and hard to break. The seed coat has a leather quality. It has a bean taste after chewing.

别称:又名挟剑豆、刀豆子、大刀豆、关刀豆等。

Byname:Xiejian Dou,Daodou Zi,Dadao Dou,Guandan Dou

功效:温中下气,益肾补元。

Efficacy:Warming spleen-stomach to guid qi downward,tonifying kidney to invigorate premordial energy.

主治病症:脾胃虚寒,呃逆、呕吐、腹胀、腹泻等;肾阳虚弱,腰痛、疝气胀痛、面色苍白等。

Indication:Spleen-stomach insufficiency-cold, hiccup, vomiting, abdominal distension, diarrhea;kidney yang deficiency,lumbago,gas-pain hernia,chills with cold limbs,pale face.

性味归经：性温，味甘。入胃、大肠、肾经。

Medicinal properties：Warm in property and sweet in flavor；enters the stomach，large intestine and kidney meridians.

用量用法：内服煎汤服或煮食，每日 6～30 g。

Usage and dosage：6～30 g is decocted or cooked daily for internal use.

进补应用：

Application in nourishment：

1. 肾阳不足，腰痛。刀豆腰子：刀豆子 20 g，猪腰 1 个，精盐适量。将猪腰剖开，去白色筋膜部分，洗净；刀豆子洗净。然后将刀豆包在猪腰内，用线扎紧，放入锅中，加水适量，用武火煮沸后，改用文火煮熟，加精盐调味。可佐餐食用。

Deficiency in kidney yang and low back pain. Daodou with pig kidneys. 20 g daodou，one pig kidney and little refined salt. Daodou Yaozi（Sword Bean and Pig Kidney）：Slice the kidney，remove the white fascia and then wash it. Next，wash daodou，wrap them into the kidney and bind the kidney tightly then put then into the pot and add an appropriate amount of water. Stew with intense fire and then switch to slow fire to cook them thoroughly. At last add some refined salt to season the flavor. It then can be eaten together with rice，bread and so on.

2. 肺气虚寒所致的小儿咳嗽、老年咳喘 刀豆饮：刀豆子 25 g，甘草 3 g，冰糖或蜂蜜适量。将刀豆子洗净，打碎，与洗净的甘草一起放入砂锅中，加水适量，用武火煮沸后，改用文火煮沸，加冰糖或蜂蜜，调匀。每日 2 次，温服。

Coughof children and infants and the elderly caused by deficiency and coldness in lung qi. Daodou Yin（Sword Bean Decoction）：25 g Daodou（Sword bean），3 g Gancao（Liquorice root）and some crystal sugar or honey. Wash and mash the sword beans and then put them into an earthern pot together with washed liquorice roots；add proper amount of water and stew them with a strong fire till it boils and then switch to a slow fire；then add some crystal sugar or honey and stir them evenly. Take it warmly，twice a day.

3. 肺气虚寒所致的头昏头痛、鼻塞流涕 刀豆散：刀豆 500 g。将刀豆洗净，用文火焙，研为细末，每日 1 次，每次 9 g，用酒送服。

Dizziness and headache caused by cold and deficiency in lung qi. Daodou San（Sword Bean Powder）：500 g Daodou（Sword bean）. Wash it and bake it dry with a slow fire and then grind it into powder. Take it once a day，9 g at a time and take it with wine.

4. 脾胃虚寒，胃痛呃逆，呕吐，腹痛腹泻；肾阳不足，腰痛，怯寒。刀豆粥：刀豆 15 g，粳米 50 g，生姜 2 片。将刀豆洗净，捣碎（或炒研末），与淘净的粳米、生姜一起放入砂锅中，加水适量，用武火煮沸后，改用文火熬煮成稀粥。每日早晚餐，温热服食。若用于呃逆，可加大剂量。

Coldness and deficiency in both spleen and stomach，stomachache with hiccup，vomit and abdomen pain with diarrhea；deficiency in kidney yang，low back pain and aversion to cold. Daodou Zhou（Sord Bean Porridge）：15 g Daodou（Sword bean），50 g nonglutinous rice and 2 slices of ginger. First，wash and mash the sword beans（or grind it after being fried），put it into an eartheln pot with washed nonglutinous rice and ginger and then add proper amount of water. Stew it with a strong fire till it boils and switch to a slow fire to stew them into porridge. Eat it at breakfast and supper daily and take it warmly. If it is used for hiccup, a larger dose is permitted.

注意事项：刀豆性温，胃热甚者慎服。

Notes：Daodou is warm in nature, thus people with excessive stomach heat should take it cautiously.

31. 海参 Sea Cucumber

Haishen(Holothurian)

形态特征：本品为刺参科动物或其他种海参的全体。

Morphology：The whole body of animals of Fam. Stichopodidae or other kinds of Holothurian.

别称：根据海参品种不同，又有刺参、梅花参、瓜参之称。

Byname：It is called Cishen, Meihua Shen and Guashen according to different species.

功效：补肾益精，养血润燥。

Efficacy：Tonifying kidney to increase sperm, moisturizing dryness by nourishing blood.

主治病症：肾精亏虚，阳痿遗精，小便频数，腰酸乏力等；阴血亏虚，形体消瘦，潮热咳嗽，咯血，消渴，大便秘等。

Indication：Deficiency of kidney – essence, impotence and seminal emission, frequent urination, waist soreness and weakness; deficiency of yin–blood, magersucht, cough with hectic fever, hemoptysis, wasting thirst, constipation.

性味归经：性温，味咸。入心、肝、肾经。

Medicinal properties：Warm in property and salt in flavor; enters the heart, liver and kidney meridians.

用量用法：内服煎汤、煮食或入丸剂。

Usage and dosage：It is used in decoction, cooked food or pill preparations for internal use.

进补应用：

Application in nourishment：

1. 精血亏虚，肾气不足，面色无华，头晕耳鸣，腰膝酸软，疲倦乏力，阳痿早泄，遗精尿频。海参粥：海参30 g，粳米100 g。将初加工好的海参切碎，加水煮烂。粳米淘洗干净，与海参一并放在砂锅内。加入清水，先用武火煮沸，再用文火煎熬20~30 min，以米熟烂为度。早晨空腹食用。

Deficiency in essence and blood. Insufficiency of kidney qi, lusterless complexion, dizziness and tinnitus, soreness and weakness of waist and knees, lassitude, Impotence, premature ejaculation or nocturnal emissions and frequent urination.

Haishen Zhou(Sea Cucumber Porridge):30 g sea cucumber and 100 g nonglutinous rice. First, slice the raw sea cucumber and boil it in water till it becomes tender, then wash the rice and put it into an earthern pot together with the sea cucumber; add some water and stew it with a strong fire till it boils and then switch to a slow fire to boil it about 20 ~ 30 minutes till the rice is well-cooked. Take it with an empty abdomen in the morning.

2. 肝肾阴虚,头晕耳鸣,咽干,心烦,腰膝酸软,大便秘结。冰糖炖海参:海参 25 g,冰糖 50 g。将海参洗净切碎,放入碗内,加入适量清水,隔水蒸 20 ~ 60 min,以海参熟烂为度。将冰糖加少量清水,煮熬成糖汁,倒入海参汤内。饮汤,食海参。

Yin deficiency of both liver and kidney, dizziness and tinnitus, dry throat, vexation and soreness and weakness of waist and knees, or constipation.

Bingtang Dun Haishen(Crystal Sugar Stewed with Sea Cucumber):25 g sea cucumber,50 g crystal sugar. First wash and slice the sea cucumber, put it into a bowl and add an appropriate amount of water. Then steam it for about 20 ~ 60 minutes till the sea cucumber is well-cooked. Next, dissolve crystal into some water and then boil it till it becomes sugar juice. Then pour the sugar juice into sea cucumber soup. Then drink the soup and eat the sea cucumber.

3. 肾气虚弱,阳痿遗精,小便频数;阴血亏虚,右肋隐痛,小便短黄,心烦易怒,低热口干,肌肤萎黄,大便秘结。海参膏:海参 500 g,珍珠层粉 30 g,蜂蜜 250 g,白糖 500 g。将海参洗净,切成细块,放在砂锅内,加入适量清水,用文火熬至溶化。加入蜂蜜、白糖、珍珠层粉,继续煎熬,搅拌均匀,收膏停火即成。晾凉后,盛人瓶内备用。每次服豆匙,每日 3 次,开水冲服。

Deficiency in kidney qi, Impotence, nocturnal emissions and frequent urination; deficiency in yin blood, and dull pain in right flank, scanty dark urine, vexation and being irritable, with low fever and thirst, witheringly yellow skin and constipation. Haishen Gao (Sea Cucumber Paste):500 g sea cucumber,30 g nacre powder,250 g honey,500 g white sugar. First wash and slice sea cucumber, put it into marmite and add a moderate amount of water. Then stew it with slow fire till it dissolve. Then put honey, white sugar, nacre powder into it, continue stewing and mix them even. Turn off the fire when it becomes ointment. After the ointment becomes cool, fill it into a bottle for reserve. Three times one day. Each time dissolve one spoon into boiled water and take it.

4. 阴血亏虚,头晕耳鸣,疲乏无力,便秘等;癌症患者用作辅助治疗。虾子海参:海参 150 g,虾子 15 g,肉汤 500 g,姜、葱、料酒、猪油、精盐、酱油、淀粉、味精适量。将海参洗净切碎。虾子清洗干净,放在碗中入适量清水和料酒,上笼蒸 10 min 左右。将锅烧热,放入猪油,投入姜片、葱段,煸炒后捞起,加料酒,再加入肉汤和食盐、酱油,放入海参和虾子。先用武火煮沸,再用文火煨成浓汁,用淀粉勾芡,加味精调味。当菜食用。

Deficiency in yin blood, dizziness and tinnitus, lassitude, constipation etc. People with cancer use it as auxiliary treatment. Xiazi Haishen(Shrimp Roe and Sea Cucumber):150 g sea cucumber,15 g shrimp roe,500 g broth, ginger, onion, cooking wine, lard, refined salt, soy sauce, starch and monosodium glutamate. First wash and slice the sea cucumber, then wash the shrimp roe and put it into a bowl, add moderate amount of water and cooking wine and then steam it in the steamer for about 10 minutes. Next, warm the pot and pour some lard and put some ginger, onion, fish them up after stir-frying. And then pour the broth and refined salt, soy sauce, shrimp roe and sea cucumber. First stew it with intense fire and then change to slow fire to simmer it into heavy gravy. At last, thicken the soup with the mixture of starch and water and then add some monosodium glutamate. Take it as a dish.

注意事项：凡脾虚腹泻，痰多者忌食。

Notes：It is contraindicated for people with spleen deficiency, diarrhea and excessive phlegm.

32. 鳖肉 Turtle Flesh

Bierou

形态特征：为鳖科动物中华鳖的肉。

Morphology：The flesh of Trionyx sinensis Wiegmann. (Fam. Trionychidae)

别称：又名团鱼肉、甲鱼肉、元鱼肉等。

Byname：Tuanyu Rou, Jiayu Rou, Yuanyu Rou

功效：滋阴凉血，益气升提。

Efficacy：Nourishing yin and cooling blood, benefiting vital energy.

主治病症：肝肾阴虚，头晕眼花，腰膝酸软，遗精；脾虚气陷，脱肛，身倦乏力，饮食减少；冲任不固，月经量多色淡，淋漓不尽等。

Indication：Liver kidney yin insufficiency, dizziness and poor eye sight, sour-weak waist and knee, spermatorrhea; sinking of qi due to deficiency of the spleen, proctoptosis, lack of power, poor eating, deficiency of thoroughfare and conception vessel, high-volume and light-color menstrual blood, successive dripping wet.

性味归经：性平，味甘。入肝、肾、经。

Medicinal properties：Neutral in property and sweet in flavor; enters the liver and kidney meridians.

用量用法：煮食或入丸剂。

Usage and dosage：It is cooked or used in pill preparations for internal use.

进补应用：

Application in nourishment：

1. 阴血亏虚，骨蒸潮热，颧红盗汗，心烦失眠，痔疮便血，男子遗精，女子崩漏、带下；脾虚气陷，气短懒言，疲乏无力，肛门直肠脱垂。红烧甲鱼：鳖1000 g，鸡翅2副，火腿50 g，蘑菇10 g，鸡清汤1500 ml，食盐、料酒、酱油、胡椒粉、白糖、味精各适量。将鳖宰杀，洗净，切成肉块，鸡翅切成两段，火腿切成厚片，蘑菇洗净。将以上各味一并放入砂锅里，加入鸡清汤和食盐、酱油、胡椒粉、白糖。先用武火煮沸,再用文火炖煮 2 h 左右,待鳖肉熟烂后停火,酌加少量味精,佐餐食用。

Deficiency in yin blood, bone-steaming tidal fever, red cheekbone and night sweating, vexation and insomnia, hemorrhoids with blood stool, nocturnal emissions for male, or uterine bleeding and leucorrhea for female; qi collapse caused by spleen deficiency, hard breathing and laziness to speak, lassitude or rectal prolepses.

Hongshao Jiayu (Turtle Braised with Soy Sauce): 1000 g turtle, two pairs of chicken wings, 50 g ham, 10 g mushroom, 1500 ml chicken consomme, and some salt, cooking wine, soy sauce, pepper, white sugar and monosodium glutamate. First kill, wash and slice the turtle and cut one chicken wing into two sections, cut the ham into thick pieces, and then wash the mushroom. Put all the above ingredients into an earthern pot and then put in the chicken consomme, salt, soy sauce, pepper and white sugar. First stew it with intense fire till it boils and switch to slow fire to continue stewing for about 2 hours. Turn off the fire till the turtle flesh is well-cooked, add some monosodium glutamate and then eat it together with food.

2. 肾阴亏虚,头晕耳鸣,潮热盗汗,腰膝酸软,多梦健忘。团鱼汤:团鱼 500 g,羊肉 250 g,草果 3 g,姜片、胡椒粉、食盐、味精各适量。将鳖宰杀、洗净,切成小块;羊肉洗净切块,与鳖肉一并放入砂锅内。加入生姜和清水。先用武火煮沸,再用文火炖煮 2 h 左右,待肉熟烂后停火。酌加少量食盐、胡椒粉、味精,佐餐食用,吃肉、喝汤。也可用补髓汤:取鳖 1 只,猪脊髓 200 g,葱、姜、胡椒粉、味精各适量。将鳖宰杀洗净,猪脊髓洗净,两味均切成块,一并放入砂锅中加入清水和姜、葱、胡椒粉。先用武火煮沸,再用文火炖煮 2 h 左右,待肉熟后停火。酌加味精,佐餐食用,吃肉喝汤。

Dificiency in kidny yin, dizziness and tinnitus, tidal fever and night sweating, soreness and weakness in waist and knees and forgettery and dreaminess.

Tuanyu Tang(Soft-shelled Turtle Soup): 500 g soft-shelled turtle, 250 g mutton, 3 g Caoguo(Tsaoko cardamon), and some ginger, pepper, salt and monosodium glutamate. First kill the turtle, wash it clean and cut it into small pieces, then wash the mutton clean and cut it into pieces; put them both into an earthern pot; then add some ginger and water; boil them with a strong fire and then stew it with a slow fire for about 2 hours til the turtle flesh is well-cooked. According to one's taste, add some salt, pepper, monosodium glutamate. Then it can be eaten with rice or bread etc.

In addition, Busui Tang(Marrow-enriching Decoction) has the same effect. 1 turtle, 200 g pig's spine marrow, some onion, ginger, pepper powder and monosodium glutamate. First get the turtle slaughtered and washed. Then cut turtle and pig's spine marrow into slice and then put them into one marmite with some water, ginger, onion, pepper powder added. First stewing the decoction with intense fire and then boil it with slow fire for about 2 hours. Turn off the fire till the flesh is well-cooked. add some monosodium glutamate in accordance with one's favor. Take it together with food; eat the meat and drink the soup.

3. 阴液不足,口干咽燥,低热不退。二母元鱼:鳖 500 g,贝母 5 g,知母 5 g,前胡 5 g,

柴胡5 g,杏仁5 g。食盐、料酒各适量。将鳖宰杀、洗净,切成块。放在大碗内,将五味中药洗净,装入纱布袋内,扎紧袋口,也放入锅内,加入适量的黄酒和食盐,再加入清水,没过肉块,放在蒸锅中蒸炖1 h左右,以鳖肉熟烂为度。趁热分顿食用。

Deficiency in yin essence,thirst and dry throat,persistent low fever.

Ermu Yuanyu(Turtle Stewed with Fritillaria and Anemarrhena):500 g turtle,5 g Beimu(Fritillaria bulb),5 g Zhimu(Common anemarrhena rhizome),5 g Qianhu(Hogfennel root),5 g Chaihu(Chinese thorowax root),5 g apricot kernels and some salt and cooking wine. First get turtle killed,washed,and cut into slice and then put in a big bowl. Then get the five drugs washed and wrapped in a gauze bag and bind the bag tightly and also put it in the bowl and added some rice wine,salt and water to immerse the flesh;then put it in a steamer to stew it for about 1 hour till the meat is well-cooked. Take it in several doses while it is still warm.

注意事项:鳖肉性滋腻,感冒初期或寒湿内盛者忌用。不宜与猪肉、兔肉、鸭肉、鸡蛋、克莱、芥菜、薄荷同食。

Notes:Turtle flesh is too greasy in property,thus is contraindicated for people with a common cold at the beginning phrase and people with excessive internal cold and dampness. It is improper to be eaten with pork,rabbit meat,duck meat,eggs,clay,mustard and Bohe(Peppermint).

33. 柿子 Persimmon

Shizi

形态特征:为柿科植物柿的果实。

Morphology:The fruit of persimmon. (Fam. Ebenaceae)

功效:清热润肺,生津止渴,涩肠止泻。

Efficacy:clearing heat and moisturizing lung,promoting fluid production to quench thirst,antidarrhea with astringent.

主治病症:肺热阴亏,咳嗽痰黄等;热伤胃阴,热病后期低热不退,口干口渴等。

Indication:lung-heat yin deficiency,cough with yellow phlegm;thermal injury of stomach-yin,successive low-grade fever in the late pyreticosis,dry mouth and thirst.

性味归经:性寒,味甘、涩。入肺、胃、大肠经。

Medicinal properties:Cold in property;sweet and astringent in flavor;enters the lung,stomach and large intestine meridians.

用量用法:内服可生食或做成柿饼食用。

Usage and dosage:It is eaten raw or taken after being dried.

进补应用:胃阴不足,烦渴口干;肺热阴,咳嗽痰多。青柿汁蜜膏:青柿子1000 g,蜂蜜适量。将柿子洗净,去柄,切碎捣烂,以洁净纱布绞取汁液,放入锅内,以文火熬至稠黏时,加入2份蜂蜜,再煎到稠黏如蜜时停火,每次1汤匙,每日2次,沸水冲服。

Application in nourishment：

Deficiency in stomach yin, polydipsia and thirst; yin deficiency caused by lung heat and cough with copious phlegm.

Qingshizhi Migao(Green Persimmon Honey Paste) : 1000 g green persimmon, and some honey. Wash green persimmons clean, remove its stalks, cut them into pieces and smash them, twist juice with a clean gauze, put them into a pot, add spoons of honey, and decoct them again with a small fire until they become dense and sticky like the honey. Take one spoon of it at a time, 2 times daily, together with boiling water.

注意事项：柿性偏寒，凡脾胃虚寒、脾虚泄泻、痰湿内盛、外感咳嗽、疟疾等均不宜食用。空腹时不宜食大量未成熟或未去皮的柿子，否则易发生柿石症，食柿后饮白酒、热水或菜汤更易发生本病。此外，柿子含鞣酸，能抑制肠液分泌，并可与食物中铁质结合而妨碍铁的吸收，故便秘以及缺铁性贫血患者不宜食柿。民间有忌与螃蟹同食之说。

Notes：Persimmon is a little cold in property, thus it is unsuitable for people with spleen and stomach cold and deficiency, spleen deficiency and diarrhea, excessive internal phlegm−dampness, exogenous cough or malaria. Besides, it is not proper to take lots of immature or unpeeled persimmons, otherwise it may cause persimmon bezoar. Drinking liquor, hot water or vegetable soup are more apt to cause persimmon bezoar. In addtion, persimmons include tannic acid, which can refrain the secretion of intestinal juice and integrate with iron in the food, which consequently hinder the iron absorption. Thus, people who suffer from constipation and iron−deficiency anemia had better not eat any persimmon. There is also a folk saying that persimmon should avoid being eaten with crabs.

34. 大枣 Chinese Jujube

Dazao(Fructus jujubae)

形态特征：熟时深红色，果肉味甜，核两端锐尖。

Morphology：Dark red when ripe, with sweet flesh and sharp sides on the stone.

别称：红枣、干枣、枣子、干赤枣、胶枣、南枣、白蒲枣、半官枣、刺枣

Byname：Hongzao, Ganzao, Zaozi, Gan Chizao, Jiaozao, Nanzao, Baipu Zao, Banguan Zao, Cizao

性味归经：味甘，性温。归脾、胃。

Medicinal properties：Sweet in flavor and warm in property; enters the spleen and stomach meridians.

功效：补中益气、养血安神，调营卫；和药性

Efficacy：Strengthening the middle warmer and benefiting vital energy, nourishing blood and tranquilization, regulating ying−wei, neutralizing nature of drug.

主治病症：脾胃虚弱；气血不足；食少便溏；倦怠乏力；心悸失眠；妇人脏躁；营卫

不和。

Indication：Weakness of the spleen and stomach, insufficiency of vital energy and blood, poor eating and loose stool; tiredness and weak; palpitation and insomnia; hysteria of woman, ying-wei disharmony.

用法用量：内服：煎汤,9 ~ 15 g。

Usage and dosage：9 ~ 15 g is used in decoction for internal use.

35. 绿豆 Mung Bean

Lùdou(Vigna Radiatus(L.)Wilczek)

形态特征：豆科菜豆属植物绿豆的种子。以色浓绿而富有光泽、粒大整齐、形圆、煮之易酥者品质最好。

Morphology：The seed of mung bean (Vigna Radiatus (L.) Wilczek) (Fam. Phaseoleae). Products of the best quality are dark green, lustrous, with big and neat granules, round shape and are easily softened when boiled.

别称：又名植豆、文豆、青小豆

Byname：Zhidou, Wendou, Qing Xiaodou

性味归经：甘,寒,入心、胃经。

Medicinal properties：Sweet in flavor and cold in property; enters the heart and stomach meridians.

功效：清热解毒,消暑利水。

Efficacy：Clearing away the heat-evil and expelling superficial evils, removing summer-heat to alleviate water retention.

主治病症：用于暑热烦渴,疮毒痈肿等症,主治：暑热烦渴;感冒发热;霍乱吐泻;痰热哮喘;头痛目赤;口舌生疮;水肿尿少;疮疡痈肿;风疹丹毒;药物及食物中毒。

Indication：Polydipsia due to summer-heat, sore and carbuncle; cold with fever; cholera with vomiting and diarrhea; asthma with heat phlegm; headache and conjunctival congestion; sore in tongue and mouth; oliguresis due to dropsy; sores ulceration and carbuncle swelling; rubella and erysipelas; drug or food poisoning.

用法用量：内服：煎汤,15 ~ 30 g,大剂量可用 120 g;研末;或生研绞汁。外用：适量,研末调敷。

Usage and dosage：15 ~ 30 g is used in decoction for internal use; or 120 g used in large dosage; it is ground into powder or twisted into juice; or proper amount of it is ground into power for external application.

注意事项：绿豆性寒凉,素体阳虚、脾胃虚寒、泄泻者慎食。

Notes：It is cold in property, thus people with yang deficiency, deficient and cold spleen and stomach and diarrhea should take it carefully.

36. 芦蒿 Seleng Wormwood

Luhao(Artemisia Selengensis)

形态特征:为菊科植物蒌蒿的全草。叶有茎,互生,羽状深裂,叶背密生灰白色细毛。小头状花絮,呈淡黄色,果实为瘦果。

Morphology:The whole grass of Louhao (Artemisiaselengensis) (Fam. Asteraceae). There are Leaves on the stem, alternate, with pinnate deep cleft and densely gray hair on the back. Small capitulum, faint yellow; its fruit is achene.

别称:蒌蒿、水艾、香艾、水蒿、藜蒿、泥蒿、蒿苔、龙艾、龙蒿、狭叶青蒿

Byname:Louhao, Shui'ai, Xiang'ai, Shuihao, Lihao, Nihao, Haotai, Long'ai, Longhao, Xiaye Qinghao

性味归经:性凉,味甘。归肝,脾胃经。

Medicinal properties:Cold in property and sweet in flavor; enters the liver, spleen and stomach meridians.

功效:利膈开胃,平抑肝火,全草入药,有止血、消炎、镇咳、化痰之效。

Efficacy:Benefiting diaphragm and promoting appetite, restraining hepatic fire; (whole herb)stopping bleeding, eliminating inflammation, relieving cough, dissipating phlegm.

主治病症:主治食欲不振,胃气虚弱、浮肿及河豚中毒等病症,以及预防牙病、喉病和便秘等

Indication:Poor appetite, stomach qi deficiency, edema and tetrodotoxin, preventing odontopathy, laryngopathy and constipation.

用法用量:嫩茎叶可凉拌、炒食。根状茎可腌渍。内服:煎汤,5～10 g

Usage and dosage:The tender stems and leaves are dressed with sauce to be eaten cold or fried to be taken; the rhizome is pickled to be taken; or 5 ~ 10 g used in decoction for internal use.

注意事项:脾胃虚寒者不宜食用过量。

Notes:People with deficient and cold spleen and stomach should not take it too much.

37. 白果 Ginkgo Seed

Baiguo(Semen Ginkgo)

形态特征:为银杏科植物银杏的干燥成熟种子。秋季种子成熟时采收,除去肉质外种皮,洗净,稍蒸或略煮后,烘干。略呈椭圆形,一端稍尖,另端钝,表面黄白色或淡棕黄色,平滑,具2～3条棱线。中种皮(壳)骨质,坚硬。内种皮膜质,种仁宽卵球形或椭

圆形。

Morphology：The dry ripe seed of ginkgo（Semen Ginkgo）（Fam. Ginkgoaceae）. The seed is ripe and collected in autumn. Remove the meat testa, wash the seeds, steam or boil slightly, and dried. The seed is oval and slightly pointed at one end, blunt the other side; the surface is yellowish-white or pale tan, smooth, with 2－3 ridges. The mesosperm is bone-like and hard; the endopleura is membranous; the kernel is broad ovoid or oval.

别称：银杏,鸭脚子、灵眼、佛指甲、佛指柑。

Byname：Yinxing,Ya Jiaozi,Lingyan,Fo Zhijia,Fozhi Gan

性味归经：甘、苦、涩,小毒。入肺、肾经

Medicinal properties：Sweet,bitter and astringent in flavor;slightly toxic;enters the lung and kidney meridians.

功效：敛肺定喘;止带缩尿

Efficacy：Astringing lung for relieving asthma,stopping leucorrhea and arresting polyuria.

主治病症：哮喘痰嗽;白带;白浊;遗精;尿频;无名肿毒;皶鼻;癣疮。

Indication：Asthma and cough with phlegm;leucorrhea;gonoblennorrhea;spermatorrhea;frequent micturition;unknown swelling toxin;rosacea;tinea.

用法用量：内服:煎汤,3～9 g;或捣汁。外用:适量,捣敷;或切片涂。

Usage and dosage：3～9 g is used in decoction or smashed into juice for internal use; proper amount of it is smashed or sliced for external application.

注意事项：1、有实邪者忌服。2、生食或炒食过量可致中毒,小儿误服中毒尤为常见。

Notes：1. It is contraindicated for people with excess syndrome. 2. Overuse of the raw or stir-baked drugs may cause poisoning. Chidren's poisoning due to wrong taking are more common.

38. 无花果 Fig

Wuhua Guo（Ficus Carica L. ）

形态特征：可食部分是由花托肥大而成的聚合果。

Morphology：The edible part is the acheme formed by the bulged torus.

别称：天仙果、明目果、映日果等。

Byname：Tianxian Guo,Mingmu Guo,Yingri Guo

性味归经：甘;凉。归肺;胃;大肠经

Medicinal properties：Sweet in flavor and cold in property;enters the lung,stomach and large intestine meridians.

功效：清热生津;健脾开胃;解毒消肿。

Efficacy：Removing heat to promote salivation;strengthening spleen and promoting appetite;detumescence by detoxification.

主治病症:主咽喉肿痛;燥咳声嘶;乳汁稀少;肠热便秘;食欲不振;消化不良,泄泻痢疾;痈肿;癣疾。

Indication:Sore – swelling throat; dry cough and hoarseness; lack of breast milk; constipation due to enteric fever; poor appetite; dyspepsia, diarrhea and dysentery, carbuncle swelling, tinea.

用法用量:内服:煎汤,1~2两;或生食1~2枚。外用:煎水洗、研末调敷或吹喉。

Usage and dosage:1 ~ 2 liang(a unit of weight, which is equal to 50 g) is used in decoction;1 ~ 2 pieces are eaten raw; or it is decocted for washing, ground into powder for external application or sprayed into the throat.

39. 生姜 Fresh Ginger

Shengjiang(Rhizoma Zingiberis Recens)

形态特征:为姜科植物姜的根茎。

Morphology:The rhizome of ginger (Rhizoma Zingiberis Recens) (Fam. Zingiberaceae).

别称:老姜、大姜

Byname:Laojiang, Dajiang

性味归经:辛,微温。入肺经、脾经、胃经。

Medicinal properties:Pungent in flavor and slightly warm in property; enters the lung, spleen and stomach meridians.

功效:解表散寒、温中止呕、温肺止咳、化痰止咳,解毒。

Efficacy:Relieving exterior syndrome to expel cold, warming the spleen–stomach to arrest vomiting, warming lung to relieve cough, neutvalizing pois on in fish and crob phlegm and relieving cough, detoxication.

主治病症:外感风寒及胃寒呕逆等证。

Indication:Affection of exotenous wind–cold, vomiting due to stomach cold.

用法用量:煎服,3~9 g,或捣汁服。

Usage and dosage:3 ~ 9 g is used in decoction or smashed into juice to be taken.

注意事项:阴虚火旺、目赤内热者,或患有痈肿疮疖、肺炎、肺脓肿、肺结核、胃溃疡、胆囊炎、肾盂肾炎、糖尿病、痔疮者,都不宜长期食用生姜。

Notes:It is unsuitable to be taken for a long time for people with yin deficiency and excessive fire, red eyes and internal heat; or people with swollen welling–abscess and clove sores, pneumonia, pulmonary abscess, tuberculosis, gastric ulcer, cholecystitis, pyelonephritis, diabetes or hemorrhoids.

40. 葱白 Scallion White

Congbai (Allium fistulosum)

形态特征：为百合科葱属植物的葱全草。通常簇生、全体具辛臭，折断后有辛味之黏液。须根丛生，白色。鳞茎圆柱形，先端稍肥大，鳞叶成层，白色，上具白色纵纹。叶基生，圆柱形，中空。

Morphology：The whole grass of Green Onion (Allium fistulosum) (Fam. Liliaceae). Usually clustered, smelly, with pungent mucus when broken; fibrous roots tufted, white; cylindrical bulb, with slightly plump apex; layers of scale leaves, white, with upper white longitudinal lines; basal leaves, cylindrical, with hollow center.

别称：葱茎白、葱白头。

Byname：Congjing Bai, Congbai Tou

性味归经：味辛；性温。归肺经；胃经。

Medicinal properties：Pungent in flavor and warm in property; enters the lung and stomach meridians.

功效：发表；通阳；解毒；杀虫

Efficacy：Relieving exterior syndrome; activating yang; detoxication; killing parasites.

主治：感冒风寒；阴寒腹痛；二便不通；痢疾；疮痈肿痛；虫积腹痛；阴毒腹痛，小儿盘肠内钓，妇人妊娠溺血，通乳汁，散乳痈，利耳鸣，涂犬毒组安置。

Indication：Common cold and wind cold; abdominal pain due to cold pathogen; difficulty in urine and stool; dysentery; carbuncle and sore; abdominal pain due to parasitic infestation; abdominal pain due to yin evil, pediatric intestines tangle, pregnancy with bleeding, lactogenesis, eliminating mammary abscess, relieving tinnitus, eliminating dog toxin.

用法用量：内服：煎汤，9～15 g；或酒煎。煮粥食，每次可用鲜品 15～30 g。外用：适量，捣敷，炒熨，煎水洗，蜂蜜或醋调敷。

Usage and dosage：9～15 g is used in decoction or decocted in wine; 15～30 g is used fresh every time to cook porridge; proper amount of it is smashed, fried for external application, or decocted for washing, or mixed with honey or vinegar for external application.

注意事项：表虚多汗者忌服。服地黄、常山人，忌食葱。

Notes：It is contraindicated for people with exterior deficiency and profuse sweating. Besides, it is incompatible with the rehmannia root (Radix Rehmanniae) and the antifeverile dichroa root (Radix Dichroae).

41. 香菜 Coriander

Xiangcai

形态特征：为伞形科植物鞠荽的全草。以色泽青绿，香气浓郁，质地脆嫩，无黄叶、烂叶者为佳。

Morphology：The whole grass of Ju Sui（Fam. Umbelliferae）. Products with bluish green color, heavy fragrance, crisp and tender texture, no yellow and broken leaves have the best quality.

别称：又名芫荽、盐荽、胡荽、香荽、延荽、漫天星等

Byname：Yansui, Yansui, Husui, Xiangsui, Yansui, Mantian Xing

性味归经：辛，温。归肺、胃经。

Medicinal properties：Pungent in flavor and warm in property; enters the lung and stomach meridians.

功效：发表透疹，开胃消食，祛风，散寒，胜湿，去翳，通鼻塞。

Efficacy：Relieving superficies to promote eruptions, promoting appetite and digestion, dispelling wind-evil, dispelling cold, eliminating dampness, removing nephelium, removing nasal obstruction.

主治病症：麻疹不透，饮食不消，纳食不佳。治感冒，寒哮，喉痹，百日咳，疹气腹痛，阿米巴痢，疟疾，疳泻，鼻渊，鼻息肉，目翳涩痒，臁疮，疥癣，跌打。

Indication：Measles without adequate eruption; indigestion, poor eating; cold, cold-induced asthma, sore throat, whooping cough, cholera abdominal pain, Ameba dysentery, malaria, malntrition diarrhea, thick rhinorrhea, nasal polyps, unsmooth and itching nephelium, ecthyma, mange, injury from fall.

用法用量：煎服，3～6 g。外用适量，或捣汁或捣烂塞鼻、研末搐鼻或捣敷。

Usage and dosage：3～6 g is used in decoction orally; or smashed into juice or ground into powder to fill into the nose or for external application.

注意事项：热毒壅盛而疹出不畅者忌服。

Notes：It is contraindicated for people with exuberant heat toxin and inhibited emergence of papules.

42. 芦荟 Aloe

Luhui（Aaloe）

形态特征：为百合科芦荟属植物芦荟的地上部分。芦荟叶簇生，呈座状或生于茎顶，

叶常披针形或叶短宽,边缘有尖齿状刺。

Morphology:The ground part of Aloe（Fam. Liliaceae）. The aloe leaves are clustered, rosulate or acrogenous on the stem top, often lanceolate, short and wide, with sharp teeth-like spikes on the margin.

性味归经:苦、寒。归肝、胃、大肠经。

Medicinal properties:Bitter in flavor and cold in property; enters the liver, stomach and large intestine meridians.

功效:清热通便,清肝除烦,杀虫消疳

Efficacy:Removing heat to loosen bowels, clearing liver to wipe out annoyance, killing parasites to recover from malntrition.

主治:肝火头痛,目赤肿痛,烦热惊风,热结便秘,虫积腹痛,小儿疳积,湿疮疥癣,痔瘘。

Indication:Headache due to hepatic fire, sore conjunctival congestion, infantile convulsion due to feverish dysphoria, constipation caused by accumulation of heat, abdominal pain due to parasitic infestation, pediatric malnutritional stagnation, damp sores, mange, hemorrhoids and fistula.

用法用量:内服:研末入胶囊,0.5 至 1.5 g;或入丸、散;不入汤剂。外用:适量,研末敷。

Usage and dosage:0.5 ~ 1.5 g is ground into powder and filled into the capsule, or used in pill or powder preparations, not in decoction; proper amount of it is ground into powder for external application.

注意事项:有慢性腹泻患者也当禁用。体质虚弱者和少年儿童不要过量食用,否则容易发生过敏。孕经期妇女严禁服用,患有痔疮出血、鼻出血的患者勿服。

Notes:It is contraindicated for people with chronic diarrhea. People with weak constitution and children should not take it too much, otherwise they would suffer from allergy. Besides, it is contraindicated for women in pregnancy and menstruation, people with hemorrhoids and bleeding, or nasal hemorrhage.

43. 木瓜 Common Gloweringqince Fruit

Mugua（Fructus Chaenomelis）

形态特征:为蔷薇科植物贴梗海棠的干燥近成熟果实。果实多呈纵剖成对半的长圆形,外表面紫红色或红棕色,有不规则深皱纹;剖面边缘向内卷曲,果肉红棕色,中心部分凹陷,棕黄色。种子扁长三角形,多脱落,质坚硬。气微清香,以质坚实、味酸者为佳。

Morphology:The near-ripe fruit of Tiegeng Haitang（Chaenomelesspeciosa）（Fam. Rosaceae）. The longitudinally half-and-half ripped fruit appears oblong, with purple red or reddish brown outside surface and irregular deep wrinkles; the section margin curves inward;

reddish brown flesh, concave center, brown yellow color; the seed is flat triangular, mostly shed, with hard texture; slightly aromatic. Products with solid texture and sour taste have the best quality.

别称：楙、木瓜实、铁脚梨、秋木瓜、酸木瓜、木瓜海棠、光皮木瓜、木瓜花、木梨、木李、榠楂、文冠果、文官果。

Byname：Mao, Mugua Shi, Tiejiao Li, Qiu Mugua, Suan Mugua, Mugua Haitang, Guangpi Mugua, Mugua Hua, Muli, Muli, Mingzha, Wenguan Guo, Wenguan Guo

性味归经：酸，温。归肝、脾经

Medicinal properties：Sour in flavor and warm in property; enters the liver and spleen meridians.

功效：舒筋活络，和胃化湿。

Efficacy：Relaxing and activating the tendons, regulating stomach and dissipating dampness.

主治病症：风湿痹症，脚气水肿，吐泻转筋。

Indication：Rheumatic arthralgia, beriberi and hydrops, vomiting, diarrhea and spasm of muscle.

用法用量：煎服，6~9 g；或入丸、散。外用：煎水熏洗。

Usage and dosage：6~9 g is used in decoction, pill or powder preparations; or decocted for external smoking or washing.

注意事项：内有郁热，小便短赤者忌服。

Notes：It is contraindicated for people with internal stagnant heat and scanty dark urine.

44. 玉米须 Corn Stigma

Yumi Xu

形态特征：为禾本科植物玉蜀黍的花柱和柱头。雌小穗密集成纵行排列于粗壮的穗轴上，颖片宽阔，先端圆形或微凹，外稃膜质透明。

Morphology：The style and stigma of maize (Fam. Poaceae). The female spikelets are densely arranged longitudinally on the thick spike stalks, with wide peristachyum, round or slightly concave apex, membranous and transparent lemma.

别称：玉麦须、五蜀黍蕊、棒子毛。

Byname：Yumai Xu, Wushushu Sui, Bangzi Mao.

性味归经：甘，平。归膀胱、肝、胆经。

Medicinal properties：Sweet in flavor and neutral in property; enters the bladder, liver and gallbladder meridians.

功效：利水消肿，清肝利胆，除湿退黄。

Efficacy：Inducing diuresis to alleviate edema, clearing liver to promote the function of gallbladder, eliminating dampness and jaundice.

主治病症:水肿,黄疸。

Indication:Hydrops,jaundice.

用法用量:煎服,30~60 g。鲜者加倍。

Usage and dosage:30~60 g is used in decoction;or double dose is used fresh.

45. 花椒 Pricklyash Peel

Huajiao(Pericarpium Zanthoxyli)

形态特征:为芸香科植物花椒的干燥成熟果实。菁葖果球形,红色或紫红色,密生粗大而凸出的腺点。

Morphology:The dry ripe fruit of Chinese pricklyash((Pericarpium Zanthoxyli)(Fam. Rutaceae). The follicle is spherical, red or purple red, with dense thick and bulging glandular spots.

别称:樶、大椒、秦椒、南椒、巴椒、蓎藙、陆拨、汉椒、点椒。

Byname:Hui,Dajiao,Qinjiao,Nanjiao,Bajiao,Tangyi,Lubo,Hanjiao,Dianjiao

性味归经:辛;性温;小毒 归脾经、胃、肾经;

Medicinal properties:Pungent in flavor and warm in property;enters the spleen, stomach and kidney meridians.

功效:温中止痛,除湿止泻,杀虫止痒。

Efficacy:Warming the spleen-stomach to relieve pain, eliminating dampness to check diarrhea, killing parasites to relieve itching.

主治病症:脾胃虚寒之脘腹冷痛,寒湿泄泻、虫积腹痛、风寒湿痹;阴痒带下;湿疹皮肤瘙痒。

Indication:Crymodynia in gastric cavity and abdomen due to insufficiency of spleen-yang,diarrhea due to cold-dampness, abdominal pain due to parasitic infestation; pudendum pruritus and morbid leucorrhea;skin pruritus due to eczema.

用法用量:内服:煎汤,3~6 g;或入丸、散。外用:适量,煎水洗可含漱;研末调敷。

Usage and dosage:3~6 g is used in decoction, pill or powder preparations; or proper amount of it is decocted for washing or gargling;or it is ground into powder for external application.

注意事项:阴虚火旺者忌服。孕妇慎服。

Notes:It is contraindicated for people with yin deficiency and excessive fire. Pregnant women should take it cautiously.

46. 鸡内金 Chicken's Gizzard-skin

Ji Neijin(Endothelium Corneum Gigeriae Galli)

形态特征:为雉科动物家鸡的干燥沙囊内壁。本品呈不规则囊片状,略卷曲。大小不一,完整者长约 3.5 cm,宽约 3 cm,厚约 0.5 cm。表面黄色、黄绿色或黄褐色,薄而半透明,有多数明显的条棱状波纹。质脆,易碎,断面角质样,有光泽。气微腥,味微苦。

Morphology: The dry inner gizzard of chicken (Gallus gallus domesticus)(Fam. Phasianidae). Irregular, caplet-like, slightly curved; sizes variable; complete ones about 3.5 cm long, 3 cm wide and 0.5 cm thick; surface yellow, yellowish green or yellowish brown, thin and nearly transparent, with numerous obvious prismatic wavy ripples; texture crisp, easily broken; section keratoid, lustrous; slightly fishy and bitter.

别称:鸡肶胵里黄皮、鸡肶胵、鸡肫内黄皮、鸡肫皮、鸡黄皮、鸡食皮、鸡合子、鸡中金、化石胆、化骨胆。

Byname: Jipichi Lihuangpi, Ji Pichi, Jidun Neihuangpi, Jidun Pi, Jihuang Pi, Jishi Pi, Ji Hezi, Ji Zhongjin, Huashi Dan, Huagu Dan

性味归经:味甘;性平。归脾;胃;肾;膀胱经。

Medicinal properties: Sweet in flavor and neutral in property; enters the spleen, stomach, kidney and bladder meridians.

功效:健脾消食;涩精止遗;消症化石。

Efficacy: Invigorating spleen to promote digestion, astringing essence and checking seminal emission, eliminating geloses and calculus.

主治:消化不良;饮食积滞;呕吐反胃;泄泻下痢;小儿疳积;遗精;遗尿;小便频数;泌尿系结石及胆结石;症瘕经闭;喉痹乳蛾;牙疳口疮。

Indication: Dyspepsia, food stagnation, vomiting and regurgitation, diarrhea, pediatric malnutritional stagnation, spermatorrhea, enuresis, frequent urination, urinary calculi, gallstone, menischesis due to geloses in the body, sore throat and throat moth, ulcerative gingivitis and aphthae.

用法用量:内服:煎汤,3~10 g;研末,每次 1.5~3 g;或入丸、散。外用:适量,研末调敷或生贴。

Usage and dosage: 3~10 g is used in decoction, or 1.5~3 g is used in ground powder, or used in pills or powder; proper amount of it is ground into powder for external application or directly applied without being processed.

注意事项:脾虚无积者慎服。

Notes: It is contraindicated for people with spleen deficiency and no accumulation and stagnation.

47. 槟榔 Areca Seed

Binglang(Semen Arecae)

形态特征:为棕榈科植物槟榔 的干燥成熟种子。呈扁球形或圆锥形。表面淡黄棕色或淡红棕色,具稍凹下的网状沟纹。质坚硬,断面可见棕色种皮与白色胚乳相间的大理石样花纹。

Morphology:The dry ripe seed of Binglang (Semen Arecae)(Fam. Arecaceae). It is flat spherical or conical. The surface is yellowish brown or reddish brown, with slightly recessed mesh grooves. It is hard and the section has marble sample patterns with brown seed skin and white endosperm.

别称:仁频、宾门、宾门药饯、白槟榔、橄榄子、洗瘴丹、大腹槟榔、槟榔子、青仔、槟榔玉、榔玉。

Byname:Renpin, Binmen, Binmen Yaojian, Bai Binglang, Ganlan Zi, Xizhang Dan, Dafu Binglang, Binglang Zi, Qingzai, Binglang Yu, Langyu

性味归经:味苦;辛;性温。归胃经;大肠经。

Medicinal properties:Bitter and pungent in flavor;warm in property;enters the stomach and large intestine meridians.

功效:驱虫,消积,下气,行水,截疟。

Efficacy:Killing parasites, removing food retention, descending qi, moving water, stopping malaria.

主治病症:虫积;食滞;脘腹胀痛;泻痢后重;脚气;水肿;疟疾。

Indication:Intestinal parasitosis, dyspeptic retention, gas pains in gastric cavity and abdomen, difficult in dysentery, beriberi, hydrops, malaria.

用法用量:内服:煎汤,6～15 g,单用杀虫,可用60～120 g;或入丸、散。

Usage and dosage:6～15 g is used in decoction, or 60～120 g is used singly to kill insects, or used in pills or powder.

注意事项:脾虚便溏或气虚下陷者忌用;孕妇慎用。

Notes:It is contraindicated for people with spleen deficiency and loose stool, or people with collapse due to qi deficiency. Besides, pregnant women should use it cautiously.

48. 莱菔子 Radish Seed

Laifu Zi(Raphanus Sativus L.)

形态特征:为十字花科植物萝卜的干燥成熟种子。炒莱菔子:取净莱菔子,置锅内用文火炒至微鼓起,并有香气为度,取出,放凉。

Morphology: The dry ripe seed of radish(Raphanus sativus L)(Fam. Cruciferae). Fried radish seed Choose some clean radish seeds, put them into a pot, fry them with a slow fire till they bulge a little and become fragrant. Take them out and cool them.

别称:萝卜子、萝白子、芦菔子、菜头子。

Byname: Luobo Zi, Luobai Zi, Lufu Zi, Caitou Zi

性味归经:味辛;甘;性平。归脾、胃经;肺经;大肠经。

Medicinal properties: Pungent and sweet in flavor; neutral in property; enters the spleen, stomach, lung and large intestine meridians.

功效:消食导滞,降气化痰。

Efficacy: Promoting digestion to disperse stagnation, depressing qi to dissipate phlegm.

主治病症:食积气滞;脘腹胀满;腹泻;下痢后重;咳嗽多痰;气逆喘满。

Indication: Food accumulation and qi stagnation, diarrhea, difficult in alo laxata, cough with excessive phlegm, qi regurgitating and dyspneal fullness.

用法用量:内服:煎汤,5~10 g;或入丸、散,宜炒用。外用:适量,研末调敷。

Usage and dosage: 5~10 g is used in decoction, pill or powder preparations; or proper amount is ground into powder for external application.

注意事项:中气虚弱者慎服。

Notes: People with weak middle qi should take it carefully.

49. 蜂蜜 Honey

Fengmi(Mel)

形态特征:为蜜蜂科昆虫中华蜜蜂或意大利蜜蜂所酿的蜜。为浓稠液体,白色,淡黄色至黄褐色,味极甜。

Morphology: The honey of Chinese bee or Italian bee. It is thick liquid; white, faint yellow or yellowish-brown; very sweet taste.

别称:石蜜、石饴、食蜜、蜜、白蜜、白沙蜜、蜜糖、沙蜜、蜂糖。

Byname: Shimi, Shiyi, Shimi, Mi, Baimi, Baisha Mi, Mitang, Shami, Fengtang

性味归经:味甘;性平。归脾经;胃经;肺经;大肠经。

Medicinal properties: Sweet in flavor and neutral in property; enters the spleen, stomach, lung and large intestine meridians.

功效:调补脾胃;缓急止痛;润肺止咳;润肠通便;润肤生肌;解毒。

Efficacy: Regulating and tonifying spleen and stomach, relaxing tension and relieving pain, moistening lung to arrest cough, loosening bowel to relieve constipation, moistening skin to promote tissue regeneration, detoxication.

主治病症:脘腹虚痛;肺燥咳嗽;肠燥便秘;目赤;口疮;溃疡不敛;风疹瘙痒;水火烫

伤;手足(皲)裂。

Indication:Asthenia – pain in gastric cavity and abdomen, xeropulmonary cough, constipation due to intestine dryness, conjunctival congestion, aphthae, unhealing ulcer, itching rubella, burn due to hot liquid or fire, chapping in hand and foot.

用法用量:内服:冲调,15～30 g;或入丸剂、膏剂。外用:适量,涂敷。

Usage and dosage:15～30 g is mixed with water, or used in pill or paste preparations;or proper amount is used for external application.

注意事项:痰湿内蕴、中满痞胀及大便不实者禁服。

Notes:It is contraindicated for people with phlegm – damp brewing internally, central fullness and abdominal distention, or people with loose stool.

50. 乌梅 Smoked Plum

Wumei(Fructus Mume)

形态特征:为蔷薇科植物梅的干燥近成熟果实。呈类球形或扁球形,直径1.5～3cm。表面乌黑色或棕黑色,皱缩不平,基部有圆形果梗痕。果核坚硬,椭圆形,棕黄色,表面有凹点;种子扁卵形,淡黄色。气微,味极酸。

Morphology:The dry and nearly ripe fruit of smoked plum(Fructus Mume)(Fam. Rosaceae). It is a kind of spherical or flat spherical, 1.5– 3 cm in diameter. The surface is black or dark brown, wrinkled, with round fruit stalk marks at the base. The fruit stone is hard, oval, tan, and with pits on the surface; the seed is flat oval, pale yellow, light smell, and very sour taste.

别称:梅实、熏梅、桔梅肉、梅、春梅。酸梅、黄仔、合汉梅、干枝梅

Byname:Meishi, Xunmei, Jumei Rou, Mei, Chunmei, Suanmei, Huangzi, Hehan Mei, Ganzhi Mei

性味归经:味酸;性平。归肝经;脾经;肺经;肾经;胃经;大肠经。

Medicinal properties:Sour in flavor and neutral in property;enters the liver, spleen, lung, kidney, stomach and large intestine meridians.

功效:敛肺止咳,涩肠止泻,止血,生津,安蛔。

Efficacy:Astringing lung to stop cough, antidarrhea with astringent, stopping bleeding, body fluid regeneration, relieving ascaris colic.

主治:久咳;虚热烦渴;久疟;久泻;痢疾;便血;尿血;血崩;蛔厥腹痛;呕吐;钩虫病。

Indication:Chronic cough, excessive thirst due to deficiency heat, chronic malaria, chronic diarrhea, dysentery, hematochezia, hemuresis, profuse uterine bleeding, abdominal pain due to ascarid faint, vomiting, ancylostomiasis.

用法用量:内服:煎汤,0.8～1.5 钱;或入丸、散。外用:煅研干撒或调敷。

Usage and dosage:0.8～1.5 qian(a unit of weight equal to 5 grams)is used in decoction, pill or powder preparations; or calcined into powder for external application.

注意事项:有实邪者忌服,胃酸过多者慎服。

Notes: It is contraindicated for people with excess syndrome. People with gastroxia should take it cautiously.

51. 南瓜子 Pumpkin Seed

Nangua Zi(Semen Cucurbitae)

形态特征:种子扁圆形,长1.2~1.8 cm,宽0.7~1 cm。表面淡黄白以至淡黄色,两面平坦而微隆起,边毋稍有棱,一端略尖,先端有珠孔,种脐稍突起或不明显。除去种皮,有黄绿色薄膜状胚乳。子叶2枚,黄色,肥厚,有油性。气微香,味微甘。以颗粒饱满、色黄白者为佳。

Morphology: The seed flat round, 1.2~1.8 cm long and 0.7~1 cm wide; surface light yellowish white to light yellow; two sides flat but slightly bulging, with slight ridges on the edge; one tip slightly sharp, with apex micropyle, prominent or unobvious umbilici; yellowish green membranous endosperm inside the episperm; cotyledon 2 pieces, yellow, fleshy, oily, slightly fragrant, slightly sweet. Products with full granules and yellowish white color have the best quality.

别称:南瓜仁、白瓜子、金瓜米、金瓜子、窝瓜子、倭瓜子。

Byname: Nangua Ren, Bai Guazi, Jin Guami, Jin Guazi, Wo Guazi, Wo Guazi

性味归经:味甘;性平。归大肠经。

Medicinal properties: Sweet in flavor and neutral in property; enters the large intestine meridian.

功效:杀虫,下乳,利水消肿。

Efficacy: Killing parasites, promoting lactation, inducing diuresis to alleviate edema.

主治:绦虫;蛔虫;血吸虫;钩虫;蛲虫病;产后缺乳;手足浮肿;百日咳;痔疮。

Indication: Tapeworm, lumbricus, blood fluke, hookworms, enterobiasis, lack of breast milk postpartum, edema in hand and foot, whooping cough, haemorrhoids.

用法用量:内服:煎汤,30~60 g;研末或制成乳剂。外用:适量,煎水熏洗。

Usage and dosage: 30~60 g is used in decoction, powdered or made into the milky preparation; proper amount is decocted for external smoking or washing.

注意事项:多食壅气滞膈。

Notes: Taking it too much may cause qi stagnation in the diaphragm.

52. 昆布 Kelp or Tangle

Kunbu（Thallus Eckloniae）

形态特征：为海带科植物海带或翅藻科植物昆布的干燥叶状体。藻体橄榄褐色，干后为暗褐色。成熟后革质呈带状

Morphology：The dry thallus of Kelp or Tangle（Thallus Eckloniae）（Fam. Laminariaceae）. The frond is olive-brown, or dark brown when dried; leathery and belt-like when ripe.

别称：纶布、海昆布。

Byname：Lunbu, Hai Kunbu.

性味归经：咸；寒；无毒。归肝经；胃经；肾经；脾经。

Medicinal properties：Salt in flavor and cold in property; nontoxic; enters the liver, stomach, kidney, and spleen meridians.

功效：消痰软坚，利水退肿。

Efficacy：Dispelling phlegm to soften abdominal mass, alleviating water retention for detumescence.

主治：瘰疬；瘿瘤；噎膈；疝，脚气水肿。

Indication：Scrofula, gall, cardiac spasm, hernia, beriberi and edema.

用法用量：内服：煎汤，5～15 g；或入丸、散。

Usage and dosage：5～15 g is used in decoction, pill or powder preparations for internal use.

注意事项：脾胃虚寒蕴湿者忌服。

Notes：It is contraindicated for people with deficent and cold spleen and stomach with brewing damp.

53. 麦芽 Germinated Barley

Maiya（Fructus Hordei Germinatus）

形态特征：为禾本科植物大麦的成熟果实经发芽干燥而得。呈梭形。表面淡黄色，背面为外稃包围，具 5 脉；腹面为内稃包围。除去内外稃后，腹面有 1 条纵沟。须根数条，纤细而弯曲。质硬，断面白色，粉性。

Morphology：The ripe fruit of barley´s（Hordeum vulgare L.）（Fam. Poaceae）dried sprout. It is spindle-like; the surface is pale yellow and covered by lemma on the back, with 5 veins on it; the segmental venter is covered by glumelle. Removing the lemma, there is a longitudinal groove on the segmental; several fibrous roots, slender and curving. It is hard and its section is white, powdery.

别称：大麦蘖、麦蘖、大麦毛、大麦芽。

Byname：Damai Nie, Mainie, Damai Mao, Damai Ya.

性味归经：甘；平。归脾经；胃经。

Medicinal properties：Sweet in flavor and neutral in property; enters the spleen and stomach meridians.

功效：消食化积；回乳。

Efficacy：Promoting digestion and eliminating food stagnation, terminating lactation.

主治：食积不消；腹满泄泻；恶心呕吐；食欲不振；乳汁郁积；乳房胀痛。

Indication：Food stagnation, abdominal distension diarrhea, nausea and vomiting, poor appetite, stagnation of breast milk, distending pain in breast.

用法用量：内服：煎汤，10～15 g，大剂量可用 30～120 g；或入丸、散

Usage and dosage：10～15 g is used in decoction; or 30～120 g is used in large dose; or used in pill and powder preparations.

注意事项：无积滞，脾胃虚者不宜用。凡痰火哮喘及孕妇，切不可用。

Notes：It is unsuitable for people with no accumulation and stagnation, or people with deficient spleen and stomach. Besides, it is contraindicated for people with phlegm fire and pregnant women.

54. 荷叶 Lotus Leaf

Heye(Folium Nelumbinis)

形态特征：为睡莲科植物莲的干燥叶。呈半圆形式或折扇形，展开后呈类圆形，全缘或稍呈波状，表面深绿色或黄绿色，较粗糙，被蜡质白粉，背面灰绿色，呈波状，较光滑，有粗脉 21～22 条，自中心向四周射出；中心有突起的叶柄残基。叶柄圆柱形，密生倒刺。质脆，易破碎。

Morphology：The dry leaf of lotus (Nelumbonucifera) (Fam. Nymphaeaceae). Semicircle or folding-fan like, nearly spherical after being spread, entire margin or slightly wavy; surface dark green or yellowish green, quite rough, covered with waxy white powder; back grayish green, wavy, quite smooth, with thick veins 21～22 pieces, sprayed from the center to the four directions; center with prominent residual petiole base; petiole cylindrical, covered with dense barbs; texture crisp, easily broken.

别称：蕸、莲叶、鲜荷叶、干荷叶、荷叶炭。

Byname：Xia, Lianye, Xian Heye, Gan Heye, Heye Tan.

性味归经：有清香气，味微苦，无毒。入脾经、胃经。

Medicinal properties：With faint scent; slightly bitter in flavor; nontoxic; enters the spleen and stomach meridians.

功效:有清热解暑、平肝降脂之功。

Efficacy:Clearing away summer heat and heat evil,pacifying liver and reducing blood fat.

主治:口干引饮、小便短黄、头目眩晕、面色红赤、高血压、高脂血症、清暑利湿、升发脾阳、止血、治暑湿泄泻、眩晕、水气浮肿、雷头风、吐血、衄血、崩漏、便血、产后血晕。

Indication:Dry mouth desiring water, little and yellowish urine, dizziness in eyes and head, red complexion, hypertension, hyperlipemia, clearing away the summer-heat to reduce dampness through diuresis, promoting spleen yang, hemostasis, summer heat-dampness diarrhea, dizziness, water-qi edema, headache with tinnitus, hematemesis, non-traumatic hemorrhage, uterine bleeding, hematochezia, postpartum faintness.

用法与用量:内服:煎汤(鲜者0.5~1两)5~15 g;或入丸、散。外用:捣敷、研末掺或煎水洗。

Usage and dosage:5~15 g(or 0.5~1 liang of the fresh)is used in decoction, pill or powder preparations for internal use; or smashed, ground into powder for external application; or decocted for washing.

注意事项:凡上焦邪盛,治宜清降者,切不可用。

Notes:It is contraindicated for people with the exuberant evil in the upper energizer. Those people should be treated by clearing and downbearing.

55. 粳米 Non-glutinous Rice

Jingmi

形态特征:米粒一般呈椭圆形或圆形。米粒丰满肥厚,横断面近于圆形,长与宽之比小于二,颜色蜡白,呈透明或半透明,质地硬而有韧性,煮后黏性油性均大,柔软可口。

Morphology:The rice appears ellipse or round; plump and fleshy, with nearly round cross-section; length-width ratio less than two; glastly pale, transparent or half transparent, with hard texture and tough nature; oily and sticky after being boiled; tastes soft and delicious.

性味归经:性平、味甘。归脾、胃经。

Medicinal properties:Neutral in property and sweet in flavor; enters the spleen and stomach meridians.

功效:补中益气,平和五脏,止烦渴,止泻,壮筋骨,通血脉,益精强志。

Efficacy:Strengthening the middle warmer and benefiting vital energy, pacifying viscera, stopping polydipsia, stopping diarrhea, strengthening bone and musculature, improving the circulation of blood vessels, benefiting spirit and strengthening will.

主治:泻痢、胃气不足、口干渴、呕吐、诸虚百损等。

Indication:Diarrhea and dysentery, gastric-qi insufficiency, dry mouth thirst, vomiting, consumptive diseases.

注意事项:糖尿病患者不宜多食。

Notes: People with diabetes should not take it too much.

56. 芡实 Gordon Euryale Seed

Qianshi(Ssemen Euryales)

形态特征:为睡莲科植物芡的干燥成熟种仁。种仁类圆球形,直径 5 ~ 8 mm,有的破碎成块。完整者表面有红棕色或暗紫色的内种皮,可见不规则的脉状网纹,一端约 1/3 为黄白色。胚小,位于淡黄色一端的圆形凹窝内。质地较硬,断面白色,粉性。气无,味淡。以饱满、断面白色、粉性足、无碎末者为佳。

Morphology: The dry ripe kernel of Qian(Euryale ferox) (Fam. Nymphaeaceae). Kernel spherical-like, 5 ~ 8 mm in diameter; some broken into pieces, with reddish brown or dark purple inside episperm on the surface of complete ones; irregular vein-like reticulate vessels, 1/3 of one tip yellowish white; embryo small, within the light yellow round hollowness; hard texture, white section, mealiness, with no smell and mild taste. Products which are full, with white section, full mealiness and no broken powder have the best quality.

别称:卵菱、鸡癰、鸡头实、雁喙实、鸡头、雁头、乌头、蒍子、鸿头、水流黄、水鸡头、肇实、刺莲藕、刀芡实、鸡头果、苏黄、黄实、鸡咀莲、鸡头苞、刺莲蓬实。

Byname: Luanling, Jiyong, Jirou Shi, Yanhui Shi, Jitou, Yantou, Wutou, Weizi, Hongtou, Shuiliu Huang, Shui Jitou, Zhaoshi, Ci Lian'ou, Dao Qianshi, Jitou Guo, Suhuang, Huangshi, Jizui Lian, Jitou Bao, Ci Lianpeng Shi

性味归经:甘;涩;平。脾经;肾经;心经;胃经;肝经。

Medicinal properties: Sweet, astringent in flavor and neutral in property; enters the spleen, kidney, heart, stomach and liver meridians.

功效:固肾涩精,补脾止泄。

Efficacy: Strengthening kidney, invigorating the spleen and stopping diarrhea.

主治:遗精;白浊;淋浊;带下;小便不禁;大便泄泻。

Indication: Spermatorrhea, gonoblennorrhea, morbid leucorrhea, urinary incontinence, diarrhea.

用法用量:内服:煎汤,15 ~ 30 g;或入丸、散,亦可适量煮粥食。

Usage and dosage: 15 ~ 30 g is used in decoction, pill or powder preparations; or proper amount is cooked in porridge to be taken.

注意事项:大小便不利者禁服;食滞不化者慎服。

Notes: It is contraindicated for people with inhibited defecation and urination. Besides, people with food stagnation should take it cautiously.

57. 桑葚 Mulberry

Sangshen

形态特征:为桑科植物桑的果穗。聚花果由多数小瘦果集合而成,呈长圆形,长 1~2 cm,直径 5~8 mm。黄棕色、棕红色至暗紫色;有短果序梗。小瘦果卵圆形,稍扁,长约 2 mm,宽约 1 mm,外具肉质花被片 4 枚。气微,味微酸而甜。以个大、肉厚、包紫红、糖性大者为佳。

Morphology: The cluster of mulberry (Morus alba L.) (Fam. Moraceae). Collective fruit, assembled by numerous small achenes, oblong, 1~2 cm long, 5~8 mm in diameter; yellowish brown, brown red to dark purple, with short infructescence stalk; small achenes oval, slightly flat, about 2 mm long and 1 mm wide; outside with 4 pieces of fleshy tapel; odor slight, taste slightly sour and sweet. Products which are big, fleshy, purple red with a lot of sugar have the best quality.

别称:桑实、文武实、黑椹、桑枣、桑葚子、桑粒、桑果。

Byname: Sangshi, Wenwu Shi, Heishen, Sangzao, Sangshen Zi, Sangli, Sangguo.

性味归经:甘、酸,寒。入肝、肾经。

Medicinal properties: Sweet and sour in flavor and cold in property; enters the liver and kidney meridians.

功效:补肝,益肾,熄风,滋液。滋阴补血、生津润燥。

Efficacy: Tonifying liver, tonifying kidney, subduing wind, nourishing body fluid. Nourishing yin and blood, generate fluids and moisturizing dryness.

主治:治肝肾阴亏,消渴,便秘,目暗,耳鸣,瘰疬,关节不利。

Indication: Kidney – liver yin – deficiency, wasting – thirst, constipation, clouded eyesight, tinnitus, scrofula, inflexible joints.

用法用量:9~15 g。

Usage and dosage: 9~15 g.

注意事项:脾胃虚寒便溏者禁服。多食致衄,孕妇忌之。

Notes: It is contraindicated for people with deficient and cold spleen and stomach and loose stool. Pregnant women shouldn't take it because overuse of it would cause bleeding.

58. 罗汉果 Grosvenor Momordica Fruit

Luohan Guo (Fructus Momordicae)

形态特征:为葫芦科植物罗汉果的干燥果实。干燥果实,圆形至长圆形,径 5~8 cm,

外表黄褐色至深棕色,较光泽,微具残留毛茸,少数有较深色的纵条纹。顶端膨大,中央有一圆形的花柱基痕,基部略狭,有果柄痕。质脆易碎,破碎后内表面黄白色,疏松似海绵状。除去中果皮,可见明显的纵脊纹 10 条。种子扁平,矩圆形或类圆形,棕色,边缘较厚,中央微凹,内有子叶 2 枚。味甜。

Morphology：The dry fruit of Luohan Guo (Fructus Momordicae) (Fam. Cucurbitaceae). The dried fruit, round to oblong, 5 ~ 8 cm in diameter；the outside yellowish brown to dark brown, quite lustrous, with residual fuzz, few with darker longitudinal stripes；the apex gibbous, with a round basal scar of the style；base slightly narrow, with stalk mark；texture crisp and easily broken；inside yellowish white when broken, sponge-like loose；10 obvious longitudinal ridge lines within the middle pericarp；seed flat, oblong or nearly round, brown, with thicker margin, concave center and 2 pieces of cotyledon；sweet in taste. Products which are round, complete, big, solid, without sound when shaken, with yellowish brown color have the best quality.

别称:拉汗果、假苦瓜、光果木鳖、金不换、罗汉表、裸龟巴。

Byname：Lahan Guo, Jia Kugua, Guangguo Mubie, Jin Buhuan, Luohan Biao, Luo Guiba

性味归经:味甘;性凉。肺经;大肠经。

Medicinal properties：Sweet in flavor and cold in property；enters the lung and spleen meridians.

功效:清肺利咽;化痰止咳;润肠通便。

Efficacy：Clearing lung and relieving sore-throat, dissipating phlegm and stopping cough, loosening bowel to relieve constipation.

主治:咳嗽;咽喉炎;扁桃体炎;急性胃炎;便秘。

Indication：Cough with phlegm due to lung heat, laryngopharyngitis, tonsillitis, acute gastritis, constipation.

用法用量:内服:煎汤,15 ~ 30 g,或炖肉;或开水泡。

Usage and dosage：15 ~ 30 g is used in decoction, or stewed with the meat, or infused in the hot water to be taken.

注意事项:脾胃虚寒者忌服。

Notes：It is contraindicated for people with deficient and cold spleen and stomach.

59. 薄荷 Peppermint

Bohe(Herba Menthae)

形态特征:为唇形科植物薄荷的干燥地上部分。上表面深绿色,下表面灰绿色,两面均有柔毛,下表面在扩大镜下可见凹点状腺鳞。茎上部常有腋生的轮伞花序,花萼钟状,先端 5 齿裂,萼齿狭三角状钻形,微被柔毛;花冠多数存在,淡紫色。揉搓后有特殊香气,味辛、凉。以叶多、色绿、气味浓者为佳。

别称：苏薄荷、水薄荷、鱼香草、人丹草、蕃荷菜、野薄荷、夜息香、南薄荷、水薄荷、鱼香菜、狗肉香、水益母、接骨草、土薄荷、人丹草、野仁丹草、苏薄荷、五香等。

Byname：The dry ground part of Bohe（Herba Menthae）（Fam. Labiatae）. Su Bohe, Shui Bohe, Yuxiang Cao, Rendan Cao, Fanhe Cai, Ye Bohe, Yexi Xiang, Nan Bohe, Shui Bohe, Yuxiang Cai, Gourou Xiang, Shui Yimu, Jiegu Cao, Tu Bohe, Rendan Cao, Ye Rendancao, Su Bohe, Wuxiang, etc.

性味归经：辛，凉。入肺经、肝经。

Medicinal properties：Pungent in flavor and cold in property; enters the lung and liver meridians.

功效：疏散风热，清利头目，利咽透疹，疏肝行气。

Efficacy：Dispelling wind and heat, benefiting head and eyes, relieving sore-throat and promoting eruptions, soothing liver and promoting qi.

主治：疏风、散热、辟秽、解毒、外感风热、头痛、咽喉肿痛、食滞气胀、口疮、牙痛、疮疥、瘾疹、温病初起、风疹瘙痒、肝郁气滞、胸闷胁痛。

Indication：Expelling wind, dissipating heat, avoiding dirty, detoxication, affection of exogenous wind-heat, headache, sore and swelling throat, dyspeptic retention and gaseous distention, aphtha, toothache, scabies, urticant eruptions, onset of seasonal prevalent diseases, itching rubella, stagnation of qi due to depression of the liver, dyspnea with pain in ribs.

用法与用量：内服：煎汤（不宜久煎），4~20 g；或入丸、散。

Usage and dosage：4~20 g is decocted（not too long）, or used in pill or powder preparations.

注意事项：阴虚血燥，肝阳偏亢，表虚汗多者忌服。

Notes：It is contraindicated for people with yin deficiency, dry blood, hyperactive liver yang, exterior deficiency and profuse sweating.

60. 菊花 Chrysanthemum Flower

Ju Hua（Flos Chrysanthemi）

形态特征：为菊科植物菊的干燥头状花序。

Morphology：The dry capitulum of Ju Hua（Flos Chrysanthemi）（Fam. Asteraceae）.

别称：帝女花、甘菊花、白菊花、黄甘菊、药菊、白茶菊、茶菊、怀菊花、滁菊、毫菊、杭菊、贡菊。

Byname：Dinǔ Hua, Gan Juhua, Bai Juhua, Huang Ganju, Yaoju, Baicha Ju, Chaju, Huai Juhua, Chuju, Haoju, Hangju, Gongju.

性味归经：辛，甘，苦，微寒。归肺、肝经。

Medicinal properties：Pungent, sweet and bitter in flavor and slightly cold in property; enters the lung and liver meridians.

功效:疏风散热,清肝明目,平抑肝阳,清热解毒。

Efficacy:Expelling wind to dissipate heat,clearing liver to improve eyesight,calming liver yang,clearing away the heat evil and expelling superficial evils.

主治:用于风热感冒,头痛眩晕,目赤肿痛,眼目昏花,疮痈肿毒。

Indication:Wind-heat type common cold,headache and dizziness,red eye with pain and swelling,dim eyesight,sore and carbuncle with swelling toxin.

用法用量:煎服,5~9 g。疏散风热用黄菊花,平肝、清肝明目用白菊花

Usage and dosage:5~9 g is used in decoction;yellow chrysanthemum flowers are used to dispell wind and heat;white chrysanthemum flowers are used to calm the liver,clear the liver and improve the eyesight.

注意事项:气虚胃寒,食少泄泻之病,宜少用之。

Note:People with qi deficiency and stomach coldness and decreased food intake and diarrhea had better not use it.

61. 橘皮 Orange Peel

Ju Pi

形态特征:为芸香科植物橘的干燥果皮。完整的果皮常剖成4瓣,每瓣多呈椭圆形,在果柄处连在一起。有时破碎分离,或呈不规则形的碎片状。外表面鲜橙红色、黄棕色至棕褐色,有无数细小而凹入的油室;内表面淡黄白色,海绵状,并有短线状的维管束(橘络)痕,果蒂处较密。质柔软,干燥后质脆,易折断,断面不平。以皮薄、片大、色红、油润、香气浓者为佳。

Morphology:The dry pericarp Orange(Fam. Rutaceae). The complete peel is usually divided into 4 parts, each appears oval and combines at the stalk; sometimes broken and separated, or appears like irregular broken pieces; outer surface bright orange red, yellowish brown to brown, with numerous fine and excavated oil cavity; inside light yellowish white, sponge-like, with short string-like marks of vascular bundles(orange vessels), dense at the fruit base; texture soft, brittle when dried, easily broken, with uneven sections; those fruits with thin peel, big pieces, red color, lubrication and fragrance are the best.

别称:橘皮、贵老、红皮、黄橘皮、广橘皮、新会皮、红橘、大红袍、川橘。

Byname:Jupi,Guilao,Hongpi,Huangjupi,Guang Jupi,Xin Huipi,Hongju,Da Hongpao,Chuanju.

性味归经:辛苦,温。入脾经、肺经。

Medicinal properties:Pungent in flavor and warm in property;enters the spleen and lung meridians.

功效:理气调中,燥湿化痰。

Efficacy:Regulating qi and adjusting the middle energizer,drying dampness to eliminate phlegm.

主治：治胸腹胀满，不思饮食，呕吐哕逆，咳嗽痰多。亦解鱼、蟹毒。

Indication：Distension in chest and abdomen, anorexia, vomiting and non – productive vomiting, cough with excessive phlegm, neutralizing poison in fish and crab.

用法用量：内服：煎汤，6~10 g；或入丸、散。

Usage and dosage：6 ~ 10 g is used in decoction, pill or powder preparations for internal use.

注意事项：1、气虚及阴虚燥咳患者不宜。2、吐血症慎服。

Note：1. Contraindicated for people with qi deficiency or yin deficiency due to dry cough. 2. People with hematemesis should take it cautiously.

62. 赤小豆 Rice Bean

Chi Xiaodou（Semen Phaseoli）

形态特征：为豆科植物赤小豆或赤豆的干燥成熟种子。呈圆柱形而稍扁，种皮赤褐色或紫褐色，平滑，微有光泽。质坚硬，不易破碎，除去种皮，可见两瓣乳白色子仁。嚼之有豆腥味。

Morphology：The dry ripe seed of rice been or red been（Fam. Leguminosae sp. ）It is cylindrical, slightly flattened, the seed coat russet or puce, smooth, slightly shiny. It is hard, hard to break；removing the skin, there are two milk white bean halves. It has a bean taste after chewing.

别称：红豆、野赤豆。

Byname：Hong Dou, Ye Chidou

功效：除热毒，散恶血，消胀满，利小便，通乳。

Efficacy：Eliminating pyretic toxicity, dispelling extravasated blood, dispelling distention and fullness.

主治：赤小豆含有较多的皂角甙，可刺激肠道。因此它有良好的利尿作用，能解酒、解毒，对心脏病和肾病、水肿均有益。它含有较多的膳食纤维，具有良好的润肠通便、降血压、降血脂、调节血糖、解毒抗癌、预防结石、健美减肥的作用。赤小豆是富含叶酸的食物。产妇，乳母多吃赤小豆有催乳的功效。

Indication：It has much gledinin which stimulates intestinal tracts, so it has the functions of diuresis, alleviating a hangover, neutralizing poison, and benefiting heart diseases, nephrosis and edema. It has much dietary fiber which can loosen bowel to relieve constipation, lower blood pressure, regulate blood sugar, neutralize poison, fight cancer, prevent calculus, keep shape and lose weight.

性味归经：酸、平。入心、小肠经。

Medicinal properties：Sour in flavor and neutral in property；enters the heart and small intestine meridians.

用量用法:煮食,煎汤或研末服。

Usage and dosage:It is cooked,decocted or ground into powder for internal use.

注意事项:赤小豆煮汁食之通利力强,消肿通乳作用甚效。但久食赤小豆则令人黑瘦结燥;阴虚而无湿热者及小便清长者忌食赤小豆。

Note:Cooked juice of the rice bean is effective in urine freeing,swelling dispersing and milk freeing. But long-term intake of it makes a person black,thin with dry bound stool. It's contraindicated for people with yin deficiency without damp heat or people with clear abundant urine.

63. 淡竹叶 Lophatherum Herb

Dan Zhuye(Herba Lophatheri)

形态特征:为禾本科植物淡竹叶的干燥茎叶。茎呈圆柱形,有节,表面淡黄绿色,断面中空。叶鞘开裂。叶片披针形,有的皱缩卷曲;表面浅绿色或黄绿色。叶脉平行,具横行小脉,形成长方形的网格状,下表面尤为明显。

Morphology:The dry stem leaf of Dan Zhuye (Herba Lophatheri)(Fam. Poaceae).
The stem is cylindrical, with nodules on it, yellowish green surface, and hollow section. The leaf sheath is chapped craze. The leaf blade is lanceolate, some is wrinkled and curling; the surface pale green or yellow-green. The leaf veins are parallel, transverse and tiny, forming a rectangular grid, particularly especially the lower surface.

功效:清热除烦、利尿通淋。

Efficacy:Clearing heat to eliminate restlessness,inducing diuresis for treating strangurtia.

主治:热病烦渴,口舌生疮,牙龈肿痛,小儿惊啼,肺热咳嗽,胃热呕哕,小便赤涩淋浊。

Indication:Heat diseases and polydipsia,sores in the mouth and tongue,sore pain in the gum,pediatric terrified crying,cough with lung heat,vomiting and non-productive vomiting due to stomach heat,and hot urination with strangury-turbidity.

性味归经:味甘、淡,性寒;归心、肺、胃、膀胱经。

Medicinal properties:Sweet and mild in flavor;cold in property;enters the heart,lung, stomach and bladder meridians.

注意事项:体虚有寒者、孕妇禁服。

Notes:It is contraindicated for people with deficient and cold syndrome and pregnant women.

64. 淡豆豉 Fermented Soybean

Dan Douchi(Semen Sojae Preparatum)

形态特征：为豆科植物大豆的成熟种子的发酵加工品。呈椭圆形，略扁。表面黑色，皱缩不平。质柔软，断面棕黑色。

Morphology: The fermentation processed products of the ripe seed of soybean (Fam. Leguminosae). It is oval, and slightly flat; the surface is black and wrinkled. It is soft, and its section is dark brown.

功效：疏散解表，宣郁除烦。

Efficacy: Evacuating and relieving exterior syndrome, eliminating depression and restlessness.

主治：外感表症，恶寒发热，胸中烦闷，虚烦不眠，口舌生疮。

Indication: Diseases caused by exogenous pathogenic factor, heat effusion and aversion to cold, restlessness in mind, agrypnia due to deficient dysphoria, sores in mouth and tongue.

性味归经：味苦、甘、辛，性凉；归肺、胃经。

Medicinal properties: Bitter, sweet and pungent in flavor; cold in property; enters the lung and stomach meridians.

用量用法：内服：煎汤，5~15 g；或入丸剂。外用：适量，捣敷；或炒焦研末调敷。

Usage and dosage: 5~15 g is used in decoction, pill or powder preparations; or proper amount is smashed, or stir-baked to brown or powdered for external application.

注意事项：胃虚易呕者慎服。

Notes: It should be taken cautiously by people with deficient stomach, nausea and vomiting.

65. 薏苡仁 Coix Seed

Yiyi Ren(Semen Coicis)

形态特征：为禾本科植物薏苡的干燥成熟种仁。呈宽卵形或长椭圆形。表面乳白色，光滑，偶有残存的黄褐色种皮。背面圆凸，腹面有 1 条较宽而深的纵沟。质坚实，断面白色，粉性。

Morphology: The dry ripe seeds of Coix lacryma-jobi L. var. ma-yuan (Roman.) Stapf. (Fam. Gramineae). It is broad ovate or long oval; the surface is milk white and smooth, with occasional remaining tan skin. It is convex round on the back and the front have a wide and deep longitudinal groove. It is solid, its section is white and powdery.

功效：利水消肿、健脾去湿、舒筋除痹、清热排脓。

Efficacy：Inducing diuresis to alleviate edema, strengthening spleen and removing dampness, soothing sinew to eliminate arthralgia spasm, removing heat to eliminate pura.

主治：脾虚腹泻，肌肉酸重，关节疼痛，水肿，脚气，白带，肺脓疡，肠痈。

Indication：Diarrhea due to spleen asthenia, sore and stiff muscles, arthralgia, edema, beriberi, leucorrhea, lung abscess and intestinal abscess.

性味归经：甘、淡、凉。归脾、胃、肺经。

Medicinal properties：Sweet, mild in flavor and cold in property; enters the spleen, stomach and lung meridians.

用量用法：内服：煎汤，10～30 g；浸酒，煮粥，做羹。

Usage and dosage：10～30 g is used in decoction, or infused in wine, cooked in porridge or made into soup for internal use.

注意事项：本品力缓，宜多服久服。脾虚无湿，大便燥结及孕妇慎服。

Notes：It is moderate in property, thus should be taken in large dose for a long time. And it should be taken cautiously by people with spleen deficiency, no dampness, dry stool and pregnant women.

66. 小茴香 Fennel

Huixiang(Foeniculum Vulgare Mill.)

形态特征：为伞形科植物茴香的干燥成熟果实。为双悬果，呈圆柱形，有的稍弯曲。表面黄绿色或淡黄色，两端略尖，顶端残留有黄棕色突起的柱基，基部有时有细小的果梗。分果呈长椭圆形，背面有纵棱 5 条，接合面平坦而较宽。

Morphology：The dry ripe fruit of Huixiang (Foeniculum Vulgare Mill) (Fam. Umbelliferae). It is mericarp, cylindrical and slightly curved. The surface is yellow-green or pale yellow, slightly pointed at both ends, there is a yellow brown raised column base on the top, sometimes with small stem on it. Its schizocarps are long oval with 5 longitudinal edges on the back; the joint surface is flat and wide.

功效：开胃进食，理气散寒，有助阳道

Efficacy：Promoting appetite, regulating qi and eliminating coldness, benefiting male sexual function.

主治：中焦有寒，食欲减退，恶心呕吐，腹部冷痛；疝气疼痛，睾丸肿痛；脾胃气滞，脘腹胀满作痛。

Indication：Cold in the middle energizer, anorexia, nausea and vomiting, coldness and pain in the abdomen, hernia with pain, testicular swelling and pain, qi-stagnation in spleen and stomach, and distension, fullness and pain in gastric cavity and abdomen.

性味归经：味辛，性温。归肾、膀胱、胃经。

Medicinal properties：Pungent in flavor and warm in property；enters the kidney，bladder and stomach meridians.

用量用法：作调味品,煎汤,或入丸、散剂。

Usage and dosage：It is used to flavor，or used in decoction，pill or powder preparations.

注意事项：有实热、虚火者不宜。

Notes：It is contraindicated for people with excessive heat and deficient fire.

67. 肉桂 Cassia Bark

Rougui（Cortex Cinnamomi）

形态特征：为樟科植物肉桂的干燥树皮。呈槽状或卷筒状。外表面灰棕色,稍粗糙,有的可见灰白色的斑纹；内表面红棕色,略平坦,划之显油痕。质硬而脆,易折断,断面不平坦,外层棕色而较粗糙,内层红棕色而油润,两层间有 1 条黄棕色的线纹。气香浓烈。

Morphology：The dry bark of Rougui（Cortex Cinnamomi）（Fam. Lauraceae）. It has a groove or drum shape；the outside surface is gray brown，relatively rough，with some visible grease stripes after scratch. It is hard and brittle，easily broken；the section is not flat；the outer layer is brown and slightly rough，the inner is red brown，oily and moist；there is a yellow brown line between the two layers. It has a strong fragrant smell.

功效：补火助阳,引火归源,散寒止痛,温通经脉。

Efficacy：Supplying fire to strengthen yang，letting the fire back to its origin，eliminating cold to stop pain，activating blood to promote menstruation.

主治：用于阳痿、宫冷、心腹冷痛、虚寒吐泻、经闭、痛经。

Indication：Impotence，cold womb，cold pain in chest and abdomen，vomiting and diarrhea due to yang deficiency cold，menischesis，dysmenorrheal，warming meridians to promote of blood circulation.

性味归经：性大热,味辛、甘。归肾、脾、心、肝经

Medicinal properties：Extremely hot in property；pungent and sweet in flavor；enters the kidney，spleen，heart and liver meridians.

用量用法：内服:煎汤,3~6 g；或入丸、散。外用:适量,研末调敷；或炒热温熨。

Usage and dosage：3~6 g is used in decoction，pill or powder preparations for internal use；or proper amount is ground into powder for external application；or stir-baked for warm pressing externally.

注意事项：阴虚火旺者禁服。

Notes：It is contraindicated for people with yin deficiency and effulgent fire.

68. 桑叶 Mulberry Leaf

Sangye(Folium Mori)

形态特征:为桑科植物桑的干燥叶。本品多皱缩、破碎。完整者有柄,叶片展平后呈卵形或宽卵形;先端渐尖,基部截形、圆形或心形,边缘有锯齿或钝锯齿,有的不规则分裂。上表面黄绿色或浅黄棕色。

Morphology:The dry leaf of mulberry(Morus alba L.)(Fam. Moraceae). Most of the product is wrinkled and broken;a complete leaf has handle and the leaf blade is ovate if spread out ; the apex is acuminate; the base has a truncation, round or cordate shape, with sawtooth or blunt sawtooth margin, and some has irregular cracks. The upper surface is yellow-green or yellow brown.

功效:疏散风热,清肺润燥,清肝明目。

Efficacy:Dispelling wind and heat,clearing lung and moisturizing dryness-syndrome.

主治:风热感冒,肺热燥咳,头晕头痛,目赤昏花。

Indication:Wind-heat type common cold, dry cough due to lung heat, dizziness and headache,conjunctival congestion with dim eyesight.

性味归经:味苦;甘;性寒。归肺经,肝经。

Medicinal properties:Bitter and sweet in flavor;cold in property;enters the lung and liver meridians.

用量用法:内服:煎汤,4.5~9 g;或入丸、散。外用:适量,煎水洗或捣敷。

Usage and dosage:4.5~9 g is used in decoction,pill or powder preparations;or proper amount is decocted for washing or smashed for external application.

注意事项:桑葚含脂肪酸,过量食用对消化道可产生刺激症状。

Notes:With fatty acid,it may stimulate the digestive tube if taken too much.

69. 苦瓜 Balsam Pear

Kugua(Momordica Charantia L.)

形态特征:为葫芦科苦瓜属植物苦瓜的瓜、根、藤及叶入药。呈椭圆形或矩圆形,全体皱缩,弯曲,果皮浅灰棕色,粗糙,有纵皱或瘤状突起。中间有时夹有种子或种子脱落后留下的孔洞。

Morphology:Kugua′s(Momordica Charantia L.)(Fam. Cucurbitaceae) melon, root, vines and leaves used as medicine. The plant is oval or oblong, all wrinkled and curved; the fruit skin is shallow ash brown, rough, with longitudinal wrinkles or strumae; sometimes with holes in the middle after seeds falling off.

性味归经：苦，寒。归脾、胃、心、肝经。

Medicinal properties：Bitter and cold in property；enters the spleen，stomach，heart and liver meridians.

功效：清热祛心火，解毒，明目，补气益精，止渴消暑，治痈。

Efficacy：Clearing heat and eliminating heart fire，detoxication，improving eyesight，invigorating vital energy and benefiting essence，quenching thirst to relieve summer heat，treating carbuncle.

主治：中暑、暑热烦渴、暑疖、痱子过多、目赤肿痛、痈肿丹毒、烧烫伤、少尿等病症。

Indication：Heat stroke，polydipsia due to summer hotness，summer suppurative boil，miliaria，conjunctival congestion with swelling and pain，carbuncle swelling with erysipelas，burn and scald，and oliguria.

用量用法：内服：煎汤，6～15 g，鲜品 30～60 g；或煅存性研末。外用：适量，鲜品捣敷；或取汁涂。

Usage and dosage：6～15 g is used in decoction，or 30～60 g used fresh，or calcined into powder for internal use；proper amount is applied fresh externally or applied with the juice.

注意事项：脾胃虚寒者不宜生食，食之令人吐泻腹痛。孕妇不宜。

Notes：People with deficient and cold spleen and stomach should not eat it raw，because taking it may cause vomit，diarrhea and abdominal pain. Pregnant women shouldn't take it.

70. 酸枣仁 Spine Date Seed

Suanzao（Semen Ziziphi Spinosae）

形态特征：为鼠李科植物酸枣的干燥成熟种子。呈扁圆形。表面紫红色，平滑有光泽。一面较平坦，中间有 1 条隆起的纵线纹；另一面稍凸起。

Morphology：The dry ripe seed of Suanzao（Semen Ziziphi Spinosae）（Fam. Rhamnaceae）. It is oval and purple on the surface；smooth on one side，and a uplift ordinate lines in the middle；side slightly raised on the other side.

性味归经：性平，味甘酸；归肝，心经。

Medicinal properties：Neutral in property；sweet and sour in flavor；enters the liver and heart meridians.

功效：养肝、宁心、安神。

Efficacy：Nourishing liver，soothing mind，calming the nerves.

主治病症：神经衰弱、心烦失眠、多梦、盗汗、易惊。

Indication：Neurastheria，insomnia due to restlessness，dreaminess，night sweat and hyperarousal.

用量用法：冲服 3～6 g。煎汤，炒香，捣为散。

Usage and dosage: 3 ~ 6 g is mixed with water, decocted, stir-baked, or smashed into powder for internal use.

注意事项：一般人群均可食用，心脏病患者尤其适合食用。

Notes: It is edible for general people, especially for heart disease patients.

71. 山楂 Hawthorn Fruit

Shanzha(Fructus Crataegi)

形态特征：为蔷薇科植物山里红或山楂的干燥成熟果实。为圆形片，皱缩不平。外皮红色，具皱纹，有灰白小斑点。果肉深黄色至浅棕色。

Morphology: The dry ripe fruit of hawthorn (Fructus Crataegi) (Fam. Rosaceae). It is round piece, wrinkled; the outer skin is red, with wrinkles and grey spots on it; the fruit meet is dark yellow to light brown.

性味归经：味甘、性、微温酸。入脾、胃、肝经。

Medicinal properties: Sweet and sour in flavor; slightly warm in property; enters the spleen, stomach and liver meridians.

功效：消食化积，行气散瘀，化浊、降脂。

Efficacy: Relieving food stagnation to promote digestion, promoting qi and eliminating stasis to activate blood circulation.

主治病症：肉食积滞、胃脘胀满、泻痢腹痛、瘀血经闭、产后瘀阻、心腹刺痛、疝气疼痛、高脂血症。

Indication: Meat stagnation, distention and fullness in gastric cavity, diarrhea and dysentery with abdominal pain, haemostasis menischesis, postpartum stasis, stabbing pain in epigastrium and abdomen, hernia with pain, hyperlipemia.

用量用法：煎服，10 ~ 15 g，大剂量 30 g。

Usage and dosage: 10 ~ 15 g is used in decoction; or 30 g is used in large dose.

注意事项：脾胃虚弱而无积滞者或胃酸分泌过多者慎用。

Notes: It should be taken cautiously by people with weak spleen and stomach, no accumulation and stagnation or people with too much gastric acid.

72. 女贞子 Glossy Privet Fruit

Nǔ Zhenzi(Fructus Ligustri Lucidi)

形态特征：为木犀科植物女贞的干燥成熟果实。呈卵形、椭圆形或肾形。表面黑紫色或灰黑色，皱缩不平，基部有果梗痕或具宿萼及短梗。体轻。外果皮薄，中果皮较松软,易剥离,内果皮木质,黄棕色,具纵棱,破开后种子通常为1粒,肾形,紫黑色,油性。

Morphology: The dry ripe fruit of Nǚ Zhen (Glossy Privet) (Fam. Oleaceae). It is ovate, and the surface is dark purple or gray, black colored and wrinkled; there are stem scars, calyx or short stalks on the base; weight light. The outer fruit skin is thin, mesocarp is soft, easy stripping, and endocarp woody, yellow brown, with longitudinal edge; usually has one seed in it, kidney-like, violet black, and oily.

性味归经:甘;苦;性凉;入肝、肾经。

Medicinal properties: Sweet and bitter in flavor; cold in property; enters the liver and kidney meridians.

功效:补益肝肾;乌须明目

Efficacy: Reinforcing liver benefiting kidney, blackening beard and improving eyesight.

主治病症:头昏目眩;腰膝酸软;遗精;耳鸣;须发早白;骨蒸潮热;目暗不明。

Indication: Lightheadedness, sour-weak waist and knees, spermatorrhea, tinnitus, early whitened beard and hair, osteopyrexia and fever, dim eyesight.

用量用法:内服:煎汤,6～15 g;或入丸剂。外用:适量,敷膏点眼。

Usage and dosage: 6～15 g is used in decoction or pill preparations; or proper amount is made into paste for external application on eyes.

注意事项:脾胃虚寒泄泻及阳虚者忌服。

Notes: It is contraindicated for people with deficient and cold spleen and stomach, diarrhea and yang deficiency.

73. 槐花 Pagodatree Flower

Huaihua (Flos Sophorae)

形态特征:为豆科植物槐的干燥花及花蕾。本品皱缩而卷曲,花瓣多散落。完整者花萼钟状,黄绿色;花瓣5,黄色或黄白色。

Morphology: The dry flower and bud of Huai (Sophora japonica Linn.) (Fam. Leguminosae). The product is wrinkled and curled, petals usually scattered. A complete flower has a bell-shaped calyx, with yellow green color; 5 petals, yellow or yellow-white color.

性味归经:味苦、性微寒,归肝、大肠经。

Medicinal properties: Bitter in flavor and slightly cold in property; enters the liver and large intestine meridians.

功效:凉血止血,清肝泻火。

Efficacy: Cooling blood to stop bleeding, clearing liver to reduce fire.

主治病症:肠风便血,痔血,血痢,尿血,血淋,崩漏,吐血,衄血,肝火头痛,目赤肿痛,喉痹,失音,痈疽疮疡。

Indication：Hematochezia, hemorrhoid blood, hematodiarrhoea, hemuresis, stranguria complicated by hematuria, uterine bleeding, hematemesis, non-traumatic hemorrhage, headache due to hepatic fire, conjunctival congestion with swelling and pain, sore throat, carbuncle abscess and sores ulceration.

用量用法：煎服,10~15 g,外用适量。

Usage and dosage：10~15 g is used in decoction；or proper amount is applied externally.

注意事项：糖尿病人最好不要多吃。消化系统不好及过敏性体质的人慎食。

Notes：It is unsuitable to be taken too much by diabetes patients. Besides, it should be taken cautiously by people with poor digestive system and allergies.

74. 广藿香 Ageratum

Guang Huoxiang（Pogostemon cablin）

形态特征：为唇形科植物广藿香的全草。本品茎略呈方柱形,多分枝,枝条稍曲折；表面被柔毛；质脆,易折断,断面中部有髓；老茎类圆柱形,被灰褐色栓皮。叶对生,皱缩成团,展平后叶片呈卵形或椭圆形；两面均被灰白色茸毛；先端短尖或钝圆,基部楔形或钝圆,边缘具大小不规则的钝齿。

Morphology：The whole grass of Guang Huoxiang（Pogostemon cablin）（Fam. Labiatae）. Its stems are slightly square column shape, much branched, and the branches slightly curled；the surface covered with pilose, fragile, easily broken；central section myelinated；old stems are cylindrical-like, covered with taupe cork. Leaves are opposite, shrinked, and are ovate or elliptic after flattening. Both sides were covered with pale pastel；the apex is acute or obtuse, base is cuneate or obtuse, there are some irregular blunt sawtooth on the margin.

性味归经：味辛；性微温。入肺、脾、胃经。

Medicinal properties：Pungent in flavor and slightly warm in property；enters the lung, spleen and stomach meridians.

功效：祛暑解表；化湿和胃。

Efficacy：removing summer-heat to relieve superficies, dissipating hygrosis to restore stomach.

主治病症：夏令感冒,寒热头痛,胸脘痞闷,呕吐泄泻,妊娠呕吐,鼻渊,手、足癣。

Indication：Cold in summer, cold-fever headache, glomus oppression in chest and gastric cavity, vomiting and diarrhea, vomiting of pregnancy, nasosinusitis, tinea of feet and hands.

用量用法：内服：煎汤,6~10 g；或入丸、散。外用：适量,煎水；或研末搽。

Usage and dosage：6~10 g is used in decoction, pill or powder preparations；or proper amount is decocted for washing or ground into powder for external application.

注意事项：阴虚血燥者不宜用。

Notes：It is unsuitable for people with yin deficiency and blood dryness.

75.金银花 Honeysuckle Flower

Jinyin Hua（Flos Lonicerae）

形态特征：本品为忍冬科植物忍冬的干燥花蕾或带初开的花。呈棒状，上粗下细，略弯曲。表面黄白色或绿白色（贮久色渐深），密被短柔毛。花萼绿色，先端 5 裂，裂片有毛。

Morphology：The dry buds or open flowers of Rendong（Lonicera Japonica）（Fam. Caprifoliaceae）. It is stick like, the upper part is thicker than the lower part, and slightly bent. The surface is yellowish-white or green white（the color is darker during storage）, covered with densely pubescent. The calyx is green, with 5 lobes, the lobes are hairy。

性味归经：甘，微苦，清香，辛，寒。归肺、胃、心、大肠经。

Medicinal properties：Sweet and slightly bitter in flavor；with faint scent；pungent and cold in property；enters the lung, stomach, heart and large intestine meridians.

功效：清热解毒，凉散风热。

Efficacy：Clearing away the heat evil and expelling superficial evils, cooling wind heat.

主治病症：痈肿疔疮，喉痹，丹毒，热毒血痢，风热感冒，温病发热。

Indication：Carbuncle swelling and furuncle, sore throat, erysipelas, toxic-heat red dysentery, wind-heat type common cold, warm-evil-induced seasonal prevalent diseases with fever.

用量用法：煎服，6~15 g。

Usage and dosage：6~15 g is used in decoction.

注意事项：脾胃虚寒及气虚疮疡忌用。

Notes：It is contraindicated for people with deficient and cold spleen and stomach and people with qi deficiency, sores and boils.

76.蒲公英 Dandelion

Pugongying（Herba Taraxaci）

形态特征：为菊科植物蒲公英、碱地蒲公英或同属数种植物的干燥全草。呈皱缩卷曲的团块。根呈圆锥形，多弯曲；表面棕褐色，抽皱；根头部有棕褐色或黄白色的茸毛，有的已脱落。叶基生，多皱缩破碎，完整叶片呈倒披针形，绿褐色或暗灰色，先端尖或钝，边缘浅裂或羽状分裂，基部渐狭，下延呈柄状，下表面主脉明显。花冠黄褐色或淡黄白色。有的可见多数具白色冠毛的长椭圆形瘦果。

Morphology：The whole dry grass of dandelion, alkali land dandelion, or congeneric species plant (Fam. Asteraceae). It is shrinking curly briquette. The root is conical and usually bending; the surface is tan, wrinkled; the root head have brown or yellowish white fuzz, some have fallen off. The leaves are basal, usually shrunken and broken; complete leaves are oblanceolate, green, brown or dark gray, its apex are acute or obtuse, with shallow split or pinnate cracks on the edge; the base is gradually narrow, the decurrent is handle shaped, the main veins obvious on the lower surface. Corolla is brown or yellowish white. Some has mostly long oval achene with white pappus on it.

性味归经：甘,微苦,寒。归肝,胃经。

Medicinal properties：Sweet and slightly bitter in flavor; cold in property; enters the liver and stomach meridians.

功效：清热解毒,消肿散结,利湿通淋。

Efficacy：Clearing away the heat-evil and expelling superficial evils, subsiding swelling and removing stasis, reducing dampness through diuresis and dredging stranguria.

主治病症：乳痈内痈,痈肿疔毒;热淋涩痛,湿热黄疸。肝火上炎引起的目赤肿痛。

Indication：Internal mammary abscess, carbuncle swelling and furunculosis, heat strangury with pain, jaundice with damp-heat pathogen, conjunctival congestion with swelling and pain caused by hyperpyrexia of liver.

用量用法：煎服,9~15 g。外用鲜品适量,捣敷或煎汤熏洗患处。

Usage and dosage：9 ~ 15 g is used in decoction; or proper amount of fresh drug is smashed for external application or decocted for external smoking or washing.

注意事项：阳虚外寒、脾胃虚弱者忌用。用量过大,可致缓泻。

Notes：It is contraindicated for people with yang deficiency and external cold, or people with weak spleen and stomach. It may cause chronic diarrhea after being taken too much.

77. 胖大海 Boat-fruited Sterculia Seed

Pang Dahai (Semen Sterculiae Lychnophorae)

形态特征：为梧桐科植物胖大海的干燥成熟种子。呈纺锤形或椭圆形。先端钝圆,基部略尖而歪,具浅色的圆形种脐,表面棕色或暗棕色,微有光泽,具不规则的干缩皱纹。外层种皮极薄,质脆,易脱落。中层种皮较厚,黑褐色,质松易碎,遇水膨胀成海绵状。嚼之有黏性。

Morphology：The dry ripe seed of Pang Dahai (Semen Sterculiae Lychnophorae) (Fam. Sterculiaceae). It is spindle or oval in shape. The apex is obtuse, and the base is slightly pointed and slanting; it has light round hilum, brown or dark brown on the surface, slightly shiny, and with irregular shrunk wrinkles. The outer layer of seed skin is very thin, brittle, easy to fall off. The middle seed skin is thick, dark brown, loose and fragile. It expands in water. It is sticky when chewing.

性味归经：味甘；淡；性凉；有小毒。归肺、大肠经。

Medicinal properties：Sweet and mild in flavor；cold in property；slightly toxic；enters the lung and large intestine meridians.

功效：清热润肺，利咽解毒，润肠通便。

Efficacy：Clearing heat and moisturizing lung, relieving sore – throat and detoxication, loosening bowel to relieve constipation.

主治病症：肺热声哑，干咳无痰，咽喉干痛，热结便闭，头痛目赤。

Indication：Lung – heat hoarseness, dry cough without phlegm, dry and sour throat, constipation due to accumulation of heat, headache and conjunctival congestion.

用量用法：1～2 枚，沸水泡服或煎服。

Usage and dosage：1～2 pieces are infused in hot water or decoction for internal use.

注意事项：脾虚寒泻者慎服。有感冒者禁用。

Notes：It should be taken carefully by people with spleen deficient and cold and diarrhea. Besides, it is contraindicated for people with common cold.

78. 白扁豆 White Hyacinth Bean

Bai Biandou（Semen Dalichoris Album）

形态特征：为豆科植物扁豆的干燥成熟种子。呈扁椭圆形或扁卵圆形，表面淡黄白色或淡黄色，平滑，略有光泽。质坚硬。种皮薄而脆，子叶2。嚼之有豆腥气。

Morphology：The dry ripe seeds of Biandou（Purple Haricot）（Fam. Leguminosae）. It is flat oval or ovoid, the surface is yellowish white or pale yellow, smooth, and slightly shiny; hard and the seed skin is brittle, cotyledons. It has a bean taste after chewing.

性味归经：甘，微温。归脾、胃经。

Medicinal properties：Sweet in flavor and slightly warm in property；enters the spleen and stomach meridians.

功效：补脾和中，化湿，消暑。

Efficacy：Invigorating the spleen and regulating the middle warmer，dissipating dampness，relieving summer heat.

主治病症：脾胃虚弱、食欲不振、大便溏泻、白带过多、暑湿吐泻、胸闷腹胀。

Indication：Weakness of the spleen and stomach，poor appetite，loose stool，leukorrhagia，summer heat–dampness vomiting and diarrhea，chest oppression and abdominal distension.

用量用法：煎服，10～15 g。炒后可使健脾止泻作用增强，故用于健脾止泻及作散剂服用时宜炒用。

Usage and dosage：10～15 g is used in decoction. It is also used to strenghthen the spleen，check diarrhea after being stir–baked as a powder preparation.

79. 决明子 Cassia Seed

Jueming Zi(Semen Cassiae)

形态特征:为豆科植物决明或小决明的干燥成熟种子。略呈菱方形,两端平行倾斜。表面绿棕色或暗棕色,平滑有光泽。一端较平坦,另端斜尖,背腹面各有 1 条突起的棱线,棱线两侧各有 1 条斜向对称而色较浅的线形凹纹。质坚硬,不易破碎。种皮薄,子叶 2。

Morphology:The dry ripe seed of Jueming(Cassia obtusifolia L.) or Xiao Jueming (Cassia tora L.)(Fam. Leguminosae). It is rhombic, both ends Leaning slightly in parallel. The surface is green brown or dark brown, smooth and glossy. One side is flat, the other end is tilted and sharp, and both sides have a bumps ridge on the back, with an oblique symmetrical shallow line beside the ridge respectively. It is not easy to break. The seed skin is thin; 2 cotyledons.

性味归经:苦,微寒。归肝、大肠经。

Medicinal properties:Bitter in flavor and slightly cold in property;enters the liver and large intestine meridians.

功效:清热明目,润肠通便。

Efficacy:Clearing heat to improve eyesight,loosening bowel to relieve constipation.

主治病症:目赤涩痛,羞明多泪,头痛眩晕,目暗不明,大便秘结。

Indication:Conjunctival congestion with pain, photophobia and excessive tearing, headache and dizziness,constipation.

用量用法:内服:煎汤,9~15 g。

Usage and dosage:9~15 g is used in decoction for internal use.

注意事项:孕妇忌服,泄泻和血压低者慎用。

Notes:It is contraindicated for pregnant women and should be carefully used by people with diarrhea and low blood pressure.

80. 马齿苋 Purslane Herb

Machi Xian(Herba Portulacae)

形态特征:为马齿苋科植物马齿苋的干燥地上部分。本品多皱缩卷曲,常结成团。茎圆柱形,表面黄褐色。叶对生或互生,倒卵形,绿褐色。花小,黄色。

Morphology:The ground part of Machi Xian (Portulaca oleracea L.)(Fam. Portulacaceae). The product is usually wrinkled and curly, often forming a lump. The stem is cylindric, and brown on the surface; the leaves are opposite, obovate and green brown; the flower is small and yellow.

性味归经：性寒，味甘酸；入心、肝、脾、大肠经。

Medicinal properties: Cold in property; sweet and sour in flavor; enters the heart, lung, spleen and large intestine meridians.

功效：清热解毒，利水去湿，散血消肿，除尘杀菌，消炎止痛，止血凉血。

Efficacy: Clearing away the heat-evil and expelling superficial evils, alleviating water retention to remove dampness, dispelling blood stasis to subside swelling, dedusting and sterilization, eliminating inflammation to stop pain, cooling blood to stop bleeding.

主治病症：痢疾，肠炎，肾炎，产后子宫出血，便血，乳腺炎等病症。

Indication: Dysentery, enteritis, nephritis, postpartum metrorrhagia, hematochezia, mastitis.

用量用法：内服：煎汤，10~15 g，鲜品 30~60 g；或绞汁。外用：适量，捣敷；烧灰研末调敷；或煎水洗。

Usage and dosage: 10~15 g is used in decoction, or 30~60 g is used fresh, or twisted to make juice for internal use; or proper amount is smashed, charred into powder for external application, or decocted for washing.

注意事项：凡脾胃虚寒，肠滑作泄者勿用。

Notes: It is contraindicated for people with deficient cold spleen and stomach and diarrhea.

81. 紫苏叶 Perilla Stem

Zisu (Caulis Perillae)

形态特征：为唇形科植物紫苏的干燥叶（或带嫩枝）。本品叶片多皱缩卷曲、破碎，完整者展平后呈卵圆形。两面紫色或上表面绿色，下表面紫色，疏生灰白色毛。叶柄紫色或紫绿色。质脆。

Morphology: The dry leaf (or twig) of Zisu (Caulis Perillae) (Fam. labiatae). The leaf is usually wrinkled, curly and broken; the complete leaf is ovoid after flattening. The surface is purple on either sides, or green upperside, and purple on the lower side, having thin grey fuzz occasionally. The petiole is purple or purplish green, brittle.

性味归经：辛，温。归肺、脾经。

Medicinal properties: Pungent in flavor and warm in property; enters the lung and spleen meridians.

功效：发汗解表，理气宽中，解鱼蟹毒。

Efficacy: Inducing sweat and dispelling exogenous evils, regulating qi and loosening the middle energizer, neutralizing poison in fish and crab.

主治病症：风寒感冒，头痛，咳嗽，胸腹胀满，鱼蟹中毒。

Indication：Wind-cold type of common cold, headache, cough, distention and fullness in chest and abdomen, poisoned by eating fish and crab.

用量用法：煎服，5~9克，不宜久煎。

Usage and dosage：5~9 g is used in decoction, without being decocted for too long.

注意事项：凡脾胃虚寒，肠滑作泄者勿用。

Notes：It is contraindicated for people with deficient cold spleen and stomach and diarrhea.

82. 三七 Sanchi

Sanqi(Radix Notoginseng)

形态特征：为五加科植物三七的干燥根和根茎。主根呈类圆锥形或圆柱形。表面灰褐色或灰黄色，有断续的纵皱纹和支根痕。顶端有茎痕，周围有瘤状突起。体重，质坚实，断面灰绿色、黄绿色或灰白色，木部微呈放射状排列。

Morphology：The dry root and rhizome of Sanqi (Radix Notoginseng) (Fam. Araliaceae). The taproot is conical or cylindrical; its surface is beige or yellowish gray, with intermittent longitudinal wrinkles and root marks. There are stem scars on the top, and strumaes on the surround. It is heavy, solid; the section is sage green, yellow-green or pale; the xylem ranges roughly in a radial pattern.

性味归经：味甘，微苦；性温。归肝、胃、心、肺、大肠经。

Medicinal properties：Sweet and slightly bitter in flavor; warm in property; enters the liver, stomach, heart, lung and large intestine meridians.

功效：止血，散血，定痛。

Efficacy：Stopping bleeding, activating blood, relieving pain.

主治病症：跌扑瘀肿，胸痹绞痛；血瘀经闭；痛经；产后瘀血腹痛；疮痈肿痛。

Indication：Swelling with blood stasis by falling, pectoral stuffiness pain, obstruction in the intestine, blood – stasis menostasis, menalgia, postpartum abdominal pain with blood stasis, carbuncle with swelling and pain.

用量用法：煎汤，3~9 g；研末，1~3 g；或入丸、散。外用：适量，磨汁涂；或研末调敷。

Usage and dosage：3~9 g is used in decoction; or 1~3 g is ground into power for use; or used in pill or powder preparations; proper amount is ground into juice or powder for external application.

注意事项：孕妇忌用。

Notes：It is contraindicated for pregnant women.

83. 五味子 Chinese Magnoliavine Fruit

Wuwei Zi(Fructus Schisandrae Chinensis)

形态特征：为木兰科植物五味子的干燥成熟果实。呈不规则的球形。表面红色、紫红色或暗红色，皱缩，显油润；有的表面呈黑红色或出现"白霜"。果肉柔软，种子1~2，肾形，表面棕黄色，有光泽，种皮薄而脆。

Morphology：The fruit of Wuwei Zi (Fructus Schisandrae Chinensis) (Fam. Schisandraceae). It is irregular spherical; the surface is red, purple or dark red, wrinkled, oily and moist; some surface is black or has "hoar-frost". The pulp is soft; 1 ~ 2 seeds, kidney-like, tan, glossy on the surface; the seed skin is thin and brittle.

性味归经：温；酸、甘；归肺、心、肾经。

Medicinal properties：Warm in property; sour and sweet in flavor; enters the lung, heart and kidney meridians.

功效：收敛固涩，益气生津，补肾宁心。

Efficacy：Restraining and astringency, benefiting vital energy and promoting the production of body fluid, invigorating the kidney and calming mind.

主治病症：久嗽虚喘，梦遗滑精，遗尿尿频，久泻不止，自汗，盗汗，津伤口渴，短气脉虚，内热消渴，心悸失眠。

Indication：Chronic cough with dyspnea due to deficiency, nocturnal emission and spermatorrhea, enuresis and frequent micturition, chronic diarrhea, spontaneous perspiration, night sweat, thirst due to the damage of body fluid, short breath and weak pulse, wasting-thirst due to internal heat, palpitation and insomnia.

用量用法：内服：煎汤，3~6 g；研末；每次1~3 g；熬膏；或入丸、散。外用：研末掺；或煎水洗。

Usage and dosage：3 ~ 6 g is used in decoction; or 1 ~ 3 g is used in paste, pill or powder preparations; or ground into powder for external application or decocted for washing.

注意事项：外有表邪，内有实热，或咳嗽初起、痧疹初发者忌服。

Notes：It is contraindicated for people with external pathogen and internal excessive heat, or cough or measles at the initial stage.

84. 巴戟天 Morinda Root

Baji Tian(Radix Morindae Officinalis)

形态特征：为茜草科植物巴戟天的干燥根。本品为扁圆柱形，略弯曲，长短不等。表面灰黄色或暗灰色,有的皮部横向断离露出木部;质韧,断面皮部厚,紫色或淡紫色,易与木部剥离;木部坚硬,黄棕色或黄白色。

Morphology：The dry root of Baji Tian（Radix Morindae Officinalis）（Fam. Rubiaceae）. The product is flat cylindrical, slightly curved, and differ in length. The surface is gray yellow or dark gray, some cortex breaks horizontally and reveals the xylem; It is tough and the cortex on the section is thick, purple or lavender, easy to peel from the xylem; the xylem is hard, yellowish brown or yellowish-white.

性味归经:辛、甘,微温。归肝、肾经。

Medicinal properties：Pungent and sweet in flavor; slightly warm in property; enters the liver and kidney meridians.

功效:补肾助阳,祛风除湿,强筋壮骨。

Efficacy：Reinforcing kidney to strengthen yang, dispelling wind and eliminating dampness, strengthening bones and muscles.

主治病症:肾虚阳痿;遗精早泄;少腹冷痛;小便不禁;宫冷不孕;风寒湿痹;腰膝酸软;风湿之气。

Indication：Impotence due to deficiency of the kidney, spermatorrhea and premature ejaculation, cold-pain in lower abdomen, urinary incontinence, dysgenesia due to cold worm, anemofrigid-damp arthralgia, sour-weak waist and knees, rheumatism in limbs.

用量用法:内服:煎汤,6～15 g;或入丸、散;亦可浸酒或熬膏。

Usage and dosage：6～15 g is used in decoction, pill or powder preparations for internal use; it is also infused in wine or used in paste preparation.

注意事项:阴虚火旺者忌服。

Notes：It is contraindicated for people with yin deficiency and excessive fire.

85. 白豆蔻 White Cardamon Fruit

Bai Doukou（Fructus Ammomi Rotundus）

形态特征:为姜科植物白豆蔻的果实。略呈圆球形,具不显着的钝三棱。外皮黄白色,光滑,一端有小突起,一端有果柄痕;两端的棱沟中常有黄色毛茸。果皮轻脆,易纵向裂开,内含种子20～30粒。

Morphology：The fruit of Bai Doukou（Fructus Ammomi Rotundus）（Fam. Zingiberaceae）. It is roughly spherical and unobvious blunt triangular in shape. The cortex is yellowish-white, smooth, with small bumps on one side and peduncle mark on the other end; the carinal canal on both ends has some yellow fuzz on it. The fruit peel is crispy, usually has longitudinal crack, containing 20～30 seeds.

性味归经:辛、大温。归脾胃,大肠经。

Medicinal properties：Pungent in flavor and extremely warm in property; enters the spleen, stomach and large intestine meridians.

功效：化湿行气，温中止呕。

Efficacy：Dissipating dampness and promoting qi, warming the spleen – stomach to arrest vomiting.

主治病症：气滞，食滞，胸闷，腹胀，嗳气，噎膈，吐逆，反胃，疟疾。

Indication：Qi stagnation, dyspeptic retention, dyspnea, abdominal distension, ructation, cardiac spasm, vomiting due to adverse rising of gastric qi, regurgitation, malaria.

用量用法：内服：煎汤，3~10 g；或入丸、散。

Usage and dosage：3 ~ 10 g is used in decoction, pill, powder preparations for internal use.

注意事项：阴虚血燥而无寒湿者忌服。

Notes：It is contraindicated for people with yin deficieny and blood dryness without cold – dampness.

86. 菟丝子 Dodder Seed

Tusi Zi(Semen Cuscutae)

形态特征：为旋花科植物南方菟丝子或菟丝子的干燥成熟种子。本品呈类球形。表面灰棕色至棕褐色，粗糙，种脐线形或扁圆形。质坚实，不易以指甲压碎。

Morphology：The dry ripe seed of Tusi Zi (Cuscuta chinensis Lam.) or Nanfang Tusi Zi (Cuscuta australis)(Fam. Convolvulaceae). It is spherical; its surface is ash brown to brown, rough; its hilum is linear or oblate; solid, not easy to crush with nail.

性味归经：味辛、甘，性平；归肝、肾、脾经。

Medicinal properties：Pungent and sweet in flavor; slightly warm in property; enters the liver, kidney and spleen meridians.

功效：补肝肾，益精髓，明目。

Efficacy：Tonifying liver and kidney, benefiting essence – marrow, improving eyesight.

主治病症：腰膝酸痛，遗精，消渴，尿有余沥，目暗。

Indication：Sore – aching waist and knees, spermatorrhea, wasting – thirst, dribbling after urination, dim eyesight.

用量用法：内服：煎汤，15~25 g；或入丸、散。外用：炒研调敷。

Usage and dosage：15 ~25 g is used in decoction, pill or powder preparations for internal use; or stir – baked for external application.

注意事项：孕妇、血崩、阳强、便结、肾脏有火、阴虚火动，六者禁用。

Notes：It is contraindicated for pregnant women, or people with metrorrhagia, penis ultroerection, coprostasis, kidney fire, yin deficiency stirring fire.

87. 远志 Thinleaf Milkwort Root

Yuanzhi(Radix Polygalae)

形态特征：为远志科植物远志或卵叶远志的干燥根。本品呈圆柱形，略弯曲。表面灰黄色至灰棕色，有较密并深陷的横皱纹、纵皱纹及裂纹。质硬而脆，易折断，断面皮部棕黄色，木部黄白色，皮部易与木部剥离。

Morphology：The dry root of Yuanzhi (Polygala tenuifolia Willd.) or Luanye Yuanzhi (Polygala sibirica L.) (Fam. Polygalaceae). The product is cylindrical, slightly bent; the surface is yellowish gray to brown, with dense and deep horizontal lines, vertical wrinkles and cracks. Its quality is hard and brittle, easily broken; the cortex on the section is tan; the xylem is yellowish-white, easily stripping from the cortex.

性味归经：苦、辛，微温。归心、肾、肺经。

Medicinal properties：Bitter and pungent in flavor; slightly warm in property; enters the heart, kidney and lung meridians.

功效：安神益智，祛痰，消肿。

Efficacy：Calming nerves and improving intelligence or wisdom, expelling phlegm, subsiding swelling.

主治病症：心肾不交引起的失眠多梦，健忘惊悸，神志恍惚，咳嗽痰多，疮疡肿毒，乳房肿痛。

Indication：Insomnia and dreaminess due to incoordination of heart yang and kidney yin, morbid forgetfulness and shock, staring spells, cough with excessive phlegm, sores ulceration and swelling toxin, swelling and pain in breast.

用量用法：内服：煎汤，30～100 g；浸酒或入丸、散。外用：适量，研末酒调敷。

Usage and dosage：30～100 g is used in decoction, wine, pill or powder preparations for internal use; or proper amount is ground into powder and mixed with wine for external application.

注意事项：心肾有火，阴虚阳亢者忌服。

Notes：It is contraindicated for people with heart and kidney fire, yin deficiency and yang hyperactivity.

88. 玫瑰花 Rose Flower

Meigui Hua(Flos Rosae Rugosae)

形态特征：本品为蔷薇科植物玫瑰的干燥花蕾。本品略呈半球形或不规则团状。花托半球形,与花萼基部合生;萼片5,披针形,黄绿色或棕绿色,被有细柔毛;花瓣多皱缩,展平后宽卵形,呈覆瓦状排列,紫红色,有的黄棕色。

Morphology：The dry bud of rose(Fam. Rosaceae). The product is roughly hemispherical or irregular lump in shape; the receptacle is hemispherical, connected with calyx base connately; 5 sepals, lanceolate, yellowish green or brown and with thin pubescence on it; petals usually wrinkles, shrivel, wide oval in shape after flattening, ranges in imbricate structure; purple or yellow brown in color.

性味归经：甘、微苦,温。归肝、脾经。

Medicinal properties：Sweet and slightly bitter in flavor;warm in property;enters the liver and spleen meridians.

功效：解郁,和血,止痛。行气解郁。

Efficacy： Relieving qi depression,harmonizing blood,relieving pain.

主治病症：肝胃气痛,食少呕恶,月经不调,跌扑伤痛。

Indication：Hepatogenous gastralgia,poor eating and vomiting,menoxenia,hurt by falling.

用量用法：泡茶,煎汤,或浸酒、熬膏服。

Usage and dosage：It is used to make tea, decoction, wine and paste preparations for internal use.

注意事项：阴虚有火者勿服。

Notes：People with yin deficiency and fire should not take it.

89. 桑白皮 White Mulberry Root－bark

Sang Baipi(Cortex Mori)

形态特征：为桑科植物桑的干燥根皮。本品呈扭曲的卷筒状、槽状或板片状,长短宽窄不一。外表面白色,有的残留橙黄色或棕黄色鳞片状粗皮;内表面黄白色,有细纵纹。体轻,易纵向撕裂,撕裂时有粉尘飞扬。

Morphology：The dry root skin of mulberry(Morus alba L.) (Fam. Moraceae). The product is twisted barrel, groove or plate－like shaped, different in length or width; the outer surface is white, some has residual orange yellow or tan scaly coarse skin; the inner surface is yellowish－white, with fine longitudinal grain on it;light weight; easy to tear longitudinally; dust floats when tearing it.

性味归经：甘寒,入肺经。

Medicinal properties：Sweet in flavor and cold in property;enters the lung meridian.

功效：泻肺平喘,利水消肿。

Efficacy：Removing heat from lung and relieving asthma, inducing diuresis to alleviate e-dema.

主治病症：肺热咳喘,面目浮肿,小便不利等症。

Indication: Cough and dyspnea due to lung heat, facial edema, difficulty in micturition.

用量用法:煎服,5~15 g。泻肺利水,平肝清火宜生用;肺虚咳嗽宜蜜炙用。

Usage and dosage: 5 ~ 15 g is used in decoction; it is used raw to drain the lung, promote the diuresis, calm the liver and clear the fire; and it is used after being stir-baked with honey to treat the cough due to the lung deficiency.

注意事项:肺寒无火及风寒咳嗽禁服。

Notes: It is contraindicated for people with lung cold, no fire or cough due to wind cold.

90. 党参 Tangshen

Dangshen(Radix Codonopsis)

形态特征:为桔梗科植物党参、素花党参或川党参的干燥根。呈长圆柱形。表面灰黄色,根头部有多数疣状突起;根头下有致密的环状横纹;支根断落处常有黑褐色胶状物。

Morphology: The dry root of tangshen, suhua tangshen or sichuan dangshen (Fam. Campanulaceae). It is long cylindrical; the surface is gray yellow; the root head has many verrucous protrusions, and some dense ring horizontal stripes under the root head; there is usually some dark brown jelly on rootlet broken place.

性味归经:性平,味甘、微酸。归脾、肺经。

Medicinal properties: Neutral in property; sweet and slightly sour in flavor; enters the spleen and lung meridians.

功效:补中益气,健脾益肺。

Efficacy: Strengthening the middle warmer and benefiting qi, strengthening spleen and benefiting lung.

主治病症:脾肺虚弱,气短心悸,食少便溏,虚喘咳嗽,内热消渴。

Indication: Asthenia in lung and spleen, short breath and palpitation, poor eating and loose stool, cough and dyspnea due to deficiency, wasting-thirst due to internal heat.

用量用法:内服:煎汤,6~15 g;或熬膏、入丸、散。生津、养血宜生用;补脾益肺宜炙用。一日 15~30 g。煎汤,煎膏滋,入粥、饭、菜肴。

Usage and dosage: 6 ~ 15 g is used in decoction, paste, pill or powder preparations for internal use; it is used raw to generate fluids and nourish the blood, or used after being stir-baked with adjuvant; 15 ~ 30 g is used daily in decoction, paste, porridge, rice or dish, etc.

注意事项:实证、热证禁服;正虚邪实证,不宜单独应用。

Notes: It is contraindicated for people with excessive and heat syndrome; it also should not be applied alone to treat excessive deficiency syndrome.

91. 益母草 Motherwort Herb

Yimu Cao(Herba Leonuri)

形态特征:为唇形科植物益母草的新鲜或干燥地上部分。茎表面灰绿色或黄绿色;体轻,质韧,断面中部有髓。叶片灰绿色,多皱缩、破碎,易脱落。轮伞花序腋生。

Morphology: The fresh or dry ground part of Yimu Cao (Herba Leonuri) (Fam. Labiatae). The stem surface is sage green or yellowish green; light weight; the section is myelinated; leaves are gray-green, usually wrinkled, broken and easy to fall off; verticillaster; axillary.

性味归经:味辛;苦。入心、肝、膀胱经。

Medicinal properties: Pungent and bitter in flavor; enters the heart, liver and bladder meridians.

功效:活血,祛瘀,调经,消水。

Efficacy: Activating blood circulation, removing blood stasis, regulating menstruation, removing water stagnation.

主治病症:月经不调,胎漏难产,胞衣不下,产后血晕,瘀血腹痛,崩中漏下,尿血,泻血,痈肿疮疡。

Indication: Menoxenia, dystocia due to pregnant vaginal bleeding, retention of placenta, postpartum faintness, abdominal pain due to stagnant blood, metrorrhagia and metrostaxis, hemuresis, diarrhea with blood, carbuncle swelling and sores ulceration.

用量用法:10~30 g,煎服;鲜品 12~40 g。或熬膏,入丸剂、外用适量捣敷或煎汤外敷。

Usage and dosage: 10~30 g is used in decoction, or 12~40 g is used fresh, or made into the paste or pill preparation; proper amount is smashed or decocted for external application.

注意事项:孕妇禁用。无瘀滞及阴虚血少者忌。

Notes: It is contraindicated for pregnant women, or people without stagnation, people with yin deficiency and few blood.

92. 苦丁茶 Ilex

Kuding Cha (Ilex latifolia Thunb.)

形态特征:主要为冬青科植物枸骨和大叶冬青的叶。叶片呈卵圆形,先端短尖,基部圆形,上面光滑,革质而厚。

Morphology: The leaf of Chinese Holly and broadleaf holly (Fam. Aquifoliaceae). The blade is oval, apex acute, base rounded, smooth, leathery and thick in quality.

性味归经:甘;苦;寒。入肝、肺、胃。

Medicinal properties:Sweet and bitter in flavor; cold in property; enters the liver, lung and stomach meridians.

功效:疏风清热;明目生津。

Efficacy:Expelling wind and clearing heat, improving eyesight and generating body fluid.

主治病症:风热头痛;齿痛;目赤;聤耳;口疮;热病烦渴;泄泻;痢疾。

Indication:Headache due to wind-heat evil, toothache, conjunctival congestion, purulent ear, aphtha, excessive thirst due to heat-evil-caused disease, diarrhea and dysentery.

用量用法:内服:煎汤,3~9 g;或入丸剂。外用:适量,煎水熏洗,或涂搽

Usage and dosage:3~9 g is used in decoction or pill preparation; or proper amount is decocted for external smoking, washing or applying treatments.

注意事项:风寒感冒者,虚寒体质者,慢性胃肠炎患者,经期女性及新产妇不宜服用。

Notes:It is unsuitable for people with common cold due to wind-cold, deficient and cold constitution, chronic gastro-enteritis, or women in menstruation or new lying-in women.

93. 佛手 Finger Citron

Foshou(Fructus Citri Sarcodactylis)

形态特征:为芸香科柑橘属植物佛手的干燥果实。为类椭圆形的薄片,常皱缩或卷曲。顶端稍宽,常有 3~5 个手指状的裂瓣。外皮黄绿色或橙黄色。果肉浅黄白色,散有凹凸不平的线状或点状维管束。

Morphology:The dry fruit of Foshou (Fructus Citri Sarcodactylis) (Fam. Rutaceae). It is oval-like sheet, often wrinkled or curly. The top is slightly wider, with 3- 5 finger shaped cracks. The cortex is yellow-green or orange-yellow. The pulp is yellow white, scattered with uneven line or dot vascular bundles.

性味归经:辛、苦、酸,温。归肝、脾、肺经。

Medicinal properties:Pungent, bitter and sour in flavor; warm in property; enters the liver, spleen and lung meridians.

功效:疏肝理气,和胃止痛。

Efficacy:Soothing liver and regulating qi, regulating stomach to stopping pain.

主治病症:肝胃气滞,胸胁胀痛,胃脘痞满,食少呕吐。

Indication:Stagnation of liver-qi and stomach-qi, distention and pain in chest and ribs, fullness in gastric cavity, poor eating and vomiting.

用量用法:内服:煎汤,3~9 g;外用:适量,捣敷。

Usage and dosage:3~9 g is used in decoction for internal use; or proper amount is smashed for external application.

注意事项：阴虚有火，无气滞症状者慎服。

Notes：People in yin deficiency with fire and without qi stagnation should use it cautiously.

94. 桔梗 Platycodon Root

Jiegeng(Radix Platycodonis)

形态特征：为桔梗科植物桔梗干燥根。呈圆柱形，表面淡黄白色至黄色，不去外皮者表面黄棕色至灰棕色。有的顶端有较短的根茎或不明显，其上有数个半月形茎痕。质脆，断面不平坦，形成层环棕色，皮部黄白色，有裂隙，木部淡黄色。

Morphology：The dry root of Jiegeng (Radix Platycodonis) (Fam. Campanulaceae). It is cylindrical, the surface yellowish white to yellow, and yellow brown to grey brown with cortes. Some root has short or unobvious rhizome and several semilune shaped stem scars on the top. It is brittle; the section is not flat; the cambium ring is brown; the cortex is yellow-white, having cracks; the xylem is light yellow in color.

性味归经：味苦；辛；性平。归肺；胃经。

Medicinal properties：Bitter and pungent in flavor; neutral in property; enters the lung and stomach meridians.

功效：开宣肺气，祛痰排脓。

Efficacy：Facilitating lung qi, expelling phlegm and discharging pus.

主治病症：外感咳嗽，咽喉肿痛，肺痈吐脓，胸满胁痛，痢疾腹痛。

Indication：Cough caused by exogenous pathogenic factor, sore and swelling in throat, lung abscess with pus vomition, fullness in chest and pain in ribs, dysentery with abdominal pain.

用量用法：内服：煎汤，3~10 g；或入丸、散。外用：适量，烧灰研末敷。

Usage and dosage：3~10 g is used in decoction, pill or powder for internal use; or proper amount is charred into powder for external application.

注意事项：阴虚久嗽、气逆及咳血者忌服。

Notes：It is contraindicated for people with yin deficiency, chronic cough, qi counterflow and hemoptysis.

95. 香薷 Chinese Mosla

Xiangru(Herba Moslae)

形态特征：为唇形科植物石香薷或江香薷的干燥地上部分。本品基部紫红色，上部黄绿色或淡黄色，全体密被白色茸毛。茎方柱形。叶对生，多皱缩或脱落，暗绿色或黄绿色,边缘有 3～5 疏浅锯齿。穗状花序顶生及腋生。

Morphology: The dry ground part of Shi Xiangru or Jiang Xiangru (Fam. Labiatae). The base of the product is amaranth; the upper part is yellow-green or pale yellow, covered with the densely white fuzz entirely. The stem is square; the leaves are opposite, wrinkled, or fallen off, dark green or yellow-green, with 3～5 shallow sawtooth on the edge. it is pica; acrogenous and axillary.

性味归经:味辛甘,性温。归肺、胃、脾经。

Medicinal properties: Pungent and sweet in flavor; warm in property; enters the lung, stomach and spleen meridians.

功效:发汗解表,化湿和中,利水消肿。

Efficacy: Inducing sweat and dispelling exogenous evils, dissipating dampness and regulating the middle warmer, inducing diuresis to alleviate edema.

主治病症:发汗解暑,行水散湿,温胃调中。治夏月感寒饮冷,头痛发热,恶寒无汗,胸痞腹痛,呕吐腹泻,水肿,脚气。

Indication: Sweating to relieve summer-heat, activating body fluid to eliminate dampness, warming stomach and regulating the middle warmer, feeling cold in summer, headache and fever, chills without sweat, fullness in chest and abdominal pain, vomiting and diarrhea, edema and beriberi.

用量用法:内服:煎汤,5～15 g,或研末。

Usage and dosage: 5～16 is used in decoction or ground into powder for internal use.

注意事项:火盛气虚,阴虚有热者禁用。

Notes: It is contraindicated for people with excessive fire, qi and yin deficiency with heat syndrome.

96. 肉豆蔻 Nutmeg

Rou Doukou (Semen Myristicae)

形态特征:为肉豆蔻科植物肉豆蔻的干燥种仁。呈卵圆形或椭圆形。表面灰棕色或灰黄色,有时外被白粉(石灰粉末)。全体有浅色纵行沟纹和不规则网状沟纹。质坚,断面显棕黄色相杂的大理石花纹,宽端可见干燥皱缩的胚,富油性。

Morphology: The dry seed of Rou Doukou (Semen Myristicae) (Fam. Myristicaceae). It is ovoid or elliptic; the surface is gray brown or yellowish gray, sometimes covered with white powder (lime powder) outside. All the seeds have light longitudinal grooves and irregular mesh grooves. It is Strong, and the section has brown-yellow hue of marbling pattern; shrunk embryo appears on the wider end, oily.

性味归经:味辛、微苦,性温,有小毒,归脾、胃、大肠、肾经,芳辣香燥,可散可涩。

Medicinal properties: Pungent and slightly bitter in flavor; warm in property; slightly toxic;enters the spleen, stomach, large intestine and kidney meridians;aromatic, pungent and dry;with scattering and astringent actions.

功效:温中行气,涩肠止泻,开胃消食。

Efficacy:Warming the spleen – stomach to promote qi, antidarrhea with astringent, promoting appetite and digestion.

主治病症:虚泻冷痢、脘腹冷痛、呕吐。

Indication:Deficiency diarrhea and cold dysentery,coldness and pain in gastric cavity and abdomen, vomiting.

用量用法:内服:煎汤,3～6 g;或入丸、散。

Usage and dosage:3～6 g is used in decoction, pill or powder preparations for internal use.

注意事项:湿热泻痢及阴虚火旺者禁服。该品忌铜器,用量不宜过大,过量可引起中毒,出现神昏、瞳孔散大及惊厥。人服肉豆蔻粉7.5 g,可引起眩晕,甚至谵语、昏睡,大量可致死亡。

Notes:It is contraindicated for people with damp heat, diarrhea, dysentery, yin deficiency and excessive fire;it is incompatible with brass ware. It shouldn't be used too much at one time. Overuse of it can cause toxication,with symptoms of dizziness,mydriasis and convulsion. Taking 7.5 g of the powder may cause dizziness,delirium. Too much use may cause death.

97. 葛根 Kudzuvine Root

Gegen(Radix Puerariae)

形态特征:为豆科植物野葛的干燥根。呈纵切的长方形厚片或小方块。外皮淡棕色至棕色,有纵皱纹,粗糙。切面黄白色至淡黄棕色,有的纹理明显。

Morphology:The dry root of Yege(Pueraria lobata)(Fam. Leguminosae). A longitudinal cutting rectangle thick slices or small squares. Skin pale brown to brown, with longitudinal wrinkles, rough. Section yellowish–white to yellowish brown, some texture clear.

性味归经:性凉,味甘、辛。入脾、胃经。

Medicinal properties:Cold in property;sweet and pungent in flavor;enters the spleen and stomach meridians.

功效:升阳解肌,透疹止泻,除烦止温。

Efficacy:Invigorating splenic yang and relieving muscles, promoting eruptions and checking diarrhea, eliminating restlessness and relieving typhoid fever.

主治病症:伤寒、温热头痛项强,烦热消渴,泄泻,痢疾,癍疹不透,高血压,心绞痛,耳聋。

Indication:Typhoid fever, headache with stiff neck due to seasonal prevalent febrile pathogens wasting–thirst.

用量用法：内服：煎汤,5~15 g;或捣汁。外用：捣敷。

Usage and dosage：5 ~ 15 g is used in decoction or smashed into juice for internal use; or it is smashed for external application.

注意事项：脾胃虚寒者慎用

Notes：People with deficiency and cold spleen and stomach should use it carefully.

98. 覆盆子 Palmleaf Raspberry Fruit

Fupen Zi (Fructus Rubi)

形态特征：为蔷薇科植物华东覆盆子的干燥果实。为聚合果,由多数小核果聚合而成,呈圆锥形或扁圆锥形。表面黄绿色或淡棕色,顶端钝圆,基部中心凹入。宿萼棕褐色,下有果梗痕。小果易剥落,每个小果呈半月形,背面密被灰白色茸毛,两侧有明显的网纹,腹部有突起的棱线。

Morphology：The dry fruit of east China raspberry (Fam. Rosaceae). It is aggregate by many small drupelets, conical or flat cone in shape. The surface is yellow-green or pale brown; the apex is obtuse; the base is recessed in the center. The persistent calyx is tan, with stem marks. The small fruit is easy peeling, each in half moon shape, densely covered with grayish white fuzz on the back; both sides have obvious overlapping curves, and raised ridge on the center.

性味归经：甘酸,平。入肝、肾膀胱经。

Medicinal properties：Sweet and sour in flavor; neutral in property; enters the liver, kidney bladder meridians.

功效：补肝益肾,固精缩尿,明目。

Efficacy：Tonifying liver and benefiting kidney, securing essence and arresting polyuria, improving eyesight.

主治病症：阳痿早泄,遗精滑精,宫冷不孕,带下清稀,尿频遗溺,目昏暗,须发早白。

Indication：Impotence and premature ejaculation, nocturnal emission and spermatorrhea, dysgenesia due to cold womb, thin morbid leucorrhea, frequent micturition, dim eyesight, early whitened hair and beard.

用量用法：内服：煎汤,1.5~3 钱;或捣汁。外用：捣敷。

Usage and dosage：1. 5 ~ 3 qian is used in decoction or smashed into juice for internal use; or it is smashed for external application.

99. 牡蛎 Oyster Shell

Muli(Concha Ostreae)

形态特征:为牡蛎科动物长牡蛎、大连湾牡蛎或近江牡蛎 的贝壳。呈圆形、卵圆形或三角形等。右壳外面稍不平,有灰、紫、棕、黄等色。

Morphology: The shell of long oyster, dalian bay oyster or near jiang oyster (Fam. Ostreidae). It is round, ovoid or triangle in shape, etc. The outside of the right shell is a bit rough, with grey, purple, brown, yellow and other colors.

性味归经:咸,微寒。归肝、胆、肾经。

Medicinal properties: Salt in flavor and slightly cold in property; enters the liver, gallbladder and kidney meridians.

功效:平肝息风,养阴。

Efficacy: Pacifying liver and extinguishing wind, nourishing yin.

主治病症:眩晕耳鸣;惊悸失眠;瘰疬瘿瘤;症瘕痞块;自汗盗汗;遗精;崩漏;带下。

Indication: Dizziness and tinnitus, shock and insomnia, scrofula and gall, concretions and glomus lump, spontaneous perspiration and night sweat, emission, uterine bleeding, and morbid leucorrhea.

用量用法:内服:煎汤,15~30 g,先煎;或入丸、散。外用:适量,研末干撒或调敷。

Usage and dosage: 15~30 g is used in decoction, pill or powder preparations for internal use; proper amount is ground into powder to be sprayed or for external application.

注意事项:急慢性皮肤病患者忌食;脾胃虚寒,慢性腹泻便溏者不宜多吃。

Notes: It is contraindicated for patients with acute or chronic skin diseases; it should not be eaten too much by people with deficient and cold spleen and stomach, chronic diarrhea and loose stool.

方剂及药膳篇 Prescriptions

呼吸系统疾病
Respiratory diseases

感冒 Common cold

葛根汤
Gegen Tang
Kudzuvine Root Decoction

【药物组成】 葛根6 g,麻黄、生姜各4.5 g,炙甘草、芍药、桂枝各3 g,红枣6 颗。

【Composition】 6 g Gegen (Kudzuvine root), 4. 5 g Mahuang (Ephedra), 4. 5 g Shengjiang(Fresh ginger),3 g Zhi Gancao(Honey-fried licorice root),3 g Shaoyao(Peony),3 g Guizhi(Cassia twig) and 6 pieces of red jujubes.

【功效】 解肌生津,发汗解表。

【Efficacy】 Relieving muscles and generating body fluid, inducing sweat and dispelling exogenous evils.

【适应证】 鼻塞,汗出不畅,肌肉酸痛,发热怕冷,头痛头晕者。

【Indication】 Nasal obstruction, difficulty in sweating, muscular soreness, difficulty in moving qi, fever and chills, headache and dizziness.

气血双补方
Qixue Shuangbu Fang
Dual Supplementation Formula of Qi and Blood

【药物组成】 黄芪25 g,当归9 g,红枣10 颗。

【Composition】 25 g Huangqi(Milkvetch root),9 g Danggui(Chinese angelica) and 10 pieces of red jujubes.

【功效】 平补气血,扶正祛邪。

【Efficacy】 Mildly tonifying qi and blood, supporting body resistance and driving away evil.

【适应证】 免疫力低下,平时易患感冒者。

【Indication】　Hypoimmunity, people vulnerable to cold.

葱豉汤
Congchi Tang
Decoctionof Scallion and Fermented Soybean

【药物组成】　葱白 3 枚,豆豉 6 g。

【Composition】　3 pieces of scallion white and 6 g Fermented soybean.

【功效】　温阳发汗。

【Efficacy】　Warming ying for sweating.

【适应证】　风寒感冒初起,畏寒无汗,头痛鼻塞,体温不高者。

【Indication】　Onset of wind-cold-type common cold, chills without sweat, headache with nasal obstruction, low temperature.

黄芪姜枣汤
Huangqi Jiangzao Tang
Soup of Milkvetch, Ginger and Jujubes

【药物组成】　黄芪 15 g,大枣 15 g,生姜 3 片。以上三物加水适量,用武火煮沸,再用文火煮约 1 h 即可。吃枣饮汤。

【Composition】　15 g Huangqi(Milkvetch root), 15 g Chinese jujubes and 3 pieces of fresh ginger. Add proper amount of water, boil them with a strong fire, and then boil them with a small fire for 1 hour. Then eat jujubes and drink the soup.

【功效】　益气补虚,解表散寒。

【Efficacy】　Benefiting qi and improving asthenia, relieving exterior syndrome to dispel coldness.

【适应证】　体虚感冒者。

【Indication】　Cold due to asthenia.

羌蓝汤
Qianglan Tang
Decoction of Notopterygium and Isatis

【药物组成】　羌活 9 ~ 12 g,板蓝根 15 ~ 30 g。

【Composition】　9 ~ 12 g Qianghuo(Notopterygium) and 15 ~ 30 g Banlangen(Isatis).

【功效】　清热解毒,辛凉解表。

【Efficacy】　Clearing away the heat-evil and expelling superficial evils, dispelling the evil in the superficies with its pungent taste and cool nature.

【适应证】　发热怕冷,头痛,或者肢体酸痛,咽喉肿痛者。

【Indication】　Fever and chills, headache, or sore limbs and throat.

姜丝鸭蛋汤
Jiangsi Yadan Tang
Soup of Shredded Ginger and Duck Eggs

【药物组成】　生姜 50 g(去皮),鸭蛋 2 个,白酒 20 mL。生姜洗净去皮,切成丝,加水 200 mL 煮沸,鸭蛋去壳打散,倒入生姜汤中,稍搅,再加入白酒,煮沸即可。每日 1 次,吃蛋饮汤,顿服,可连服 3 日。

【Composition】　50 g fresh ginger (peeled), 2 duck eggs, 20 ml wine. Wash the fresh ginger clean, peel and slice it, and boil it with 200 ml water; shell and scatter the duck eggs, pour it into the ginger soup, stir and add some wine to boil. Take it once daily. Eat duck eggs and drink the soup. Take in single doses for 3 days.

【功效】　解表散寒。

ActionsRelieving the exterior syndrome and dispersing cold.

【适应证】　感冒初起者。

【Efficacy】　Indication The first stage of common cold.

【Efficacy】　Relieving exterior syndrome and dispelling coldness.

【Indication】　Onset of cold.

葱姜汤
Congjiang Tang
ScallionWhite and Ginger Soup

【药物组成】　葱白 3~5 枚,生姜 5 片,红糖适量。

【Composition】　3~5 pieces of scallion white, 5 pieces of fresh ginger and proper amount of brown sugar.

【功效】　发表散寒。

【Efficacy】　Relieving exterior syndrome to dispel coldness.

【适应证】　恶寒重,发汗轻者,雨淋水后引起的腹部冷痛。

【Indication】　Serious chills (being mild after sweating), abdominal coldness after being caught in the rain.

桑菊饮
Sangju Decoction
Decoction ofMulberry Leaves and Chrysanthemums

【药物组成】　连翘 5 g,桑叶 8 g,杏仁、桔梗、苇根各 6 g,薄荷、甘草、菊花各 3 g。

【Composition】　5 g Lianqiao (Weeping forsythia), 8 g Sangye (Mulberry leaf), 6 g apricot kernels, 6 g Jiegeng (Platycodon root), 6 g Weigen (Phragmites root), 3 g peppermints, 3 g Gancao (Liquorice root) and 3 g Juhua (Chrysanthemun flower).

【功效】　宣肺止咳,疏风清热。

【Efficacy】　Facilitating lung to stop cough, expelling wind and clearing heat.

【适应证】　风热初起,咳嗽,口渴者。

【Indication】　Onset of wind heat, cough, thirst.

咳嗽 Cough

柴朴汤
Chaipo Tang
Decoction of Thorowax and Officinal Magnolia

【药物组成】　柴胡、独活、前胡、黄芩、苍术、厚朴、陈皮、半夏曲、茯苓、藿香各6 g,甘草3 g。

【Composition】　6 g Chaihu (Chinese thorowax root), 6 g Duhuo (Pubescent angelica root), 6 g Qianhu (Hogfennel root), 6 g Huangqin (Baical skullcap root), 6 g Cangzhu (Atractylodes rhizome), 6 g Houpo (Officinal magnolia bark), 6 g Chenpi (Dried tangerine peel), 6 g Banxiaqu (Fermented pinellia), 6 g Fuling (Tuckahoe), 6 g Huoxiang (Ageratum) and 3 g Gancao (Liquorice root).

【功效】　理气止咳化痰。

【Efficacy】　Regulating qi, relieving cough and reducing sputum.

【适应证】　咳嗽痰多,伴腹胀者。

【Indication】　Cough with excessive sputum and abdominal distention.

童参麦冬饮
Tongshen Maidong Decoction
Decoction of Heterophylly Falsestarwort and Dwarf Lilyturf

【药物组成】　太子参15 g,麦冬12 g,甘草6 g。

【Composition】　15 g Taizi Shen (Heterophylly falsestarwort root), 12 g Maidong (Dwarf lilyturf tuber) and 6 g Gancao (Liquorice).

【功效】　益气止咳。

【Efficacy】　Benefiting qi and relieving cough.

【适应证】　肺虚引起的咳嗽者。

【Indication】　Cough due to lung asthenia.

六君子汤
Liujunzi Tang
Six Gentlemen Decoction

【药物组成】　白术、茯苓、陈皮、甘草各9 g,半夏12 g,人参10 g。

【Composition】　9 g Baizhu (Largehead atractylodes rhizome), 9 g Fuling (Tuckahoe), 9 g Chenpi(Dried tangerine peel),9 g Gancao(Liquorice root),12 g Banxia(Pinellia tuber)and 10 g Renshen(Ginseng).

【功效】 健脾和胃,化痰止咳。

【Efficacy】 Strengthening the spleen and stomach, dissipating phlegm and stopping cough.

【适应证】 脾胃气虚引起的咳嗽痰多者。

【Indication】 Cough with excessive phlegm due to qi-asthenia of spleen and stomach.

贝母饮
Beimu Yin
Fritillaria Decoction

【药物组成】 贝母、百合、麦冬各6 g,紫苑、桑白皮、桔梗、大黄各3 g,甘草2 g。

【Composition】 6 g Beimu(Fritillaria bulb),6 g Baihe(Lily bulb),6 g Maidong(Dwarf lilyturf tuber),3 g Ziwan(Tatarian aster root),3 g Sangbaipi(White mulberry root-bark),3 g Jiegeng(Platycodon root)and 3 g Dahuang(Rhubarb),2 g Gancao(Liquorice).

【功效】 滋阴润肺,化痰止咳。

【Efficacy】 Nourishing yin and moisturizing lung,dissipating phlegm to stop cough.

【适应证】 咽干咳嗽者。

【Indication】 Cough with dry pharynx.

甘桔汤
Ganju Tang
Decoction of Liquorice and Platycodon

【药物组成】 桔梗10 g,甘草6 g。

【Composition】 10 g Jiegeng(Platycodon root)and 6 g Gancao(Liquorice).

【功效】 宣肺化痰。

【Efficacy】 Facilitating lung and dissipating phlegm.

【适应证】 咳嗽痰多,咽喉肿痛者。

【Indication】 Cough with excessive phlegm,sore throat.

宁嗽化痰汤
Ningsou Huatan Tang
Cough-calming and Phlegm-resolving Decoction

【药物组成】 桔梗、枳壳、半夏、陈皮、前胡、葛根、茯苓、紫苏、杏仁各9 g,桑白皮、甘草各6 g,麻黄、生姜各3 g。

【Composition】 9 g Jiegeng(Platycodon root),9 g Zhike(Orange fruit),9 g Banxia (Pinellia tuber),9 g Chenpi(Dried tangerine peel),9 g Qianhu(Hogfennel root),9 g Gegen (Kudzuvine root),9 g Fuling(Tuckahoe),9 g Zisu(Perilla stem)and 9 g apricot kernels,6 g

Sangbaipi(White mulberry root-bark),6 g Gancao(Liquorice),3 g Mahuang(Ephedra)and 3 g fresh ginger.

【功效】 理气止咳化痰。

【Efficacy】 Regulating qi,stopping cough and dissipating phlegm.

【适应证】 外感风寒引起的咳嗽,鼻塞者。

【Indication】 Cough and nasal obstruction due to affection of exotenous wind-cold.

润燥益阴汤
Runzao Yiyin Tang
Dryness-moistening and Yin-boosting Decoction

【药物组成】 南沙参、北沙参各15 g,天冬、知母、玄参、生地、枸杞各12 g,百部9 g,甘草6 g。

【Composition】 15 g Nan Shashen(Fourleaf ladybell root),15 g Bei Shashen(Coastal glehnia root), 12 g Tiandong(Cochinchinese asparagus root), 12 g Zhimu(Common anemarrhena rhizome),12 g Xuanshen(Figwort root),12 g Shengdi(dried/fresh rehmannia root)and 12 g Gouqi(Chinese wolfberry),9 g Baibu(Stemona root)and 6 g Gancao(Liquorice).

【功效】 清肺祛痰,润肺止咳,滋养肝肾。

【Efficacy】 Clearing lung to dissipate phlegm,moistening lung to arrest cough,nourishing liver and kidney.

【适应证】 肺燥咳嗽见痰中带血者。

【Indication】 Xeropulmonary cough with blood phlegm.

部杏天冬汤
Buxing Tiandong Tang
Decoction of stemona,apricot Kernel and Cochinchinese asparagus

【药物组成】 炙百部、天门冬各6 g,杏仁5 g,短风茶9 g,吉祥草15 g。

【Composition】 6 g Zhi Baibu(Honey-fried Stemona root)and 6 g Tianmen Dong(Cochinchinese asparagus root),5 g apricot kernels,9 g Duanfeng Cha and 15 g Jixiang Cao(Reineckia carnea Kunth).

【功效】 清肺化痰,活血降气。

【Efficacy】 Clearing lung to dissipate phlegm, activating blood circulation and depressing qi.

【适应证】 阵发性痉挛性咳嗽者。

【Indication】 Paroxysmal and spasmodic cough.

枇杷叶露
Pipaye Lu
Loquat Leave Syrup

【药物组成】 鲜枇杷叶若干,制成露剂,日服 2～3 次,每次 60～120 g。

【Composition】 Pick some fresh loquat leaves, make them into syrup. Take it 2～3 times daily, 60～120 g every dose.

【功效】 清肺止咳。

【Efficacy】 Clearing lung to stop cough.

【适应证】 肺热咳嗽者。

【Indication】 Cough due to lung heat.

紫菀汤
Ziwan Tang
Tatarian Aster Decoction

【药物组成】 紫菀、阿胶、知母、贝母、桔梗、茯苓各 6 g,人参、五味子、甘草各 3 g。

【Composition】 6 g Ziwan(Tatarian aster root), 6 g E Jiao(Ass hide glue), 6 g Zhimu (Common anemarrhena rhizome), 6 g Beimu(Fritillaria bulb), 6 g Jiegeng(Platycodon root) and 6 g Fuling(Tuckahoe), 3 g Renshen(Ginseng), 3 g Wuweizi(Chinese magnoliavine fruit) and 3 g Gancao(Liquorice).

【功效】 养阴清热,化痰止咳。

【Efficacy】 Eliminating heat by nourishing yin, dissipating phlegm to stop cough.

【适应证】 肺虚久咳者。

【Indication】 Chronic cough due to lung asthenia.

清肺汤
Qingfei Tang
Clearing-lung Decoction

【药物组成】 麦冬、天冬、知母、贝母、橘红、黄芩、桑皮各 9 g,甘草 6 g。

【Composition】 9 g Maidong (Dwarf lilyturf tuber), 9 g Tiandong (Cochinchinese asparagus root), 9 g Zhimu(Common anemarrhena rhizome), 9 g Beimu(Fritillaria bulb), 9 g Juhong(Red tangerine peel), 9 g Huangqin(Baical skullcap root), 9 g Sangpi(White Mulberry Root-bark) and 6 g Gancao(Liquorice).

【功效】 清肺化痰,润燥止咳。

【Efficacy】 Clearing lung to dissipate phlegm, moisturizing dryness-syndrome to stop cough.

【适应证】 肺热咳嗽者。

【Indication】 Cough with lung heat.

玉竹粥
Yuzhu Zhou
Yuzhu Porridge

【药物组成】 玉竹 15 g,粳米 100 g,冰糖少许。

【Composition】 15 g Yuzhu（Fragrant solomonseal rhizome）,100 g non-glutinous rice and a little crystal sugar.

【功效】 补肺养胃,生津止渴。

【Efficacy】 Reinforcing lung and nourishing the stomach,promoting fluid production to quench thirst.

【适应证】 适用于中老年人肺阴不足,肺燥咳嗽,干咳少痰,烦渴口干,咽干舌燥等症,并有延年益寿、护肤美容的功效。

【Indication】 Being available to syndromes such as the old with lung-yin deficiency,xeropulmonary cough,dry cough with less phlegm,excessive thirst with dry mouth,dry pharynx and tongue. It also has functions as lengthening life,skin care and beautifying.

哮喘 Asthma

乌药百部汤
Wuyao Baibu Tang
Decoction ofCombined Spicebush Root and Stemona Root

【药物组成】 乌药、百部、党参各 10 g,枳实、半夏、甘草各 6 g,苏子 12 g。

【Composition】 10 g Wuyao（Combined spicebush root）,10 g Baibu（Stemona root）and 10 g Dangshen（Tangshen）,6 g Zhishi（Immature orange fruit）,6 g Banxia（Pinellia tuber）and 6 g Gancao（Liquorice root）,12 g Suzi（Perilla）.

【功效】 止咳定喘,润肺下气。

【Efficacy】 Relieving cough and asthma,moistening lung to lower qi.

【适应证】 支气管哮喘发作期患者。

【Indication】 Onset period of bronchial asthma.

鱼腥五味子平喘汤
Yuxing Wuweizi Pingchuan Tang
Antiasthmatic decoction of heartleaf houttuynia and Chinese magnoliavine fruit

【药物组成】 五味子 30 g,地龙 10 g,鱼腥草 40 g。

【Composition】 30 g Wuweizi（Chinese magnoliavine fruit）,10 g Dilong（Earthworm）and 40 g Yuxing Cao（Heartleaf Houttuynia）.

【功效】 敛肺平喘。

【Efficacy】 Astringing lung and antiasthma.

【适应证】 重度哮喘患者。

【Indication】 Serious asthma.

川贝杏仁饮
Chuanbei Xingren Yin
Decoction of Cirrhosae and Apricot Kernels

【药物组成】 川贝母 6 g,杏仁 3 g,冰糖少许。川贝母、杏仁加清水适量,用武火烧沸后将冰糖放入,转用文火煮 30 min 即可。每日睡前服 1 次。

【Composition】 6 g Chuan Beimu(Cirrhosae),3 g apricot kernels and a little crystal sugar. Decoct the cirrhosae and apricot kernels in clean water with a strong fire,then put the crystal sugar in,and then cook them with a small fire for 30 minutes. Take it one time daily before sleeping.

【功效】 清热定喘。

【Efficacy】 Clearing heat and relieving asthma.

【适应证】 气粗息涌,喉中痰鸣如吼,胸高胁胀,咳呛阵作,咳痰色黄者。

【Indication】 Thick breath,wheezy phlegm in the throat like growling,fullness in the chest and distention around the ribs,intermittent cough with yellowish phlegm.

苏子粥
Suzi Zhou
Perilla Porridge

【药物组成】 苏子 10 g,粳米 50 g,红糖适量。将苏子捣为泥与粳米、红糖同入锅内,加水煮成粥。每日早晚温服,5~7 日为 1 个疗程。

【Composition】 10 g Suzi(Perilla),50 g non-glutinous rice and proper amount of brown sugar. Put the mashed perilla,non-glutinous rice and brown sugar into a pot,add some water, and cook them into porridge. Take it warmly in the morning and evening daily,with 5~7 days taken as a treatment course.

【功效】 降气化痰,止咳定喘。

【Efficacy】 Depressing qi and eliminating phlegm,relieving cough and asthma.

【适应证】 寒哮型支气管哮喘。

【Indication】 Cold-wheezing bronchial asthma.

黄芪炖乳鸽
Huangqi Dun Ru ge
Milkvetch Root Stewed with a Young Pigeon

【药物组成】 黄芪 30 g,怀山药 30 g,茯苓 30 g,乳鸽 1 只。以上四物共放炖盅内,加水 200~250 mL,隔水炖 2 h,加入盐、味精调味。每隔 3~5 日服食 1 次,可常服。

【Composition】 30 g Huangqi(milkvetch root),30 g Huai Shanyao(Chinese yam),30 g Fuling(Tuckahoe)and a young pigeon. Put them into a stewing pot, add 200 ~ 250 ml water, and then stew them above water for 2 hours, flavor with salt and the monosodium glutamate. Take it once every 3 ~5 days constantly.

【功效】 益气补肺,固表定喘。

【Efficacy】 Benefiting qi and reinforcing lung, strengthening superficial defence and relieving asthma.

【适应证】 肺气虚型支气管哮喘。

【Indication】 Lung-qi deficiency bronchial asthma.

山药茯苓包子
Shanyao Fuling Baozi
Steamed buns stuffed with yam andTuckahoe

【药物组成】 山药粉100 g,茯苓粉100 g,面粉200 g,白糖300 g,碱适量。将山药粉、茯苓粉加水适量调成枘状,蒸半小时后,调以面粉、白糖,发酵,以猪油、青丝、红丝少许为馅,包成包子,蒸熟即可。可作早点或点心食用。

【Composition】 100 g Shanyao(Chinese yam)powder,100 g Fuling(Tuckahoe)powder, 200 g sour,300 g white sugar and proper amount of soda. Mix the yam powder and Tuckahoe powder with proper amount of water, make them into paste, steam them for half an hour, mix them with flour and white sugar, ferment and make steamed buns stuffed with little lard and pieces of orange peels dyed green and red. Take the buns as breakfast or snack.

【功效】 健脾益气化痰。

【Efficacy】 Strengthening spleen, benefiting qi and eliminating phlegm.

【适应证】 咳嗽痰多,食少脘痞,便溏,常因饮食不当而诱发者。

【Indication】 Cough with excessive phlegm, poor eating and fullness in gastric cavity, loose stool caused by improper diet.

虫草全鸭
Chongcao Quanya
Caterpillar Fungus and a Whole Duck

【药物组成】 冬虫夏草10 g,老雄鸭1只。将鸭洗净,劈开鸭头,纳入虫草8~10枚,扎紧,余下虫草与葱姜装入鸭腹内,放入蒸锅中,再注入清汤,加食盐、胡椒、绍酒,上笼蒸1~2 h。出笼后去姜、葱,加味精即可。佐餐食用。

【Composition】 10 g Dongchong Xiacao(Caterpillar fungus)and one old male duck. Wash the duck clean, cut the duck head, put in 8 ~ 10 pieces of caterpillar fungus, tie it up, put the rest caterpillar fungus, scallion and ginger into the duck's abdomen, put into the steaming pot, pour into the light soup, add salt, pepper and Shaoxing rice wine, steam for 1 ~ 2 hours, take out the ginger and scallion, add monosodium glutamate and take it together with food.

【功效】 补肾纳气定喘。

【Efficacy】 Improving inspiration by invigorating the kidney and relieving asthma.

【适应证】 短气喘促,动则为甚,吸气不利,痰吐起沫者。

【Indication】 Short and quick breath(more serious while moving), difficulty in breathing with foam phlegm.

蔗汁淮山糊
Zhezhi Huaishan Hu
Sugarcane Juice and Yam Paste

【药物组成】 怀山药 60 g,甘蔗汁 250 g。将怀山药捣烂,加甘蔗汁,放锅中隔水炖熟即成。每日早晚餐或作点心食用。

【Composition】 60 g Huai Shanyao(Chinese yam) and 250 g sugarcane juice. Smash the Huai Shanyao(Chinese yam), add sugarcane juice, stew it in the pot above water. Take it with a dinner or as a snack.

【功效】 补脾润肺,化痰止咳。

【Efficacy】 Invigorating the spleen and moisturizing lung, dissipating phlegm to stop cough.

【适应证】 脾气虚型支气管哮喘。

【Indication】 Spleen-qi-deficiency bronchial asthma.

支气管炎 Bronchitis

瓜蒌止咳汤
Gualou Zhike Tang
Cough-arresting Snakegourd Decoction

【药物组成】 瓜蒌仁 15 g,川贝母、杏仁、苏子、桑叶、麻黄各 10 g,半夏 6 g。

【Composition】 15 g Gualou Ren(Snakegourd seed), 10 g Chuan Beimu(Sichuan fritillary bulb), 10 g apricot kernels, 10 g Suzi(Perilla), 10 g Sangye(Mulberry leaf), 10 g Mahuang(Ephedra) and 6 g Banxia(Pinellia tuber).

【功效】 祛痰平喘。

【Efficacy】 Expelling phlegm and antiasthma.

【适应证】 支气管炎急性期发作,咳嗽,气喘,痰多者。

【Indication】 Acute phase of bronchitis, cough and asthma with excessive phlegm.

哮喘平一号
Xiaochuanping Yihao
Number 1 Asthma-calming Drug

【药物组成】 炙麻黄、生甘草、黄芩、陈皮各4.5 g,杏仁、前胡、桑叶、桑白皮、蒸百部各9 g,炙紫菀、海蛤粉各15 g。

【Composition】 4.5 g honey-fried Mahuang(Ephedra),4.5 g raw Gancao(Liquorice), 4.5 g Huangqin(Baical skullcap root),4.5 g Chenpi(Dried tangerine peel),9 g apricot kernels,9 g Qianhu(Hogfennel root),9 g Sangye(Mulberry leaf),9 g Sangbaipi(White mulberry root-bark),9 g steamed Baibu(Stemona root),15 g honey-fried Ziwan(Tatarian aster root)and 15 g sea clam powder.

【功效】 清肺散寒,止咳平喘。

【Efficacy】 Clearing lung and expelling coldness,stoping cough and antiasthma.

【适应证】 喘息性支气管炎属表虚而阳气不足者。

【Indication】 Asthmatic bronchitis with superficial asthenia and yang-qi deficiency.

姜汁牛肺糯米饭
Jiangzhi Niufei Nuomi Fan
GlutinousRice with Ginger and Ox Lung

【药物组成】 牛肺150~200 g,生姜汁10~15 mL,糯米适量。牛肺切块,加糯米文火焖熟,起锅时加入生姜汁即成。

【Composition】 150~200 g ox lung,10~15 ml fresh ginger and proper amount of glutinous rice. Cut the ox lung into pieces,stew it with glutinous rice on a mall fire,add ginger after cooking it.

【功效】 祛痰补肺,温暖脾胃。

【Efficacy】 Expelling phlegm and reinforcing lung,warming spleen and stomach.

【适应证】 适用于老人寒嗽日久之慢性支气管炎。

【Indication】 Chronic bronchitis with cold cough of the old.

黄芪御寒鸡
Huangqi Yuhan Ji
Cold-resisting Chicken with Milkvetch

【药物组成】 母鸡1只(重1 000 g 以上),蜜炙黄芪50 g,防风、附子、蜜炙麻黄各10 g。母鸡宰杀后去毛,剖腹,洗净,滤干,背朝下腹朝上放入瓷盆内,加水小半碗。将4味中药装入纱布袋,扎口,塞入鸡腹。鸡内脏洗净,放药袋上,淋黄酒2匙,盆不加盖,用旺火隔水蒸4 h,至鸡肉酥烂,将药袋从鸡腹中取出,挤干汁水,倒入鸡腹中,弃药渣。宜于立冬以后食用。喝鸡汁,每次3~4匙,每天2~3次,鸡肉可蘸酱油佐餐服食。

【Composition】 A hen(weighing more than 1000 g),50 g honey-fried Huangqi

（Milkvetch root），10 g Fangfeng（Ledebouriella root），10 g Fuzi（Monkshood）and 10 g honey-fried Mahuang（Ephedra）. Kill the hen，remove its hairs，cut its abdomen，wash it clean，dry it and put it into a porcelain pot，add water（less than half a bowl），put the above-mentioned drugs into a gauze bag，tie it up and stuff into the chicken abdomen；wash the internal organs of chicken clean，put on the drug bag，pour 2 spoons of rice wine，steam above water in a uncovered pot for 4 hours with a strong fire，until the chicken become softened；take the drug bag out of the chicken abdomen，wipe the juice，pour into the chicken abdomen，abandon the drug residues. Taken it after Lidong（the 19th "solar term" of the lunar calendar meaning "beginning winter" but is 45 days before the winter solstice）. Drink the chicken soup，3 ~ 4 spoons every time，2 ~ 3 times daily. Take the chicken dipped with soy sauce at dinners.

【功效】　温阳益气，固表平喘

【Efficacy】　Warming yang and benefiting qi，strengthening superficial defence amd anti-asthma.

【适应证】　适用于冬重夏轻的老年慢性支气管炎。

【Indication】　Chronic bronchitis of the old（serious in winter and mild in summer）.

紫河车炖冬虫夏草
Ziheche Dun Dongchong Xiacao
Dried Human Placemta Stewed with Caterpillar Fungus

【药物组成】　紫河车半具，冬虫夏草 10 g。紫河车漂洗干净，切块，与冬虫夏草一起炖熟，调味，饮汤食肉。

【Composition】　Half a Ziheche（Dried human placemta）and 10 g Dongchong Xiacao（Caterpillar fungus）. Rinse and wash the dried human placemta clean，cut in into pieces，stew it with caterpillar fungus，flavor it，then drink the soup and eat the meat.

【功效】　补益肺肾。

【Efficacy】　Benefiting lung and kidney.

【适应证】　适用于老年慢性支气管炎属肺肾两虚者，症见久咳喘息、身体虚弱等。

【Indication】　Lung-kidney-concurrent-insufficiency chronic bronchitis of the old with long-term cough，gasping and physical weakness.

灵芝粉蒸肉饼
Lingzhifen Zheng Roubing
Glossy Ganoderma Steamed with Meat

【药物组成】　灵芝 3 g，猪瘦肉 100 g。灵芝研末。猪肉剁成肉泥，与灵芝末拌匀后加酱油调味，隔水蒸熟，佐餐食用。

【Composition】　3 g Lingzhi（Glossy ganoderma）and 100 g lean pork. Grind the glossy ganoderma into powder；chopped the pork into muddy flesh，mix it with glossy ganoderma powder，flavor with soy sauce，steam above water until it is fully cooked. Take it together with food.

【功效】　益气养阴,安神。

【Efficacy】　Supplementing qi and nourishing yin,calming nerves.

【适应证】　适用于老年慢性支气管炎、慢性胃炎、消化不良等。

【Indication】　Chronic bronchitis,chronic gastritis and dyspepsia of the old.

核桃猪腰
Hetao Zhuyao
Walnut Kernels and Pig Kidneys

【药物组成】　猪腰500 g,核桃仁70 g,鸡蛋清2个,干淀粉50 g,生姜、葱各15 g,料酒、麻油各25 mL,精盐5 g,植物油750 mL(实耗80 mL)。将猪腰对剖,片去腰臊洗净,切十字花刀,再切成3块。核桃仁用开水泡涨,削去外皮,用刀铡成丁。生姜洗净切片,葱切段。腰片用料酒、精盐、姜片、葱拌匀入味,干淀粉用蛋清调成糊待用。锅置火上,加油,烧至六成热时,将核桃丁摆在腰花上,裹上蛋清淀粉糊下锅,逐块炸成浅黄色捞出。待全部炸完后,待油温升至八成热时,再将全部腰块倾入锅内,炸成金黄色,沥去余油,淋上麻油装盘即成。

【Composition】　500 g pig kidney,70 g walnut kernels,2 egg white,50 g dry starch,15 g fresh ginger,15 g scallion,25 mL cooking wine,25 mL sesame oil,5 g refined salt and 750 ml vegetable oil(80 ml is actually used). Split the pig kidney,remove the medulla,cut with the cross shape,and cut it into 3 pieces;soak the walnut kernels till they swell,peel them,cut into little squares;wash the fresh ginger clean and slice it,cut the scallion into sections;mix the kidney slices evenly with cooking wine,refined salt,ginger slices and scallion,cover the egg white with dry starch and blend them into paste for use;put the pot onto the fire,add oil,put the walnut kernels on the kidney slices,and put them into the pot together with the prepared paste when the oil is 60% boiled,fry them piece by piece into light yellow color and take them out;then pour all the fried kidney slices into the pot when the oil is 80% boiled,fry them into golden yellow color,drip the oil,pour the sesame oil onto them and then put them into a plate.

【功效】　补肺肾,定虚喘。

【Efficacy】　Reinforcing lung and kidney,relieving dyspnea due to deficiency.

【适应证】　适用于老年慢性支气管炎肺肾虚而致之喘咳等。

【Indication】　Chronic bronchitis of the old,dyspnea with cough due to lung−kidney asthenia.

陈皮兔肉
Chenpi Turou
Tangerine Peels Fried with Rabbit Meat

【药物组成】　净兔肉35 g,陈皮0.5 g,鲜汤10 ml,干海椒(或辣椒)1 g,植物油15 ~ 20 mL,调料适量。兔肉洗净,切2厘米方丁入碗内,加盐、料酒、葱节、植物油、姜片拌匀。

辣椒切碎。陈皮用温水浸泡 10 min,切成小方块。味精、白糖、酱油、鲜汤入碗内调成汁。炒锅加油,烧至七成热时下辣椒,炒至棕黄色,下肉炒散发白,再入陈皮、花椒、姜、葱,继续炒至肉干酥,入调好的酱油汁、醋,搅匀,放辣椒油,炒至汁收干呈棕红色,去葱、姜,装盘,再淋上香油即成。

【Composition】 35 g clean rabbit meat,0.5 g Chenpi(Dried tangerine peel),10 mL delicious soup,1 g dried hot pepper(or chili),15~20 mL vegetable oil and proper amount of flavoring. Wash the rabbit meat clean, cut it into 2 cm side length cubes, mix it with salt, cooking wine, scallion sections, vegetable oil and ginger slices; cut the chili into pieces, soak the dried tangerine peel in warm water for 10 minutes, and cut it into cubes; put the monosodium glutamate, white sugar, soy sauce and delicious soup into a bowl, mix them into juice; put oil into the cooking kettle, and put in the chili when the oil is 70% boiled, fry them into brown yellow color, put in meat, fry it into white pieces, put in dried tangerine peel, pepper, ginger and scallion, continue to fry it until the meat becomes dry and crumbly, put in the mixed soy sauce and vinegar, blend them evenly, put in the pepper oil, fry it until it becomes dry and brown red, take the scallion and ginger out, put them into a plate and pour the sesame oil onto it.

【功效】 补中益气,理气化痰。

【Efficacy】 Strengthening the middle warmer and benefiting qi, regulating qi and dissipating phlegm.

【适应证】 适用于老年慢性支气管炎咳嗽痰喘、食欲不振,亦可作为糖尿病、动脉硬化、高血压病人的膳食,并可预防衰老。

【Indication】 Chronic bronchitis of the old with cough, humid asthma and poor appetite; also being as food for the patients with diabetes, arteriosclerosis, high blood pressure; preventing aging.

肺癌 Lung Cancer

清肺解毒汤
Qingfei Jiedu Tang
Lung-clearing and Toxic-eliminating Decoction

【药物组成】 沙参、夏枯草各 15 g,麦冬、天冬、干蟾皮各 9 g,百部、葶苈子、八月札各 12 g,鱼腥草、山海螺、生薏苡仁、白毛藤、白花蛇舌草、生牡蛎各 30 g,天龙 5 g(研末分吞)。

【Composition】 15 g Shashen(Root of straight ladybell), 15 g Xiakucao(Selfheal spike),9 g Maidong(Dwarf lilyturf tuber),9 g Tiandong(Cochinchinese asparagus root),9 g dried toad skin,12 g Baibu(Stemona root),12 g Tinglizi(Lepidium seed),12 g Bayuezha (Fiveleaf akebia fruit),30 g Yuxing Cao(Heartleaf Houttuynia),30 g Shanhailuo(Lance asiabell root),30 g raw Yiyi Ren(Coix seed),30 g Baimaoteng(Solanum lyratum),30 g

Baihua Sheshecao (Oldenlandia diffusa) , raw oysters , 5 g Tianlong (Centipede) . Take the powder in several doses.

【功效】 养阴清肺,解毒散结。

【Efficacy】 Nourishing yin and clearing lung , diminishing stagnation by detoxification.

【适应证】 原发性肺癌属于阴虚痰热型者。

【Indication】 Yin-deficiency phlegm-heat type constitutional lung cancer.

加味生脉汤
Jiawei Shengmai Tang
Magnoliavine Pulse-promoting Decoction

【药物组成】 党参、麦冬、山药、熟地、贝母、沙参各9 g,五味子6 g。

【Composition】 9 g Dangshen (Tangshen) , 9 g Maidong (Dwarf lilyturf tuber) , 9 g Shanyao (Chinese yam) , 9 g Shudi (Prepared rhizome of rehmannia) , 9 g Beimu (Fritillaria bulb) , 9 g Shashen (Root of straight ladybell) and 6 g Wuwei Zi (Chinese magnoliavine fruit) .

【功效】 益气养阴,清热化痰。

【Efficacy】 Supplementing qi and nourishing yin.

【适应证】 原发性肺癌属于气阴两虚型者。

【Indication】 Qi-yin deficiency type constitutional lung cancer.

活血软坚汤
Huoxue Ruanjian Tang
Blood-activating and Hard-softening Decoction

【药物组成】 夏枯草、海藻各15 g,贝母、玄参、天花粉、赤芍、炙山甲、当归各9 g,栝楼仁12 g,红花5 g。

【Composition】 15 g Xiakucao (Selfheal spike) , 15 g kelp , 9 g Beimu (Fritillaria bulb) , 9 g Xuanshen (Figwort root) , 9 g Tianhuafen (Trichosanthes root) , 9 g Chishao (Red peony root) , 9 g stir-fried pangolin scales , 9 g Danggui (Chinese angelica) , 12 g Gualou Ren (Trichosanthes seed) and 5 g safflower.

【功效】 行气活血,化瘀软坚。

【Efficacy】 Promoting qi to activate blood , dissolving the stasis and softening hard mass.

【适应证】 原发性肺癌属于气滞血瘀型者。

【Indication】 Qi-stagnancy and blood-stasis type constitutional lung cancer.

益元化浊汤
Yiyuan Huazhuo Tang
Qi-invigorating and Turbidity-dissolving Decoction

【药物组成】 生黄芪、鸡血藤各20 g,女贞子、枸杞子、鸡内金各15 g,清半夏、茯苓、焦白术各12 g,陈皮6 g,焦三仙各9 g。

【Composition】 20 g raw Huangqi (milkvetch root), 20 g Jixueteng (Leatherleaf milletia), 15 g Nǚzhenzi(Glossy privet fruit), 15 g Gouqizi(Chinese wolfberry), 15 g Ji Neijin (Chicken's gizzard – skin), 12 g Qing Banxia (Prepared pinellia tuber), 12 g Fuling (Tuckahoe), 12 g scorched Baizhu (Largehead atractylodes rhizome), 6 g Chenpi (Dried tangerine peel) and 9 g Jiaosanxian(Charred Triplet).

【功效】 补气养阴,燥湿化痰。

【Efficacy】 Invigorating qi and nourishing yin, drying dampness to eliminate phlegm.

【适应证】 肺癌化疗有毒副反应者。

【Indication】 Poison and side reaction in lung cancer chemotherapy.

甘草雪梨煲猪肺
Gancao Xueli Bao Zhufei
Pig Lungs Stewed with Liquorice and Pears

【药物组成】 甘草5 g,雪梨两个,猪肺约250 g。梨削皮切成块,猪肺洗净切成片, 挤去泡沫,与甘草同放砂锅内。加冰糖少许,清水适量,小火熬煮3 h后服用。每日1次。

【Composition】 5 g Gancao(Liquorice root), 2 snow pears and about 250 g pig lungs. Peel the pears and cut them into pieces; wash the pig lungs clean, slice them, press out the foam, put them into an earthern pot with the liguorice root; add little crystal sugar and proper amount of clean water, stew it with a small fire for 3 hours. Take it once daily.

【功效】 润肺除痰。

【Efficacy】 Moisturizing lung and eliminating phlegm.

【适应证】 适用于咳嗽不止者。

【Indication】 Excessive cough.

五味子炖肉
Wuweizi Dun Rou
Magnoliavine Stewed with Meat

【药物组成】 五味子10 g,鸭肉或猪瘦肉适量。五味子与肉一起蒸食或炖食,并酌 情加入调料。肉、药、汤俱服。

【Composition】 10 g Wuwei Zi(Chinese magnoliavine fruit) and proper amount of duck meat or lean pork. Steam or stew the magnoliavine fruit with meat and flavor them. Take all of the meat, drug and decoction.

【功效】 补肺益肾,止咳平喘

【适应证】 适宜于肺癌肾虚型病人。

Efficacy】 Invigorating lung and kidney, relieving cough and asthma.

【Indication】 Kidney–asthenia type lung cancer.

薏米赤豆粥
Yimi Chidou Zhou
Coix and Beans Porridge

【药物组成】 薏苡米 100 g,赤小豆 50 g,大枣 20 枚,白糖适量。薏苡米、赤小豆浸泡 5 h,将赤小豆放入锅内,加水煮烂,下入薏苡米、大枣,用慢火煮至米熟,放入白糖调匀,继用慢火煮至米烂成稀粥即可。每日数次随意服食,连服 10 ~ 15 天。

【Composition】 100 g Yirenmi(Coix seed), 50 g red beans, 20 pieces of jujubes and proper amount of white sugar. Soak the coix seeds and red beans for 5 hours, then put red beans into a pot, boil them in water, then put in the coix seeds and jujubes; stew them with a slow fire until they are fully cooked, mix them with the white sugar and then continue to boil them with a slow fire to make a gruel. Take it several times daily at will, and take it continuously for 10 ~ 15 days.

【功效】 清热解毒、止血利湿。

【Efficacy】 Clearing away the heat-evil and expelling superficial evils, stop bleeding and reducing dampness through diuresis.

【适应证】 用于肺癌咳嗽痰少、色黄难咯、胸痛痰血、心烦口渴、食欲不佳者。

【Indication】 Lung cancer with syndromes as cough with less phlegm, difficulty in coughing out yellowish phlegm, pain in chest and bloody phlegm, restlessness and thirst, and poor eating.

虫草炖老鸭
Chongcao Dun Laoya
Caterpillar Fungus Stewed with Old Duck

【药物组成】 老鸭一只,冬虫夏草 10 g,杏仁 10 g,葱、姜少许,调料适量。冬虫夏草先用温水洗两遍,用少许水泡胀,捞出;杏仁用开水泡 15 min,去皮,鸭洗净。将杏仁、冬虫夏草、老鸭、葱、姜、料酒、盐、上汤、和泡虫草的水一块下入锅内,先用大火烧沸,小火煨至熟烂,后淋上香油即可。

【Composition】 An old duck, 10 g(Caterpillar fungus), 10 g apricot kernels, little scallion and ginger and proper amount of flavoring. Wash the caterpillar fungus 2 times with warm water, soak it with little water and take it out when it swells; soak the apricot kernels for 15 minutes in hot water, peel them, wash the duck clean, put the apricot kernels, caterpillar fungus, old duck, scallion, ginger, cooking wine, salt, stock and soaking water of caterpillar fungus into the pot, boil them with a big fire and then stew them with a small fire until the meat is softened, then pour the sesame oil onto it.

【功效】 补肺益肾,祛痰止咳

【Efficacy】 Invigorating lung and kidney, expelling phlegm to arrest coughing.

【适应证】 用于肺癌见有咳嗽咳痰,自汗盗汗、腰膝酸软者。

【Indication】 Lung cancer with syndromes as cough with phlegm, spontaneous perspiration and night sweat, and sour—weak waist and knees.

肺结核 Tuberculosis

疗肺宁
Liaofei Ning
Lung–healing Drug

【药物组成】 穿心莲、山海螺、百部各9 g,白及粉6 g。

【Composition】 9 g Chuanxinlian(Creat),9 g Shanhailuo(Lance asiabell root),9 g Baibu(Stemona root)and 6 g Baiji(Bletilla)powder.

【功效】 清热润肺,化痰止咳。

【Efficacy】 Clearing heat and moisturizing lung,dissipating phlegm and stopping cough.

【适应证】 肺痨(肺结核)者。

【Indication】 Tuberculosis.

双参蜜耳饮
Shuangshen Mi'er Yin
Decoction of Ginseng,Glehnia,Honey and Fungus

【药物组成】 西洋参10 g,北沙参15 g,白木耳10 g。白木耳水发后将西洋参、北沙参放入与白木耳一次加足水,武火烧热,文火慢炖,待汤稠时入蜂蜜调匀即可。可随意饮用。

【Composition】 10 g Xiyangshen(American ginseng),15 g Bei Shashen(Coastal glehnia root)and 10 g white fungus. Soften the white fungus in water, and then put the American ginseng,coastal glehnia root and the white fungus into a pot,add enough water at a time;then boil them with a big fire and stew them with a slow fire,put in honey to mix with them when the decoction becomes dense. Take it at will.

【功效】 益气养阴润肺。

【Efficacy】 Supplementing qi,nourishing yin and moisturizing lung.

【适应证】 气阴两虚型肺结核患者调理用。

【Indication】 Regulation for qi–yin deficiency pulmonary tuberculosis.

芩部丹
Qinbu Dan
Pill of Baical Skullcap and Stemona

【药物组成】 黄芩9 g,百部18 g,丹参9 g。

【Composition】 9 g Huangqin(Baical skullcap root),18 g Baibu(Stemona root)and 9 g

Danshen(Red sage root).

【功效】 清热润肺,活血抗痨。

【Efficacy】 Clearing heat and moisturizing lung,activating blood circulation against tuberculosis.

【适应证】 肺结核见潮热咳嗽者。

【Indication】 Tuberculosis with hectic fever and cough.

保肺散
Baofei San
Lung-healing Powder

【药物组成】 北沙参 12 g,云茯苓、百合、玉竹、黑芝麻、炙紫菀、蒸百部各 9 g,苦桔梗 6 g,广陈皮 5 g,粉甘草 3 g,薄荷叶 2 g,将黑芝麻洗干净炒香,其他药味烤燥,共研细末。每服 6 g,日服 3 次,以米汁或者白糖水冲服。

【Composition】 12 g Bei Shashen(Coastal glehnia root),9 g Fuling(Tuckahoe),9 g Baihe(Lily bulb),9 g Yuzhu(Dried solomanseal),9 g black sesames,9 g honey-fried Ziwan (Tatarian aster root),9 g steamed Baibu(Stemona root),6 g platycodon root,5 g Guang Chenpi(Southern dried tangerine peel),3 g shaved Gancao(Liquorice root)and 2 g peppermint leaves. Wash the black sesames clean, stir-bake them into a fragrant state, bake other ingredients dry and grind all of them into fine powder. Take 6 g in one dose,3 times daily, together with rice juice or syrup made by white sugar.

【功效】 滋阴润肺,止咳化痰。

【Efficacy】 Nourishing yin and moisturizing lung,relieving cough and reducing sputum.

【适应证】 肺结核潮热自汗、喉燥咽干者。

【Indication】 Tuberculosis with hectic fever,spontaneous perspiration and dry throat and larynx.

滋阴鳖肉汤
Ziyin Bierou Tang
Yin-nourishing Turtle Meat Decoction

【药物组成】 鳖肉 250 g,百部、地骨皮、黄芪各 15 g,生地 20 g。将鳖肉切块,百部、地骨皮、黄芪、生地装入纱布袋中,封口。把鳖肉放入沸水锅中,撇去浮沫,加入药物和姜片、葱段、黄酒。先用武火煮沸后,改用文火炖煮 1 h。去药袋,加食盐、味精调味,再煮一二沸即成。每日 1 次,佐餐食用,连食 7 ~ 10 d。

【Composition】 250 g turtle meat,15 g Baibu(Stemona root),15 g Digupi(Wofberry bark),15 g Huangqi(Milkvetch root)and 20 g Shengdi(Dried/fresh rehmannia root). Cut the turtle meat into pieces,put the stemona root,wolfberry bark,milkvetch root and the dried/ fresh rehmannia root into a gauze bag and seal its opening;put the turtle meat into boiling water, skim the floating foam,put in the drugs,ginger slices,scallion sections and rice wine;boil them with a strong fire and stew them with a small fire for 1 hour; take out the bag of drugs, flavor with salt and monosodium glutamate, then boil them one to two times. Take it once daily together with food continuously for 7 ~ 10 days.

【功效】 益气养阴,抗痨。

【Efficacy】 Supplementing qi and nourishing yin, fighting against tuberculosis.

【适应证】 气阴两虚型肺结核患者调理用。

【Indication】 Regulation for qi-yin deficiency pulmonary tuberculosis.

虫草乌鸡汤
Chongcao Wuji Tang
Decoction of caterpillar fungus and black chicken

【药物组成】 乌骨鸡200 g,冬虫夏草10 g,怀山药30 g。在砂锅中加水1500 mL,入乌骨鸡,旺火烧开,即下冬虫夏草、山药片,改用文火,1 h后即可食用,食时加食盐、味精调味。

【Composition】 200 g black chicken, 10 g Dongchong Xiacao(Caterpillar fungus) and 30 g Huai Shanyao(Chinese yam). Put 1500 mL water and the black chicken into an earthern pot, boil them with a strong fire, put the caterpillar fungus and Chinese yam slices in, use a small fire to cook them for 1 hour; then take it flavored with salt and monosodium glutamate.

【功效】 杀虫滋阴,润肺清热。

【Efficacy】 Killing parasites and nourishing yin, moisturizing lung to clear heat.

【适应证】 阴虚肺热型肺结核患者调理用。

【Indication】 Regulation for yin-deficiency lung-heat type pulmonary tuberculosis.

消化系统疾病
Digestive system diseases

口腔溃疡 Mouth Ulcers

莲子栀子汤
Lianzi Zhizi Tang
Decoction of Lotus Plumules and Cape Jasmine Fruits

【药物组成】 莲子30 g,栀子15 g,冰糖适量。

【Composition】 30 g Lianzi(Lotus plumele),15 g Zhizi(Cape jasmine fruit)and proper amount of crystal sugar.

【功效】 清泻心火。

【Efficacy】 Clearing and purging the sthenic heart-fire.

【适应证】 心脾积热引起的口疮。

【Indication】 Sores in mouth due to accumulation of heart and spleen.

半夏泻心汤
Banxia Xiexin Tang
Heart-draining decoction of pinellia

【药物组成】 半夏12 g,炙甘草、黄芩、干姜、人参各9 g,黄连3 g,红枣4枚。

【Composition】 12 g Banxia(Pinellia tuber),9 g Zhi Gancao(Honey-fried licorice root),9 g Huangqin(Baical skullcap root),9 g dried ginger,9 g Renshen(Ginseng),3 g Huanglian(Goldthread)and 4 pieces of red jujubes.

【功效】 调和寒热,和胃降逆。

【Efficacy】 Harmonizing coldness and heat,regulating stomach to calm the regurgitation。

【适应证】 口腔溃疡引起疼痛者。

【Indication】 Mouth ulcer with pain.

玄参莲枣饮
XuanshenLianzao Yin
Decoction of Figwort,Lotus Plumules and Jujubes

【药物组成】 玄参90 g,丹皮、炒枣仁各30 g,柏子仁、莲子心各9 g。用水清洗,入砂锅中,加水300 mL,小火煎煮30 min,去渣,加水再煎,滤取汁液,将两次所得药汁合并,加白糖少许,分3次服用,每日1剂。

【Composition】　90 g Xuanshen(Figwort root),30 g Danpi(Moutan bark), and 30 g stir-baked jujube kernels,9 g shelled cedar seeds and 9 g Lotus plumule. Wash them clean, put them into an earthern pot, add 300 mL water, decoct them with a small fire for 30 minutes, remove the residues, add water to decoct again, filter and keep the juice, combine the two juices, add litter white sugar, take it in three times, one dose daily.

【功效】　养阴降火。

【Efficacy】　Nourishing yin and reducing fire.

【适应证】　适用于心火过旺,口腔溃疡,口干舌红,渴欲饮冷水,经常失眠。

【Indication】　Excessive heart fire, mouth ulcer, dry mouth and red tongue, thirst disring for water, frequent insomnia.

鸭头饮
Yatou Yin
Duck Head Decoction

【药物组成】　咸鸭头 1 个,用清水浸泡干咸鸭头,洗净,放入小砂罐中,加水适量,先用大火煮沸,再改用小火慢煨 30 min 左右,1 次饮完,每日 2 次。

【Composition】　Choose a dried salty duck head, rinse it with clean water, wash it clean and put it into an earthern pot, add proper amount of water, boil it with a big fire, and then stew it with a small fire for 30 minutes. Drink all of it at a time,2 times daily.

【功效】　清热泻火。

【Efficacy】　Clearing heat and reducing fire.

【适应证】　适用于阴虚内热,或内有湿热蕴积,火热上冲,口腔溃疡,或者口舌生疮。

【Indication】　Yin asthenia generating intrinsic heat;or dampness-heat accumulation, fire heat going upward, mouth ulcer;or sores in mouth and tongue.

萝卜鲜藕汁
Luobo Xian'ou Zhi
Radish and Lotus Roots Juice

【药物组成】　生萝卜 250 g,鲜莲藕 500 g。将萝卜和藕用水洗净,于洁净器皿中捣碎烂,用消毒纱布双层绞取汁,每日数次取适量含于口中,片刻后咽下。

【Composition】　250 g fresh radish and 500 g fresh lotus roots. Wash the radish and lotus roots clean, smash them in a clean container, press out the juice with two layers of sterile gauze. Suck proper amount of it in the mouth several times daily, and then swallow it after a short while.

【功效】　养阴清热。

【Efficacy】　Eliminating heat by nourishing yin.

【适应证】　适用于阴虚火旺,口腔溃疡。

【Indication】　Asthenic yin causing excessive pyrexia, mouth ulcer.

银耳莲子羹
Yin'er Lianzi Geng
Porridge of White Fungus and Lotus Seeds

【药物组成】 银耳 25 g,莲子 50 g。用水将银耳、莲子洗干净,入锅中,加水煮至银耳熟烂,加冰糖或白糖溶化,早晚各食 1 小碗。

【Composition】 25 g white fungus and 50 g lotus seeds. Wash them clean, put them into a pot, add water to cook until the white fungus is fully cooked; melt some crystal sugar or white sugar into it. Take a small bowl of them in the morning and another small bowl in the evening.

【功效】 清热养阴。

【Efficacy】 Clearing heat and nourishing yin.

【适应证】 适用于阴虚火旺,口腔溃疡或口舌生疮。

【Indication】 Asthenic yin causing excessive pyrexia, mouth ulcer or sores in mouth and tongue.

绿豆粥
Lǜdou Zhou
Mung Porridge

【药物组成】 绿豆 100 g,粳米 150 g,白糖 15 g。绿豆、粳米用水淘洗干净,入锅中,加水适量,小火慢慢熬煮成粥,粥成时加入白糖,每日早晚作正餐服食。

【Composition】 100 g Mung beans, 150 non-glutinous rice and 15 g white sugar. Rinse the mung beans and rice, wash them clean, put them into a pot, add proper amount of water, stew them with a small fire into a porridge, then add some white sugar into the porridge. Take it at dinners daily.

【功效】 和脾胃,祛内热。

【Efficacy】 Harmonizing spleen and stomach, expelling internal heat.

【适应证】 适用于脾胃不和,食欲不振,消化力弱,经常性口腔溃疡,反复不愈。

【Indication】 Spleen-stomach disharmony, poor appetite, weak digestive power, frequent mouth ulcer.

慢性结肠炎 Chronic Colitis

温中汤
Wenzhong Tang
Center-warming Decoction

【药物组成】 党参、白术、茯苓、防风、焦神曲、焦山楂各 9 g,炮姜 3 g,炙甘草、陈皮各 6 g,白芍、秦皮各 12 g。

【Composition】　9 g Dangshen（Tangshen）, 9 g Baizhu（Largehead atractylodes rhizome）, 9 g Fuling（Tuckahoe）, 9 g Fangfeng（Ledebouriella root）, 9 g scorch-fried Shenqu（Medicated leaven）, 9 g scorch-fried hawthorns, 3 g baked ginger, 6 g Zhi Gancao（Honey-fried licorice root）, 6 g Chenpi（Dried tangerine peel）, 12 g Baishao（White peony root）and 12 g Qinpi（Ash brak）.

【功效】　健脾温中,清肠化湿。

【Efficacy】　Strengthening spleen and warming spleen-stomach, clearing intestine and dissipating dampness.

【适应证】　大便次数多且质稀薄者。

【Indication】　Frequent thin stools.

益气汤
Yiqi Tang
Qi-benefiting Decoction

【药物组成】　黄芪、薏苡仁各 12 g,党参、茯苓、血余炭、赤石脂、白芍各 10 g,白术炭、陈皮炭、柴胡、厚朴、黄连各 6 g。

【Composition】　12 g Huangqi（Milkvetch root）, 12 g Yiyiren（Coix seed）, 10 g Dangshen（Tangshen）, 10 g Fuling（Tuckahoe）, 10 g Xueyutan（Carbonized hair）, 10 g Chishizhi（Red halloysite）, 10 g Baishao（White peony root）, 6 g charred Baizhu（Largehead atractylodes rhizome）, 6 g charred tangerine peel, 6 g Chaihu（Chinese thorowax root）, 6 g Houpo（Officinal magnolia bark）and 6 g Huanglian（Goldthread）.

【功效】　补中益气,固肠止泻。

【Efficacy】　Strengthening the middle warmer and benefiting qi, strengthening intestine to check diarrhea.

【适应证】　大便带血且次数较多,伴肛门坠胀者。

【Indication】　Frequent stools with blood, distention and tenesmus.

白芍饮
Baishao Yin
Decoction of White Peony Root

【药物组成】　白芍 15 g,茯苓 20 g,白术 15 g,生姜 10 g,附子片 15 g,红糖 20 g。将附片炙好,先煮 30 min 去水,白芍、茯苓、生姜、白术洗净,切片。将以上药物放入炖锅内,加水适量,置武火上烧沸,再用文火煎煮 30 min,去渣,加入红糖搅匀即成。代茶饮用。

【Composition】　15 g Baishao（White peony root）, 20 g Fuling（Tuckahoe）, 15 g Baizhu（Largehead atractylodes rhizome）, 10 g fresh ginger, 15 g Fuzi（Monkshood）slices and 20 g brown sugar. Cook the stir-baked monkshood for 30 minutes, remove water, wash the white peony root, Tuckahoe, fresh ginger and largehead atractylodes rhizome clean, slice them and put them into a stewing pot, add proper amount of water, boil them with a strong fire, and then stew them with a small fire for 30 minutes, remove the residues, put in the brown sugar and mix them. Take it as a tea.

【功效】 消炎止泻。

【Efficacy】 Eliminate inflammation to check diarrhea.

【适应证】 对慢性结肠炎泄泻者效果较好。

【Indication】 Chronic colitis with diarrhea.

银花红薯粥
Yinhua Hongshu Zhou
Porridge of Honeysuckle and Sweet Potatoes

【药物组成】 红薯,大米,金银花,生姜。红薯切成小块或研成细粉,加入金银花(视临床症状轻重酌量)、生姜,按常法煮饭、煮粥均可。每日 3 餐均吃,要坚持吃,不少于 3 ~ 4 个月,方可逐步收效。

【Composition】 Sweet potatoes, rice, Jinyinhua (Honeysuckle) and fresh ginger. Cut the sweet potatoes into small pieces or grind them into fine powder, put in the honeysuckle (taking differnt amounts according to clinical symptoms) and fresh ginger, and cook rice or porridge as usual methods. Take it at 3 dinners daily consistenly. It will take effects after being taken for 3 ~ 4 months.

【功效】 清热解毒,调味和中。

【Efficacy】 Clearing away the heat−evil and expelling superficial evils, regulating taste and harmonizing the middle warmer.

【适应证】 对于慢性结肠炎腹胀、腹痛症状较明显者适用。

【Indication】 Chronic colitis with abdominal distention and pain

马齿苋饭
Machixian Fan
Purslane Rice

【药物组成】 马齿苋,大米。马齿苋洗净切细,和大米调和。加水常法煮饭。可早晚服食。连服 15 d 以上。

【Composition】 Purslane and rice. Wash the purslane clean and cut it into fine pieces, mix it with rice and cook them with water. Take it in the morning and evening continuously for more than 15 days.

【功效】 清热解毒,止痢止泻。

【Efficacy】 Clearing away the heat – evil and expelling superficial evils, stopping dysentery and diarrhea.

【适应证】 本方对溃疡性结肠炎急性发作时有效。

【Indication】 Acute episode of ulcerative colitis.

山药芡实扁豆糕
Shanyao Qianshi Biandou Gao
Cake of Yam, Gordon Uryale and Hyacinth Beans

【药物组成】 鲜山药,赤小豆,芡实米、白扁豆,云茯苓各 15 g。乌梅。先将赤小豆制成豆沙,加适量白糖待用;将云茯苓、白扁豆、芡实米研成细粉。加少量水蒸熟;鲜山药蒸熟 去皮,加入茯苓等蒸熟的药粉,拌匀成泥状。将药泥在盘中薄薄铺一层,再将豆沙铺一层,如此铺成六七层,成千层糕状,上锅再蒸。待熟取出。以乌梅、白糖熬成浓汁。浇在蒸熟的糕上,即可食用。

【Composition】 15 g fresh Shaoyao(Chinese yam), 15 g red beans, 15 g Qianshi(Gordon uryale), 15 g Bai Biandou(White hyacinth bean), 15 g Yun Fuling(Yunnan tuckahoe) and smoked plums. Make red beans into the bean paste, add proper amount of white sugar for use; grind the Yunnan Tuckahoe, white hyacinth beans and Gordon uyales into fine powder, add little water and steam them until they are fully cooked; steam and peel the fresh Chinese yam, put in the steamed tuckahoe powder, blend them into a mash; spread a thin layer of drug mash on the plate, then spread a layer of bean paste, then drug mash again, making a cake six or seven layers; steam the cake and take it out when it is fully cooked; stew the smoked plum and white sugar into dense juice, pour the juice onto the steamed cake, then take the cake.

【功效】 益气健脾,固涩收敛止泻。

【Efficacy】 Nourishing qi to invigorate spleen, astringing to stop diarrhea.

【适应证】 更适宜于疾病缓解期食用,急性炎症期效果稍逊。

【Indication】 Eating in the disease-free period(with less effects during acute inflammation).

消化不良 Indigestion

茯苓当归饮
Fuling Danggui Yin
Decoction of Tuckahoe and Angelica

【药物组成】 白茯苓、当归(微灸)、芍药、炙甘草各 50 g,桂皮(去粗皮)75 g。

【Composition】 50 g White Fuling(Tuckahoe), 50 g slightly fried Danggui(Chinese angelica), 50 g Shaoyao(Peony), 50 g Zhi Gancao(Honey-fried licorice root) and 75 g Guipi(raw bark removed).

【功效】 健脾化湿,温中止痛。

【Efficacy】 Invigorating spleen to eliminate dampness, warming the spleen-stomach to relieve pain.

【适应证】 脾气虚弱引起的挑食、厌食者。

【Indication】 Food preferences and anorexia due to deficiency-weakness of spleen-qi.

平胃散
Pingwei San
Stomach-calming Powder

【药物组成】 苍术 120 g,厚朴 90 g,陈皮 60 g,炙甘草 30 g,生姜 2 片,红枣 5 枚。

【Composition】 120 g Cangzhu(Atractylodes rhizome),90 g Houpo(Officinal magnolia bark),60 g Chenpi(Dried tangerine peel),30 g Zhi Gancao(Honey-fried licorice root),2 slices of fresh ginger and 5 pieces of red jujubes.

【功效】 燥湿健脾,消胀散满。

【Efficacy】 Eliminating dampness to strengthen spleen,reducing distention and fullness.

【适应证】 脾湿引起的食欲低下者。

【Indication】 Poor appetite due to spleen dampness.

麦芽丸
Maiya Wan
Malt Pills

【药物组成】 麦芽 40 g,神曲 20 g,白术、橘皮各 10 g。

【Composition】 40 g malt,20 g Shenqu(Medicated leaven),10 g Baizhu(Largehead atractylodes rhizome)and 10 g tangerine peel.

【功效】 消食化积。

【Efficacy】 Promoting digestion by dissipating food stagnation.

【适应证】 食欲不振,快嚼进食者。

【Indication】 Poor appetite and eating with fast hiccup.

茯苓和胃汤
Fuling Hewei Tang
Stomach-strengthening Tuckahoe Decoction

【药物组成】 柴胡、白术、白芍各 10 g,薄荷 7 g,茯苓 15 g。

【Composition】 10 g Chaihu(Chinese thorowax root),10 g Baizhu(Largehead atractylodes rhizome),10 g Baishao(White peony root),7 g Bohe(Peppermint)and 15 g Fuling(Tuckahoe).

【功效】 疏肝理气,健脾和胃。

【Efficacy】 Soothing liver to regulate qi,strengthening the spleen and stomach.

【适应证】 消化不良引起腹胀者。

【Indication】 Abdominal distention due to dyspepsia.

消谷丸
Xiaogu Wan
Pills for Grain Digestion

【药物组成】 神曲180 g,炒乌梅肉120 g,炮姜120 g,麦芽90 g,诸药研末炼蜜为丸。

【Composition】 180 g Shenqu(Medicated leaven),120 g stir-baked mume fruit,120 g baked ginger and 90 g malt are ground into powder,honey-fried and made into pills.

【功效】 消食和胃。

【Efficacy】 Promoting digestion and regulating stomach.

【适应证】 脾胃虚弱口中无味者。

【Indication】 Tasteless due to weakness of the spleen and stomach.

保赤万应散
Baochi Wanying San
Infant-safeguarding Red Powder

【药物组成】 鸡内金30 g,神曲、麦芽、山楂各100 g,研末用糖水调服。

【Composition】 30 g Ji Neijin(Chicken's gizzard-skin),100 g Shenqu(Medicated leaven),100 g malt and 100 g hawthorns are ground into powder and mixed with syrup.

【功效】 健脾消积。

【Efficacy】 Strengthening spleen to reduce food stagnation.

【适应证】 小儿疳积,身体瘦弱,毛发稀疏,脘腹胀满者。

【Indication】 Infantile malnutritional stagnation, thinness and weakness, sparseness of hair, distension and fullness in abdomen and gastric cavity.

酒积丸
Jiuji Wan
Pills for Wine Accumulation

【药物组成】 黄连、乌梅肉各30 g,半夏曲20 g,枳实、砂仁各15 g,杏仁9 g,巴豆霜3 g,上药为细末,蒸饼为丸,每服9 g。

【Composition】 30 g Huanglian(Goldthread),30 g smoked plums,20 g Banxiaqu(Fermented pinellia),15 g Zhishi(Immature orange fruit),15 g Sharen(Amomum fruit),9 g apricot kernels,3 g Badoushuang(Powdered croton seed). Powder the above ingredients,steam and make them into pills. Take 9 g per dose.

【功效】 清热理气,消积导滞。

【Efficacy】 Clearing heat and regulating qi,removing food retention and stagnation.

【适应证】 饮酒受伤成积,时呕痰水者。

【Indication】 Frequent injury by drinking with vomiting phlegm water.

刺梨蜜饮
Cili Miyin
Decoction of Roxburgh and Honey

【药物组成】　刺梨 200 g,蜂蜜 50 g。

【Composition】　200 g roxburgh rose and 50 g honey.

【功效】　健胃消食。

【Efficacy】　Invigorating stomach for digestion.

【适应证】　食欲不振者。

【Indication】　Poor appetite.

谷芽山楂饮
Guya Shanzha Yin
Decoction of rice sprout and hawthorn

【药物组成】　谷芽 15 g,山楂 15 g。

【Composition】　15 g Rice sprouts and 15 g hawthorns.

【功效】　调中消食,开胃健脾。

【Efficacy】　Regulating the middle warmer for digestion, promoting appetite and strengthening spleen.

【适应证】　消化不良,食欲差者。

【Indication】　Dyspepsia, poor appetite.

胃炎 Gastritis

清中消痞汤
Qingzhong Xiaopi Tang
Middle-clearing and Lump-dissipating Decoction

【药物组成】　太子参、麦门冬、丹参各 15 g,炙半夏、炒栀子、丹皮各 8 g,柴胡、甘草各 6 g,青皮 10 g。

【Composition】　15 g Taizi Shen(Heterophylly falsestarwort root),15 g Maimendong,15 g Danshen(Red sage root),8 g honey-fried Banxia(Pinellia),8 g stir-baked Zhizi(Cape jasmine fruit),8 g Danpi(Moutan bark),6 g Chaihu(Chinese thorowax root),6 g Gancao(Liquorice root)and 10 g Qingpi(Green tangerine peel).

【功效】　益胃养阴,清中消痞。

【Efficacy】　Benefiting stomach and nourishing yin, clearing the middle warmer and dissipating abdominal lumps.

【适应证】　胃炎引起的腹胀,胃部不适者。

【Indication】 Abdominal distention due to gastritis, stomach discomfort.

清胃竹茹汤
Qingwei Zhuru Tang
Stomach-clearing Bamboo Shavings Decoction

【药物组成】 竹茹、白芍各 12 g, 芦根 25 g, 蒲公英、麦冬各 15 g, 枳壳、石斛各 9 g, 薄荷、甘草各 6 g。

【Composition】 12 g Zhuru (Bamboo shavings), 12 g Baishao (White peony root), 25 g Lugen (Reed root), 15 g Pugongying (Dandelion), 15 g Maidong (Dwarf lilyturf tuber), 9 g Zhike (Orange fruit), 9 g Shihu (Dendrobium stem), 6 g Bohe (Peppermint) and 6 g Gancao (Liquorice root).

【功效】 理气止痛。

【Efficacy】 Regulating qi to alleviate pain.

【适应证】 以疼痛为主的胃炎患者。

【Indication】 Gastritis with pain.

金橘饮
Jinju Yin
Cumquat Decoction

【药物组成】 金橘 200 g, 白蔻仁 20 g, 白糖适量。金橘加水用中火烧 5 min, 再加入白蔻仁、白糖, 用小火略煮片刻即可。每日 1 剂, 或随意食之。

【Composition】 200 g cumquat, 20 g round cardamom seeds and proper amount of white sugar. Stew the cumquat with water with a middle fire for 5 minutes, put in the round cardamom seeds and white sugar, then decoct it with a small fire for a short while. Take it one dose daily, or take it at will.

【功效】 疏肝解郁, 调和脾胃。

【Efficacy】 Soothing liver to relieve depression, harmonizing spleen and stomach.

【适应证】 胃脘胀痛, 攻窜两胁, 嗳气则舒, 呕吐吞酸, 遇情志失调加重者。

【Indication】 Distention and pain in the gastric cavity effecting on ribs of both sides, being comfortable while belching, vomiting and acid regurgitation, being more serious while being in disorder of emotion-thought.

丁香姜糖
Dingxiang Jiangtang
Clove and Ginger Sugar

【药物组成】 白砂糖 50 g, 生姜末 30 g, 丁香粉 5 g, 香油适量。白砂糖加少许水, 放入砂锅, 文火熬化, 加生姜末、丁香粉调匀, 继续熬至挑起不粘手为度。另备一大搪瓷盆, 涂以香油, 将熬的糖倒入摊平。稍冷后趁软切作 50 块。

【Composition】 50 g white sugar, 30 g fresh ginger powder, 5 g clove powder and proper amount of sesame oil. Stew the white sugar with water in an earthern pot with a small fire till the sugar melt, mix it with fresh ginger powder and clove powder, then stew them till they are not sticky any more; spread the sesame oil onto the bottom of a big enamel basin, put the stewed sugar into the basin and spread it flat; cut it into 50 pieces after it cools.

【功效】 温中降逆,益气健脾。

【Efficacy】 Warming the spleen-stomach to descend adverse-rising qi, nourishing qi to invigorate spleen.

【适应证】 脘腹痞胀或隐痛,喜温喜按,食欲减退,间或泛吐清水,面黄消瘦,神疲乏力,四肢欠温,大便溏薄者。

【Indication】 Distention or pain in gastric cavity and abdomen favoring warmth and pressing, poor appetite, spit water, yellowish face and emaciation, fatigue, coldness in limbs, loose stools, loose stool.

鸡内金饼
Ji'neijin Bing
Chicken's gizzard-skin Cake

【药物组成】 鸡内金 10 g,红枣 30 g,白术 10 g,干姜 1 g,面粉 500 g,白糖 300 g。将鸡内金、红枣、白术、干姜同入锅内,加瑙水用文火煮 30 min,去渣留汁备用。将药汁倒入面粉,加白糖、发面,揉成面团,待发酵后,加碱适量,做成饼。将饼置于蒸笼上,武火蒸 15 min 后即成。早晚作点心食用,可常食。

【Composition】 10 g Ji Neijin(Chicken's gizzard-skin), 30 g red jujubes, 10 g Baizhu (Largehead atractylodes rhizome), 1 g dried ginger, 500 g flour and 300 g white sugar. Put the chicken's gizzard-skin, red jujubes, Largehead atractylodes rhizome and dried ginger into a pot, boil it with a small fire for 30 minutes, remove the residues, keep the juice for use; pour the juice into flour, add white sugar, leaven dough, rub it into a dough, add proper amount of soda after it ferments and make it into round flat cakes; put cakes on the steamer and steam them with a strong fire for 15 minutes. Take them frequently as a snack in the morning or the evening.

【功效】 消食化积,健脾益胃。

【Efficacy】 Promoting digestion to reducing food stagnation, strengthening spleen and benefiting stomach.

【适应证】 脾胃虚寒型慢性胃炎。

【Indication】 Spleen-stomach insufficiency-cold chronic gastritis.

胃及十二指肠溃疡 Gastric and Duodenal Ulcer

两和镇痛饮
Lianghe Zhentong Yin
Liver & Stomach-soothing and Pain-relieving Decoction

【药物组成】　柴胡、枳壳、佛手、厚朴各 12 g,白芍、炒香附、神曲各 15 g,甘草 6 g。

【Composition】　12 g Chaihu(Chinese thorowax root),12 g Zhike(Orange fruit),12 g Foshou(Finger citron),12 g Houpo(Officinal magnolia bark),15 g Baishao(White peony root),15 g stir-baked Xiangfu(Cyperus tuber),15 g Shenqu(Medicated leaven) and 6 g Gancao(Liquorice root).

【功效】　疏肝和胃,行滞止痛。

【Efficacy】　Soothing liver and regulating stomach,expelling stagnation to relieve pain.

【适应证】　胃及十二指肠溃疡引起节律性疼痛不适者。

【Indication】　Rhythmic pain caused by gastric and duodenal ulcer.

芪芍及草汤
Qishao Jicao Tang
Decoction of Milkvetch,Bletilla and Liquorice

【药物组成】　黄芪 25 g,海螵蛸 20 g,白及、甘松、元胡各 12 g,甘草 6 g。

【Composition】　25 g Huangqi(Milkvetch root),20 g Hai Piaoxiao(Cuttlebone),12 g Baiji(Bletilla),12 g Gansong(Spikenard),12 g Yuanhu(Corydalis tuber) and 6 g Gancao (Liquorice root).

【功效】　健脾益气,活血止痛,制酸止血。

【Efficacy】　Strengthening spleen and benefiting qi,promoting blood circulation to arrest pain,restraining acids and stopping bleeding.

【适应证】　胃及十二指肠溃疡引起的反酸、嗳气或呕血者。

【Indication】　Sour regurgitation, belching and haematemesis caused by gastric and duodenal ulcer.

黄芪建中汤
Huangqi Jianzhong Tang
Center-fortifying Milkvetch Decoction

【药物组成】　饴糖 30 g,桂枝、生姜各 9 g,黄芪 10 g,炙甘草 6 g,大枣 6 枚。

【Composition】　30 g malt extract,9 g Guizhi(Cassia twig),9 g fresh ginger,10 g Huangqi(Milkvetch root),6 g Zhi Gancao(Honey-fried licorice root),6 pieces of jujubes.

【功效】　温中补虚,缓急止痛,和里缓急。

【Efficacy】 Warming spleen – stomach and improving asthenia, relaxing tension and relieving pain, harmonizing the interior and relaxing tension.

【适应证】 中焦虚寒引起的胃及十二指肠溃疡。

【Indication】 Gastric and duodenal ulcer caused by deficiency–cold in middle energizer.

生姜木瓜汤
Shengjiang Mugua Tang
Ginger and Papaw Soup

【药物组成】 生姜 30 g,木瓜 500 g,红枣 30 枚,醋 50 mL。将上 4 味一起用砂锅文火炖熟。每日 1 剂,分 3 次食用,连服 3~4 剂。

【Composition】 30 g fresh ginger, 500 g papaw, 30 pieces of red jujubes and 50 ml vinegar. Put the above 4 ingredients into an earthern pot and stew them with a small fire. Take it in 3 times, one dose daily, 3~4 doses successively.

【功效】 健脾化瘀

【Efficacy】 Strengthening spleen and dissipating blood stasis.

【适应证】 适用于胃、十二指肠溃疡等症。

【Indication】 Gastric and duodenal ulcer.

鲜姜煨猪肚
Xianjiang Wei Zhudu
Fresh ginger stewed with pork tripe

【药物组成】 鲜姜 250 g,猪肚 1 个,酱油适量。将猪肚洗净,装入切成片的鲜姜,扎好,放砂锅内文火煨熟,去姜,猪肚切丝。猪肚丝拌酱油及调料吃,并可饮汤。每个猪肚分 3 日吃完,可连吃 10 个。

【Composition】 250 g fresh ginger, 1 pork tripe, proper amount of soy sauce. Wash the pork tripe clean, put in sliced fresh ginger, tie it up, put into the earthernware pot and stew it with a small fire, take the ginger out, slice the pork tripe. Mix the pork tripe slices with soy sauce and flavoring, eat it and drink the soup. Eat up every pork tripe within 3 days, and take 10 pork tripe successively.

【功效】 温中健脾

【Efficacy】 Warming spleen–stomach and strengthening spleen.

【适应证】 适用于胃溃疡症。

【Indication】 Gastric ulcer.

马铃薯蜜膏
Malingshu Migao
Paste of Potato and Honey

【药物组成】 鲜马铃薯 1000 g,蜂蜜适量。将鲜马铃薯洗净,用绞肉机加工捣烂,再用洁净纱布搅取汁,放锅中以大火烧沸,后改文火煎熬,浓缩至黏稠时加一倍量的蜂蜜,再煎至黏稠如膏状停火,冷却装瓶。空腹服用,每次 1 汤匙,每日 2 次,20 天为 1 个疗程。

【Composition】 1000 g fresh potatoes and proper amount of honey. Wash the potatoes clean, smash them with the meat grinder, press out the juice with clean gauze, put it into the pot and boil it with a big fire, then decoct it with a small fire, add double amount of honey when it is condensed into a sticky state, then decoct them into a sticky paste; put it into a bottle. Take it with an empty abdomen, one spoon at a time, 2 times per day, with 20 days taken as a treatment course.

【功效】 和胃调中。

【Efficacy】 Harmonizing stomach and regulating the middle energizer.

【适应证】 适用于胃、十二指肠溃疡等症。治疗中忌辣椒、葱、醋、酒等刺激性食物。

【Indication】 Gastric and duodenal ulcer (No eating pungency food as chilli, spring onion, vinegar and alcohol during treatment.).

包心菜粥
Baoxincai Zhou
Cabbage Porridge

【药物组成】 包心菜 500 g,粳米 50 g。先将包心菜水煮半小时,捞出菜后,入粳米煮粥。温热服,每日服 2 次。

【Composition】 500 g cabbage and 50 g non-glutinous rice. Boil the cabbage in water for half an hour, take the cabbage out, put in the rice to cook porridge. Take it warmly, twice per day.

【功效】 缓急止痛。

【Efficacy】 Relaxing tension and relieving pain.

【适应证】 适用于胃脘拘急疼痛,对胃、十二指肠溃疡有止痛和促进溃疡愈合作用。

【Indication】 Contracture in gastric cavity with pain (relieving pain and promoting healing of gastric and duodenal ulcer).

呃逆 Hiccup

橘皮竹茹汤
Jupi Zhuru Tang
Decoction of Tangerine Peel and Bamboo Shavings

【药物组成】 竹茹、橘皮各 12 g,生姜 9 g,甘草 6 g,大枣 5 g,人参 3 g。

【Composition】 12 g Zhuru (Bamboo shavings), 12 g Jupi (Tangerine peel), 9 g fresh ginger, 6 g Gancao (Liquorice root), 5 g jujubes and 3 g Renshen (Ginseng).

【功效】 清热化痰,止呕除烦。

【Efficacy】　Eliminating phlegm by cooling, stopping vomiting and relieving restlessness.

【适应证】　胃虚有热,呃逆干呕者。

【Indication】　Gastric asthenia with heat, hiccup and vomiturition.

降逆顺气汤
Jiangni Shunqi Tang
Adverse-lowering and qi-regulating Decoction

【药物组成】　赤芍、当归、白芍各 12 g,桃仁、枳壳、木香、苏子、郁金、炮姜各 9 g,红花、厚朴、牛膝、炒麦芽各 15 g,丹参 20 g,代赭石 30 g。

【Composition】　12 g Chishao(Red peony root), 12 g Danggui(Chinese angelica), 12 g Baishao(White peony root), 9 g Taoren, 9 g Zhike(Orange fruit), 9 g Muxiang, 9 g Suzi (Perilla), 9 g Yujin(Turmeric), 9 g baked ginger, 15 g safflowers, 15 g Houpo(Officinal magnolia bark), 15 g Niuxi, 15 g stir-baked malt, 20 g Danshen(Red sage root), 30 g Daizheshi(Red ochre).

【功效】　理气降逆。

【Efficacy】　Regulating qi and calm the adverse-rising qi.

【适应证】　顽固性呃逆者。

【Indication】　Intractable hiccup.

丁香柿蒂汤
Dingxiang Shidi Tang
Decoction of Clove and Persimmon Calyx

【药物组成】　丁香 6 g、柿蒂 9 g、人参 3 g、生姜 6 g。

【Composition】　6 g clove, 9 g Shidi(The calyx and receptacle of a persimmon), 3 g Renshen(Ginseng)and 6 g fresh ginger.

【功效】　温中降逆,益气和胃。

【Efficacy】　Warming the spleen-stomach to descend adverse-rising qi, benefiting qi and harmonizing qi.

【适应证】　胃虚有寒,呃逆不止,或恶心呕吐,得热则减者。

【Indication】　Gastric asthenia with coldness, successive hiccup; or nausea and vomiting (relieving when warmed).

快气汤
Kuaiqi Tang
Qi-regulating Decoction

【药物组成】　砂仁 250 g,香附 1000 g,甘草 125 g,诸药研末,盐汤点下。

【Composition】　250 g Sharen(Amomum fruit), 1000 g Xiangfu(Cyperus tuber)and 125 g Gancao(Liquorice root)are ground into powder and taken with salty soup.

【功效】 理气畅中,和胃降逆。

【Efficacy】 Regulating qi and opening the middle warmer, harmonizing stomach and descending adverse-rising qi.

【适应证】 胃中痰逆呕吐者。

【Indication】 Vomiting due to adverse-rising phlegm in stomach.

干姜刀豆饮
Ganjiang Daodou Yin
Ginger and Sword Bean Decoction

【药物组成】 干姜4 g,刀豆20 g,柿蒂5 个。三味入砂锅内,加清水500 mL,泡透煎至300 mL,去渣留汁待食。每日早晨,空腹乘热食用。

【Composition】 4 g dried ginger, 20 g Daodou(Sword bean) and 5 Shidi(The calyx and receptacle of a persimmon). Put them into an earthern pot, add 500 mL clean water, soak them fully and decoct them into 300 mL, filter the residues, keep the juice. Take it warmly with an empty abdomen in morning daily.

【功效】 此汤有温中止呃之功。

【Efficacy】 Warming the spleen-stomach and stopping hiccup.

【适应证】 适用于胃癌呃逆。

【Indication】 Cancer with adverse-rising hiccup.

半夏生姜茶
Banxia Shengjiang Cha
Pinellia and Ginger Decoction

【药物组成】 制半夏12 g,生姜6 g,伏龙肝200 g。先将伏龙肝打碎入锅,加清水800 mL,武火煎30 min,过滤留汁,加入半夏、生姜同煎取汁待服。代茶,温频饮。

【Composition】 12 g Zhi Banxia(Prepared pinellia), 6 g fresh ginger, and 200 g Fulonggan(Oven earth). Smash the oven earth and put it into a pot, add 800 mL clear water, decoct with a strong fire for 30 minutes, filter it, keep the juice, decoct with the pinellia and fresh ginger and take the juice for taking. Drink it as a tea warmly in several doses.

【功效】 温中化饮,降逆止呕

【Efficacy】 Warming the spleen-stomach to relieving phlegm, reducing adverse-rising qi to stop vomiting.

【适应证】 适用于胃癌的呃逆、呕吐反胃等病症。

【Indication】 Cancer with adverse-rising hiccup, vomiting with regurgitation.

胆囊炎 Cholecystitis

柴草汤
Chaicao Tang
Thorowax and Liquorice Decoction

【药物组成】 金钱草 30 g,柴胡、白芍、郁金、乌贼骨、浙贝母各 9 g,炙甘草 3 g。

【Composition】 30 g Jinqiancao(Christina loosestrife),9 g Chaihu(Chinese thorowax root),9 g Baishao(White peony root),9 g Yujin(Turmeric),9 g Guzeigu(Cuttlebone),9 g Zhe Beimu(Zhejiang Fritillary bulb) and 3 g Zhi Gancao(Honey-fried liquorice root).

【功效】 清热利湿除黄。

【Efficacy】 Clearing away heat evil, reducing dampness through diuresis and relieving jaundice.

【适应证】 慢性胆囊炎患者。

【Indication】 Chronic cholecystitis.

胆囊汤
Dannang Tang
Cholecystitis-treating Decoction

【药物组成】 生大黄、元明粉、柴胡、虎杖、枳实、半夏、黄芩、山栀子各 9 g,茵陈、对座草各 30 g。

【Composition】 9 g Sheng Dahuang (Raw rhubarb), 9 g Yuanmingfen (Refined mirabilite),9 g Chaihu(Chinese thorowax root),9 g Huzhang(Giant knotweed),9 g Zhishi (Immature orange fruit),9 g Banxia(Pinellia tuber),9 g Huangqin(Baical skullcap root),9 g Shan Zhizi(Gardenia fruit),30 g Yinchen(Capillary artemisia) and 30 g Duizuocao(Christina loosestrife).

【功效】 清热退黄。

【Efficacy】 Clearing away heat evil and relieving jaundice.

【适应证】 急性胆囊炎患者。

【Indication】 Acute cholecystitis.

利胆消黄汤
Lidan Xiaohuang Tang
Jaundice-relieving Cholagogic Decoction

【药物组成】 茵陈、败酱草、板蓝根、玉米须各 30 g,金钱草 60 g,郁金 12 g,栀子 10 g。

【Composition】 30 g Yinchen(Capillary artemisia),30 g Baijiangcao(Patrinia),30 g Banlan Gen(Isatis root),30 g corn stigma,60 g Jinqiancao(Christina loosestrife),12 g Yujin (Turmeric) and 10 g Zhizi(Cape jasmine fruit).

【功效】 清热利湿,利胆疏肝。

【Efficacy】 Clearing away heat evil to reduce dampness through diuresis, promoting the function of gallbladder and soothing liver.

【适应证】 急性胆囊炎。

【Indication】 Acute cholecystitis.

鸡内金粥
Ji'neijin Zhou
Chicken's Gizzard-skin Porridge

【药物组成】 粳米100 g,鸡内金5～6 g,白糖适量。将鸡内金用文火炒至黄褐色,研为细粉。先将粳米、白糖入锅内,加水800 ml左右,煮至粥将成时,放入鸡内金粉,再煮一沸即成。

【Composition】 100 g nonglutinous rice, 5～6 g Ji Neijin(Chicken's gizzard-skin) and proper amount of white sugar. Stir-bake chicken's gizzard-skin to yellowish brown with a small fire and grind it into powder; put the rice and sugar into a pot, add 800 ml water, put into the power of chicken's gizzard-skin, boil it into porridge.

【功效】 健脾消食。

【Efficacy】 Invigorating spleen to promote digestion.

【适应证】 慢性胆囊炎患者。

【Indication】 Chronic cholecystitis.

肝炎 Hepatitis

退黄降酶汤
Tuihuang Jiangmei Tang
Icteric Hepatitis-relieving and Enzyme-reducing Decoction

【药物组成】 茵陈30～50 g,田基黄、海金沙、蒲公英、垂盆草各20 g,板蓝根20 g,泽兰12 g,焦山楂30 g,丹参15 g。水煎服,每日1剂,10日为1疗程。

【Composition】 30～50 g Yinchen(Capillary artemisia), 20 g Tianjihuang(Japanese St. Johnswort), 20 g Haijinsha(Climing fern), 20 g Pugongying(Dandelion), 20 g Chuipencao (Stringy stonecrop), 20 g Banlan Gen(Isatis root), 12 g Zelan(Lycopus herb), 30 g scorched hawthorn fruits, 15 g Danshen(Red sage root). Take the decoction one dose daily, with 10 days taken as a treatment course.

【功效】 清热利湿,活血解毒。

【Efficacy】 Clearing away heat evil to reduce dampness through diuresis, activating blood circulation for detoxication.

【适应证】 急性黄疸型肝炎。

【Indication】 Acute icteric hepatitis.

消毒利黄汤
Xiaodu Lihuang Tang
Toxic–removing and Jaundice–eliminating Decoction

【药物组成】 川黄连 1.5 g,生山栀、炒麦芽、连翘壳各 4.5 g,淡竹叶、茵陈、赤茯苓各 6 g,生甘草、细木通、生枳壳各 2.4 g。

【Composition】 1.5 g Chuan Huanglian(Sichuan goldthread),4.5 g Sheng Shanzhi (Gardenia fruit),4.5 g Chao Maiya(Stir–baked malt),4.5 g Lianqiao Ke(Forsythia fruit),6 g Dan Zhuye(Henom bamboo leaf),6 g Yinchen(Capillary artemisia),6 g Chi Fuling(Light red tuckahoe),2.4 g raw Gancao(Liquorice root),2.4 g Ximutong(Clematis kerriana)and 2.4 g raw Zhike(Orange fruit).

【功效】 清胎毒,利黄疸。

【Efficacy】 Clearing away infantile carbuncle,reducing jaundice.

【适应证】 新生儿黄疸。

【Indication】 Infantile jaundice.

速效救黄汤
Suxiao Jiuhuang Tang
Effective Jaundice–eliminating Decoction

【药物组成】 茵陈、丹参、赤芍、麦芽各 15 g,板蓝根、茯苓、白术各 10 g,柴胡、黄芩、陈皮、甘草各 6 g,大枣 6 枚。

【Composition】 15 g Yinchen(Capillary artemisia),15 g Danshen(Red sage root),15 g Chishao(Red peony root),15 g malt,10 g Banlan Gen(Isatis root),10 g Fuling(Tuckahoe) and 10 g Baizhu(Largehead atractylodes rhizome),6 g Chaihu(Chinese thorowax root),6 g Huangqin(Baical skullcap root),6 g Chenpi(Dried tangerine peel),6 g Gancao(Liquorice root)and 6 jujubes.

【功效】 健脾利湿,解毒退黄。

【Efficacy】 Strengthening spleen to reduce dampness through diuresis,detoxication and eliminating jaundice.

【适应证】 小儿黄疸型肝炎。

【Indication】 Infantile icteric hepatitis.

二甲调肝汤
Er'jia Tiaogan Tang
Liver–regulating decoction of pangolin scales and turtle shells

【药物组成】 炒山甲、丹参、白芍、女贞子各 15 g,鳖甲、糯米根须各 24 g,三七 6 g,茵陈、田基黄各 30 g,太子参、茯苓各 18 g。

【Composition】 15 g Chao Shanjia(Pangolin scales),15 g Danshen(Red sage root),15 g Baishao(White peony root) and 15 g Nǔzhenzi(Glossy privet fruit), 24 g Biejia(Turtle shell), 24 g Nuomi Genxu(Glutinous rice root), 6 g Sanqi(Asnchi), 30 g Yinchen(Capillary artemisia), 30 g Tianjihuang(Lesser hypericum), 18 g Taizi Shen(Heterophylly falsestarwort root) and 18 g Fuling(Tuckahoe).

【功效】 活血清热消积,益气养阴。

【Efficacy】 Activating blood circulation, clearing away the heat-evil and eliminating qi stagnation, supplementing qi and nourishing yin.

【适应证】 慢性肝炎,早期肝硬化。

【Indication】 Chronic hepatitis, hepatic cirrhosis at early stage.

丹参合剂
Danshen Heji
Red Sage Mixture

【药物组成】 丹参、当归、桃仁、郁金、金银花、香附、陈皮各 9 g,败酱草 12 g,茵陈 21 g,甘草 6 g,大枣 5 枚。

【Composition】 9 g Danshen (Red sage root), 9 g Danggui (Chinese angelica), 9 g Taoren(Peach seed), 9 g Yujin(Turmeric), 9 g Jinyinhua(Honeysuckle flower), 9 g Xiangfu (nutgrass galingale rhizome) and 9 g Chenpi (Dried tangerine peel), 12 g Baijiangcao (Patrinia), 21 g Yinchen(Capillary artemisia), 6 g Gancao(Liquorice root) and 5 jujubes.

【功效】 活血祛瘀,清热解毒,疏肝利胆。

【Efficacy】 Activating blood circulation to eliminating blood stasis, clearing away the heat-evil and expelling superficial evils, soothing liver to promote the function of gallbladder.

【适应证】 传染性肝炎。

【Indication】 Infectious hepatitis.

艾叶鹌鹑蛋
Aiye Anchundan
Artemisia Leaves and Quail Eggs

【药物组成】 艾叶 10 g,鹌鹑蛋 2 个。艾叶与鹌鹑蛋同放锅内,加清水 400 ml 煮至蛋熟。去汤吃蛋,每日 1 次,5~7 d 为 1 个疗程。

【Composition】 10 g Artemisia leaves, 2 quail eggs. Put Artemisia leaves and quail eggs into the pot, add 400 ml clean water, boil them till the eggs are fully cooked. Remove the soup, eat eggs once per day, with 5~7 days taken as a treatment course.

【功效】 温阳散寒,益气补虚。

【Efficacy】 Warming yang and dispelling coldness, benefiting qi and improving asthenia.

【适应证】 脾肾阳虚型慢性肝炎、肝硬化。

【Indication】 Chronic hepatitis and cirrhosis with spleen-kidney yang deficiency.

重型消黄汤

Zhongxing Xiaohuang Tang

Decoction for treating Severe Icteric Hepatitis

【药物组成】 茵陈 90 g,生石膏、鲜茅根各 30 g,炒黄柏、炒知母、藿香、佩兰、杏仁各 9 g,赤芍、丹皮、龙胆草、泽兰各 15 g。

【Composition】 90 g Yinchen(Capillary artemisia),30 g gypsum,30 g Xian Maogen (Fresh Cogongrass rhizome),9 g stir-baked Huangbai(Phellodendron),stir-baked Zhimu (Anemarrhena),Huoxiang(Ageratum),9 g apricot kernels,15 g Chishao(Red peony root),15 g Danpi(Moutan bark),15 g Longdancao(Gentian root) and 15 g Zelan(Hirsute shiny bugleweed herb).

【功效】 清热利湿,活血解毒,芳香透表。

【Efficacy】 Clearing away the heat to reduce dampness through diuresis,activating blood circulation for detoxication,relieving exterior syndrome with fragrance.

【适应证】 重型急性传染性黄疸型肝炎。

【Indication】 Serious and infectious icteric hepatitis.

玫瑰花粥

Meiguihua Zhou

Rose porridge

【药物组成】 玫瑰花 10 g,粳米 60 g。粳米加水煮粥,粥将成时,撒入玫瑰花瓣,稍煮几沸即可。可作早餐服食。

【Composition】 10 g rose,60 g non-glutinous rice. Cook the rice and water into porridge,put into rose petals and boil it. Take it as breakfast.

【功效】 疏肝和胃。

【Efficacy】 Soothing liver and regulating stomach.

【适应证】 肝气郁结型肝炎。

【Indication】 Hepatitis with stagnation of liver-qi.

郁金清肝茶

Yujin Qinggan Cha

Liver-clearing Tea of Turmeric

【药物组成】 郁金(醋制)10 g,炙甘草 5 g,绿茶 2 g,蜂蜜 25 g。上四味,加水 1000 mL,煮 30 min,取汁即可。每日 1 剂,不拘时频频饮之。

【Composition】 10 g vinegar-processed Yujin(Turmeric),5 g Zhi Gancao(Honey-fried licorice root),2 g green tea and 25 g honey. Boil the drugs with 1000 mL water for 30 minutes and get the juice. Take one dose daily frequently.

【功效】 疏肝解郁,利湿祛瘀。

【Efficacy】 Soothing liver and relieving qi depression, eliminating dampness to remove blood stasis.

【适应证】 胁肋胀痛,疼痛走窜不定的肝炎患者。

【Indication】 Hypochondrium distending pain, hepatitis with moving pain.

肝炎药蛋
Ganyan Yaodan
Medicated Eggs for Treating Hepatitis

【药物组成】 瘦猪肉30 g,鸡骨草30 g,鸡蛋2 个,山栀根30 g。以上四味加水1000 mL,同煮至猪肉烂熟,去药渣。食肉吃蛋饮汤,5~7 d 为1 个疗程。

【Composition】 30 g lean pork, 30 g Jigucao(Canton love-pea vine), 3 eggs and 30 g Shanzhigen(Gardenia root). Cook the four ingredients with 1000 mL water, boil them until the pork is fully cooked, then remove the medicinal residues. Eat the meat and eggs, drink the soup. 5~7 days are taken as a treatment course.

【功效】 益气养血;清热解毒,降酶。

【Efficacy】 Benefiting qi and nourishing blood, clearing away the heat-evil and expelling superficial evils, lowering enzyme.

【适应证】 胁痛隐隐,口干咽燥,或右侧胁肋部疼痛,右胁腹有积块者。

【Indication】 Hypochondrium pain, dry mouth and throat; or patients with pain at the right hypochondrium and with mass at the right flank.

荸荠炖公鸡
Biqi Dun Gongji
Water Chestnut Stewed with a Cock

【药物组成】 公鸡1 只,荸荠500~1000 g。鸡和荸荠一起放清水适量,炖至鸡肉烂熟即可食用。喝汤吃鸡肉、荸荠,每周1 次。

【Composition】 A cock and 500~1000 g water chestnut. Put the cock and water chestnut into a pot, add proper amount of water, stew them till the chicken is fully cooked and edible. Drink soup, eat chicken and the water chestnut, once per week.

【功效】 补气填精,化滞消积。

【Efficacy】 Invigorating qi for essence replenishment, eliminating food stagnation.

【适应证】 肝肾阴虚型的慢性肝炎。

【Indication】 Chronic hepatitis with liver kidney yin insufficiency.

茯苓赤小豆薏米粥
Fuling Chixiaodou Yimi Zhou
Porridge of Poria, Adzuki Beans and Coix

【药物组成】 白茯苓粉20 g,赤小豆50 g,薏米100 g,白糖适量。赤小豆、薏米共煮粥,至粥成后,加茯苓粉稍煮片刻,加白糖调味。每日数次,可随意食之。

【Composition】 20 g White Fuling(Tuckahoe)powder,50 g red beans,100 g coix seeds and proper amount of white sugar. Cook the red beans and coix seeds into porridge,put in the Tuckahoe powder,boil them for a short while and flavor it with white sugar. Take it several times daily,or take it at will.

【功效】 健脾祛湿。

【Efficacy】 Strengthening spleen to eliminating dampness.

【适应证】 水湿内停型慢性肝炎、肝硬化患者。

【Indication】 Chronic hepatitis and cirrhosis with dampness stagnation.

山楂甲鱼汤
Shanzha Jiayu Tang
Decoction of Hawthorn and Turtle

【药物组成】 甲鱼1只(约500 g),生山楂30 g。将甲鱼去头,洗净,与生山楂共放砂锅内,加清水适量煮至甲鱼肉烂熟,即可食用。食肉饮汤,每周1次。

【Composition】 A turtle(about 500 g) and 30 g raw hawthorns. Remove the head of the turtle,wash it clean,put it into an earthen pot with the raw hawthorns,add proper amount of clean water,boil it till the turtle is fully cooked and edible. Eat the meat and drink the soup, once per week.

【功效】 理气活血。

【Efficacy】 Regulating qi to activate blood circulation.

【适应证】 瘀血停滞型的慢性肝炎、肝硬化患者。

【Indication】 Chronic hepatitis and cirrhosis with stagnation of blood stasis.

胆结石 Gall-stone

金钱草煎剂
Jinqiancao Jianji
Christina Loosestrife Decoction

【药物组成】 金钱草100 g加水煎煮。

【Composition】 Decoct 100 g Jinqian Cao(Christina loosestrife)with water.

【功效】 利胆排石。

【Efficacy】 Promoting the function of gallbladder and removing gallstone.

【适应证】 胆结石引起的闷胀、疼痛者。

【Indication】 Distention and pain due to gallstone.

胆道排石汤
Dandao Paishi Tang
Biliary Calculus Decoction

【药物组成】 金钱草 30 g,茵陈、郁金各 15 g,枳实、木香各 9 g,生大黄 6~9 g。

【Composition】 30 g Jinqian Cao (Christina loosestrife), 15 g Yinchen (Capillary artemisia), 15 g Yujin (Turmeric root tuber), 9 g Zhishi (Immature orange fruit) and 9 g Muxiang(Common aucklandia root) and 6~9 g Sheng Dahuang(Raw rhubarb).

【功效】 清热利湿,行气止痛,利胆排石。

【Efficacy】 Clearing away the evil-heat to reduce dampness through diuresis, promoting qi circulation to relieve pain, promoting the function of gallbladder to remove gallstone.

【适应证】 胆石症。

【Indication】 Cholelithiasis.

陈皮牛肉
Chenpi Niurou
Dried Tangerine Peel and Beef

【药物组成】 陈皮丝 50 g,牛肉 1500 g,植物油 1000 g,葱段 50 g,生姜丝 50 g,干辣椒丝 10 g,黄酒 15 g,酱油 50 g,精盐 6 g,味精 3 g,白糖 25 g,食醋、糖色、花椒、鲜汤、麻油各适量。将牛肉切成粗丝,炒锅上火,放油烧热后下牛肉丝炸干,捞出沥油。锅内留余油 50 克,放入适量花椒炸焦,捞去花椒。再放入葱段、生姜丝、陈皮丝、干辣椒丝、煸出香味后烹入黄酒、酱油和鲜汤,加入精盐、味精、白糖、食醋,把汤调成红色,调好口味,放入牛肉丝,用小火烧至汁浓稠,淋入适量麻油,盛盘晾凉即成。当菜佐餐,随意食用。

【Composition】 50 g Chenpi Si (Dried tangerine peel slices), 1500 g Beef, 1000 g vegetable oil, 50 g green onion pieces, 50 g fresh ginger slices, 10 g dried hot pepper slices, 15 g yellow wine, soy 50 g, 6 g salt, 3 g monosodium glutamate, 25 g sugar, and proper amount of vinega, caramel, wild pepper, delicacy soup and sesame oil. Cut the beef into thick slices, fry them to dry with hot oil, then fish them out and drain the oil. Leave 50 g oil in the pan, fry some wild pepper and fish them out. Fry green onion pieces, fresh ginger slices, dried tangerine peel and dried hot pepper slices until fragrant, put in yellow wine, soy, delicacy soup; mix some salt, monosodium glutamate, sugar, and vinegar in the soup to change the color into red, adjust its taste, and put beef slice into it. Cook the soup with gentle fire until it dries up, add some sesame oil. Dish off and cool it. Take casually with staple food.

【功效】 滋补脾胃,益气养血,疏利肝胆。

【Efficacy】 Tonifying spleen and stomach, benefiting qi and nourishing blood, soothing liver to promote the function of gallbladder.

【适应证】 胆石症。

【Indication】 Cholelithiasis.

白茅根炖肉

Baimao Gen Dun Rou

Cogongrass Rhizome Stew Pork

【药物组成】 鲜白茅根 50 g,猪精肉 500 g。白茅根、猪肉洗净,肉切片,白茅根切成小段一同入砂锅中,加葱、姜、清水适量,先用大火烧沸,再用小火婉至肉熟烂,除去葱、姜、白茅根,加入精盐、味精、吃肉喝汤。

【Composition】 50 g Fresh Baimao Gen(Cogongrass rhizome),500 g lean pork. Wash cogongrass rhizome and pork;slice the pork and cut cogongrass rhizome into pieces. Put them into earthen pot;add proper amount green onion,ginger and water. Boil with fire,and cook meat thoroughly with gentle fire. Remove the green onion,ginger and Baimao root;add some salt and monosodium glutamate. Eat the pork and drink the soup.

【功效】 清热利湿。

【Efficacy】 Clearing away heat evil to reduce dampness through diuresis.

【适应证】 适用于肝胆湿热,胆道结石,胁痛隐隐。

【Indication】 Dampness-heat of liver and gall,biliary calculi and pain in the flank.

大金钱草蒸猪肝

Da Jinqiancao Zheng Zhugan

Longhairy Antenoron Herb Steamed Pork Liver

【药物组成】 大金钱草 60 g,猪肝 250 g,狗宝 1.5 g。金钱草、狗宝洗净,捣碎研成细末,猪肝洗净入沸水中氽透,用凉水冲洗干净,沥去水分切成片放在碗内,撒上药末,拌匀,加葱节、姜片、清汤,入笼中蒸 30 min 左右,取出泌出汤汁,加食盐、味精调味,用以佐餐。

【Composition】 60 g Da Jinqiancao(Longhairy Antenoron Herb),250 g liver,1.5 g Goubao(Stone of a dog's gallbladder kidney or bladder). Wash the longhairy antenoron herb and stone of a dog's gallbladder kidney or bladder, smash and grind into fine power; liver washed,boil in the boiling water thoroughly,rinse in cold water,drain off the water,cut into pieces,placed in the bowl,mix with some drug powder,add green onion,ginger,light soup, steam in the cage for about 30 minutes,remove the secretion soup,add salt adn monosodium glutamate to flavor it. Take with the meal.

【功效】 疏肝利胆。

【Efficacy】 Soothing liver to promote the function of gallbladder.

【适应证】 适用于胆道结石。

【Indication】 Biliary calculi.

金钱草粥
JinqiancaoZhou
Christina Loosestrife Soup

【药物组成】 新鲜金钱草60 g,粳米50 g,冰糖15 g。金钱草洗净水煎取汁,粳米淘洗干净,倒入药汁,加水适量,煨煮成粥,入冰糖搅拌溶化,随宜服食。

【Composition】 60 g fresh Jinqiancao(Christina loosestrife),50 g Jingmi(Non-glutinous rice),15 g sugar. Wash christina loosestrife,boil and take the juice,non-glutinous rice washing clean,put in the drug juice,add proper amount of water,simmer it into porridge,mix some sugar until dissolves. Take proper amount.

【功效】 清热祛湿,利胆退黄。

【Efficacy】 Clearing away heat and dissolving dampness,promoting the function of gallbladder to cure jaundice.

【适应证】 适用于湿热蕴积于肝胆,胆道结石,肋下常痛,厌食油腻。

【Indication】 Accumulation of dampness and heat in the liver and gall,biliary calculi, pain in the flank,being tired of greasy food.

便秘 Constipation

蜂蜜饮
Fengmi Yin
Honey Drink

【药物组成】 蜂蜜15 g,加温开水调匀。

【Composition】 15 g Honey,mix with warm water.

【功效】 润肠通便,补中缓急,润肺止咳,美容养颜。

【Efficacy】 Loosening bowel to relieve constipation,strengthening the middle energizer and relaxing tension,moistening lung to arrest cough,improving looks.

【适应证】 肠燥便秘,脾胃虚弱,肺虚干咳者。

【Indication】 Intestine dryness and constipation,weakness of the spleen and stomach,dry cough due to lung asthenia.

通幽汤
Tongyou Tang
Pylorus Smoothing Soup

【药物组成】 桃仁、红花各9 g,生地、熟地黄、当归各10 g,升麻、炙甘草各6 g。

【功效】 养阴活血,滋燥通幽。

【Efficacy】 Nourishing yin to activate blood circulation,moisturizing dryness and smoothing pylorus.

【适应证】 幽门不通,噎膈便秘者。

生地、熟地黄、当归各10 g,升麻、炙甘草各

【Composition】 9 g Taoren(Peach kernel), Honghua(Safflower) each, 10 g Shengdi (Dried/fresh rehmannia root), Shu Dihuang(Prepared rehmannia root) and Danggui(Chinese angelica)(Chinese angelica) each, 6 g Shengma(Cimicifuga rhizome) and Zhi Gancao(Honey –fried licorice root) each.

【Indication】 Pylorus blockage, cardiac spasm and constipation.

油焖枳实萝卜
You Men Zhishi Luobo
Braised Immature Orange Fruit Radish

【药物组成】 枳实10 g,白萝卜、虾米适量。水煎枳实,取汁备用。将萝卜切块,用猪油煸炸,加虾米,浇药汁适量,煨至极烂,加葱、姜丝、盐适量调味即可食之。佐餐食之。

【Composition】 10 g Zhishi(Immature orange fruit), white radish and proper amount of shrimp. Boil and take immature orange fruit juice aside. Diced radish, stir–fried with lard, add the shrimp, and pour some juice, simmer it until extremely well–done, add onions, ginger, salt to spice it. Take with the meal.

【功效】 顺气通便。

【Efficacy】 Guiding qi downward and purgation.

【适应证】 大便秘结,嗳气频作,胸胁胀满,脘腹痞问,食少纳呆者。

【Indication】 Constipation, successive belching, fullness in chest and hypochondrium, mass in abdomen and gastric cavity, poor eating or anorexia.

决明炖茄子
Jueming Dun Qiezi
Cassia Seed Stew Eggplant

【药物组成】 决明子10 g,茄子2个。先将决明子加水煎煮,取汁备用。茄子油炒后,放入药汁及适量的佐料炖熟食之。佐餐食用。

【Composition】 10 g Juemingzi(Cassia Seed), 2 eggplants. First boil Cassia Seed and take the juice aside. Eggplant Fried, put the juice into it and add proper amount of seasoning. Stew unit well–done. Take with the meal.

【功效】 清热通便。

【Efficacy】 Removing heat to loosen bowels.

【适应证】 大便干结,小便短赤,面赤身热者。

【Indication】 Dry stool, oliguria with reddish urine, reddish complexion and general fever.

锁阳红糖饮
Suoyang Hongtang Yin
Songaria Cynomorium Herb Brown Sugar Drink

【药物组成】 锁阳 20 g,红糖适量。

【Composition】 Suoyang(Songaria cynomorium herb)20 g,proper amount of brown sugar.

【功效】 温阳润肠通便。

【Efficacy】 Warming yang,loosening bowel to relieve constipation.

【适应证】 阳气虚引起的排便困难者。

【Indication】 Difficult defecation due to deficiency of yang-qi.

锁蓉羊肉面
Suorong Yangrou Mian
Songaria Cynomorium Herb Cistanche Lamb Noodle

【药物组成】 锁阳 5 g,肉苁蓉 5 g,羊肉 50 g,面粉 200 g。水煎锁阳、肉苁蓉,去渣留汁,待凉,以药汁合面做面条,用羊肉汤煮面,加葱、盐等调味即成。作主食或点心食用。

【Composition】 5 g Suorong(Songaria cynomorium herb),5 g Roucongrong(Cistanche),50 g lamb,200 g flour. Boil songaria cynomorium herb and Cistanche with water, remove residue and take the juice, let cool, make dough with the juice, stew noodle with mutton soup, add onions, salt and other seasonings. Take as a staple food or snack food

【功效】 温阳通便。

【Efficacy】 Warming yang to relieve constipation.

【适应证】 大便艰涩,排出困难。小便清长,面色青白,四肢不温,喜热畏寒,腹中冷痛,或腰脊冷重者。

【Indication】 Difficult defecation; clear urine in large amounts, pale facial expression, coldness in four limbs, favoring heat and chills.

黄芪苏麻粥
Huangqi Suma Zhou
Milkvetch Root, Perilla and Fructus Cannabis Soup

【药物组成】 黄芪 10 g,苏子 50 g,火麻仁 50 g,粳米 250 g。黄芪、苏子弋火麻仁打碎,加水适量煎煮 5~10 min,取药汁备用,入粳米,以药汁煮粥。每日 1 剂,分数次食完。

【Composition】 10 g Huangqi(Milkvetch root),50 g Suzi(Perilla),50 g Huomaren(Fructus cannabis),250 g Jingmi(Non-glutinous rice). Smash milkvetch root, perilla and fructus cannabis, boil with proper amount of water for 5~10 minutes, take its juice, boil the juice with non-glutinous rice. Take one dose a day several times.

【功效】 益气润肠。

【Efficacy】　Benefiting qi to moisten intestines.

【适应证】　气虚便秘者。

【Indication】　Constipation due to deficiency of vital energy.

松核蜜汤
Songhe Mi Tang
Pine Nut Kernel, Walnuts Kernel and Honey Soup

【药物组成】　松子仁 50 g，核桃仁 50 g，蜂蜜 500 g。将松子仁、核桃仁去衣，烘干研为细末，与蜂蜜和匀即成。早晚各服 2 匙。

【Composition】　50 g Pine nut kernel, 50 g walnuts kernel, 500 g honey. Peel the pine nut kernel and the walnuts kernel, bake them dry and grind into fine powder, mix with honey throughly. Take 2 spoons once. Take twice daily in the morning and evening.

【功效】　养阴润肠。

【Efficacy】　Nourishing yin to moisten intestines.

【适应证】　血虚便秘者。

【Indication】　Constipation due to blood-deficiency.

杏仁当归炖猪肺
Xingren Danggui(Chinese angelica) Dun Zhuti
Almond and Chinese Angelica Stew Lung

【药物组成】　杏仁 15 g，当归 15 g，猪肺 250 g。将猪肺洗净切片，在沸水中汆后捞起，与杏仁、当归同放入砂锅内，加清水适量煮汤，煮熟后调味即可。每日 1 次，吃猪肺饮汤。可连续食用数日。

【Composition】　15 g Xingren(Almond), 15 g Danggui(Chinese angelica), 250 g lung. Wash and slice the lung, boiled in water for a short time and fish up. Put into the earthen with almond and Chinese angelica, add proper amount of water to cook soup and spice it. Take once a day; take the meat and soup. Take it for several days continuously.

【功效】　温通开秘。

【Efficacy】　Warming to to relieve constipation.

【适应证】　阳虚便秘者。

【Indication】　Constipation due to yang deficiency.

桑葚地黄蜜膏
Sangshen Dihuang Mi Gao
Mulberry, Dried Rehamnnia Root and Honey Cream

【药物组成】　桑葚 500 g，生地黄 200 g，蜂蜜适量。将桑葚、生地加水适量煎煮。每 30 min 取煎液 1 次，加水再煎，共取煎液 2 次。合并煎液，再以小火煎熬浓缩至较稠黏时，加蜂蜜 1 倍，至沸停火，待冷装瓶备用。每日 2 次，每次 1 汤匙；以沸水冲化。

【Composition】 500 g Sangshen(Mulberry), 200 g Sheng Dihuang(Dried rehamnnia root)and proper amount of honey. Decoct mulberry and dried rehamnnia root with water. Take the decoction every 30 minutes, add water and decoct again, take the decoction twice. Combined the decoction, and then concentrated it with gentle fire until it is viscous and sticky, add honey with the same amount and turn down the fire until it gets boiled. Install it in a bottle after it's cooled. Take twice a day, 1 tablespoon once; brew it with boiling water

【功效】 养阴清热,润肠通便。

【Efficacy】 Eliminating heat by nourishing yin, loosening bowel to relieve constipation.

【适应证】 大便干结,面色无华,头晕目眩,心悸健忘,或颧红耳鸣者。

【Indication】 Dry stool, dark facial expression, dizziness, palpitation with morbid forgetfulness; or reddish cheek and tinnitus.

麻子苏子粥
Mazi Suzi Zhou
Hempseed Perilla Porridge

【药物组成】 紫苏子50 g,大麻子50 g,洗净,研极细末,用水再研取汁150 mL,分2次煮粥啜之。

【Composition】 50 g Zisuzi(Purple perilla), 50 g Damazi(Hempseed), wash and grind them into fine powder, grind it again with water and take150 mL juice, divide it into 2 parts and decoct porridge with the juice.

【功效】 润肠通便。

【Efficacy】 Loosening bowel to relieve constipation.

【适应证】 妇人产后便秘,老人、虚人风秘者。

【Indication】 Constipation after childbirth, anemogenous constipation of the aged and people with deficiency syndrome.

腹泻 Diarrhea

车前山药汤
Cheqian Shanyao Tang
Asiatic Plantain Seed and Common Yam Rhizome Soup

【药物组成】 山药30 g,车前子12 g,车前子包煎。

【Composition】 30 g Shanyao(Common yam rhizome), 12 g Cheqianzi(Asiatic plantain seed). Asiatic plantain seed wraped and decocted.

【功效】 健脾清热,固肠止泄。

【Efficacy】 Strengthening spleen to clear away the heat, strengthening intestine to check diarrhea.

【适应证】　慢性肠炎,久而不愈,腹泻反复发作者。

【Indication】　Chronic enteritis,recurrent attacks of diarrhea.

二神丸
Ershen Wan

【药物组成】　补骨脂120 g,肉豆蔻60 g。

【Composition】　120 g Buguzhi(Psoralea fruit),60 g Roudoukou(Nutmeg).

【功效】　温脾暖胃,固肠止泄。

【Efficacy】　Warming spleen and stomach,strengthening intestine to check diarrhea.

【适应证】　五更泄泻。

【Indication】　Diarrhea before dawn.

健脾益胃散
Jian Pi Yi Wei San
Spleen and Stomach Strengthen Powder

【药物组成】　莲子肉、芡实、扁豆、薏苡仁、山药、白术、茯苓各120 g,党参60 g,临用时候可加适量白糖。

【Composition】　120 g Lotus seed pulp, Qianshi (Gordon euryale seed), Biandou (Hyacinth bean), Yiyiren (Coix seed), Shanyao (Common yam rhizome), Baizhu (Largehead atractylodes rhizome), Fuling (Tuckahoe) each, 60 g Dangshen (Tangshen) (Tangshen), add proper amount of sugar before taken.

【功效】　健脾益胃。

【Efficacy】　Strengthening spleen and benefiting stomach.

【适应证】　用于脾虚腹泻者。

【Indication】　Diarrhea due to spleen deficiency.

薯蓣汤
Shuyu Tang
CommonYam Rhizome Soup

【药物组成】　怀山药30 g,茯苓15 g,神曲10 g,红糖10 g。上药水煎顿服。每日1剂,顿服。

【Composition】　30 g Huai Shanyao(Common yam rhizome),15 g Fuling(tuckahoe),10 g Shenqu(Medicated leaven),10 g brown sugar. Decoct these drugs and take the juice. Take one dose a day and take at a draught.

【功效】　补脾渗湿止泻。

【Efficacy】　Tonifying spleen,excreting dampness to check diarrhea.

【适应证】　大便时溏时泻,迁延反复,完谷不化者。

【Indication】　Loose stool or diarrhea,poor digestion.

豆花煎鸡蛋
Douhua Jian Jidan
Flowerof Hyacinth Dolichos Fried Egg

【药物组成】 扁豆花30 g,鸡蛋2个,盐少许。将鸡蛋打入碗中与扁豆花拌匀,用油煎炒,撒盐末少许即可。每日1剂,分2次服用,可连服5~7 d。

【Composition】 30 g Biandouhua(Flower of hyacinth dolichos) ,2 eggs, a little salt. Put the egg in the bowl and mix with flower of hyacinth dolichos, fry with oil and add a little salt. Take 1 dose twice a day and take 5 to 7 days repeatedly.

【功效】 清热解毒,化湿止泻。

【Efficacy】 Clearing away the heat – evil and expelling superficial evils, dissipating dampness to check diarrhea.

【适应证】 湿热型腹泻患者。

【Indication】 Dampness–heat diarrhea.

胡萝卜汤
Huluobo Tang
Carrot soup

【药物组成】 鲜胡萝卜2个,炒山楂15 g。鲜胡萝卜与炒山楂以水煎汤,加红糖适量即可。每日1剂,可连用3~5 d。

【Composition】 Two fresh carrots, 15 g fried hawthorn. Decoct fresh carrots and fried hawthorn and take the juice, add proper amount of brown sugar. Take 1 dose a day, and take 3 to 5 days repeatedly.

【功效】 顺气消食,化积止泻。

【Efficacy】 Guiding qi downward and promoting digestion, eliminating food stagnation to check diarrhea.

【适应证】 伤食腹泻者。

【Indication】 Diarrhea due to improper dietary disorders.

三花防风茶
Sanhua Fangfeng Cha
Three Flowers and Ledebouriella Root Tea

【药物组成】 扁豆花24 g,莱莉花12 g,玫瑰花12 g,防风12 g。将上四味水煎取液,加入红糖调味代茶饮。每日1剂,不拘时频饮。

【Composition】 24 g Biandouhua(Flower of hyacinth dolichos) ,12 g jasmine flower, 12 g rose and 12 g Fangfeng(Ledebouriella root). Decoct these drugs and take the juice, add some brown sugar and take as tea. Take one dose a day and take frequently as one wish.

【功效】 抑肝扶脾止泻。

【Efficacy】 Regulating liver and spleen to check diarrhea.

【适应证】 胸胁胀闷,嗳气食少,每因抑郁恼怒或情绪紧张之时,发生腹痛泄泻者。

【Indication】 Distention and pression in chest and hypochondrium, eructation and poor appetite, diarrhea with abdominal pain due to mental depression, anger or mental tension.

山药扁豆糕
Shanyao Biandou Gao
Common yam rhizome and hyacinth bean Cake

【药物组成】 鲜山药 200 g,鲜扁豆 50 g,陈皮丝 3 g,红枣肉 500 g。

【Composition】 200 g Fresh Shanyao (Common yam rhizome), 50 g fresh Biandou (Hyacinth bean), 3 g Chenpi Si(Dried tangerine peel slices), 500 g jujube meat.

【功效】 健脾和胃,调中止泄。

【Efficacy】 Strengthening the spleen and stomach, regulating the middle energizer to check diarrhea.

【适应证】 脾虚气弱,消化力弱引起的腹泻者。

【Indication】 Deficiency of the spleen causing weakness of qi, diarrhea due to poor digestion.

鲜马齿苋粥
Xian Machixian Zhou
Fresh Purslane Porridge

【药物组成】 鲜马齿苋 50 g,粳米 50 g。将马齿苋洗净切碎,与粳米同入砂锅,加水 800 ~ 1000 mL,煮成菜粥,适当调味。可作早晚餐服食。

【Composition】 50 g Fresh Machixian(Purslane), 50 g Jingmi(Non-glutinous rice). Put chopped purslane and washed non-glutinous rice into the earthrn pot, add 800 to 1000 mL water and boil the porridge, add proper amount of spice. Take it as breakfast or supper.

【功效】 清热解毒,利湿止泻。

【Efficacy】 Clearing away the heat-evil and expelling superficial evils, to reduce dampness through diuresis, eliminating dampness to check diarrhea.

【适应证】 腹泻腹痛,泻下急迫,或泻而不爽,粪色黄褐,气味臭秽,肛门灼热者。

【Indication】 Diarrhea with abdominal pain, urgent purgation; or non-smooth diarrhea with yellowish brown stool, odor smell and burning pain in anus.

党参酒方
Dangshen Jiu Fang
Tangshen Wine

【药物组成】 党参 1 条,白酒 500 毫升。

【Composition】 One Dangshen(Tangshen), 500 ml white wine.

【功效】 补中益气,健脾止泻。

【Efficacy】 Strengthening the middle energizer and benefiting qi, strengthening spleen to check diarrhea.

【适应证】 脾虚泄泻,四肢无力,食欲不佳者。

【Indication】 Diarrhea due to spleen deficiency, weakness in limbs and poor appetite.

荔核大米粥
Lihe Dami Zhou
Litchi Seed and Rice Porridge

【药物组成】 干荔核 15 枚,山药 15 g,莲子肉 15 g,粳米 50 g。先煎前三味,去渣取汁,后下米煮成粥。可作早晚餐服食。

【Composition】 15 dried litchi seeds, 15 g Shanyao(Common yam rhizome), 15 g lotus meat, 50 g Jingmi(Non-glutinous rice). Fry the first 3 drugs, remove the dregs and take the juice, cook porridge with non-glutinous rice. Take with breakfast or supper.

【功效】 补肾健脾,温阳散寒。

【Efficacy】 Tonifying kidney and strengthening spleen, warming yang and dispelling coldness.

【适应证】 黎明之前脐腹作痛,肠鸣即泻者。

【Indication】 Abdominal pain before dawn, diarrhea with rugitus.

姜橘椒鱼羹
Jiangju Jiaoyu Geng
GingerOrange Pepper Fish Soup

【药物组成】 鲫鱼 250 g,生姜 30 g,橘皮 10 g,胡椒 3 g。生姜片、橘皮、胡椒用纱布包扎后填入鲫鱼肚内,加水适量,小火煨熟,加食盐少许调味。空腹喝汤吃鱼。

【Composition】 250 g Crucian, 30 g fresh ginger, 10 g orange peel and 3 g pepper. Wrap the fresh ginger, orange peel and pepper and put it in the crucian stomach, add proper amount of water and decoct with gentle fire, flavor it with a little salt. Eat the meat and drink soup with empty stomach.

【功效】 温中散寒,健脾利湿。

【Efficacy】 Warming the middle energizer to dispel coldness, strengthening spleen.

【适应证】 泄泻清稀,甚如水样,腹痛肠鸣者。

【Indication】 Clear diarrhea like water with abdominal pain and rugitus.

黄芪山药莲子粥
Huangqi Shanyao Lianzi Zhou
Milkvetch Root, Common Yam Rhizome and Lotus Pulp Porridge

【药物组成】 黄芪 100 g,山药 100 g,莲子肉(去心)100 g。将上三味洗净共煮粥。

可作早晚餐服食。

【Composition】 100 g Huangqi (milkvetch root) , 100 g Shanyao (Common yam rhizome) ,100 g lotus pulp(without germ). Wash these drugs and decoct for porridge. Take as breakfast or supper.

【功效】 健脾益胃止泻。

【Efficacy】 Strengthening spleen and benefiting stomach to check stomach.

【适应证】 脾虚腹泻者。

【Indication】 Diarrhea due to spleen deficiency.

荔核山药羹
Lihe ShanyaoGeng
Litchi Seed and Common Yam Rhizome Soup

【药物组成】 干荔核 15 个,山药 20 g,莲子肉 15 g,粳米 50 g。

【Composition】 15 dried litchi seeds,20 g Shanyao(Common yam rhizome) ,15 g lotus seed and 50 g Jingmi(Non-glutinous rice).

【功效】 补肾健脾,温阳散寒止痛。

【Efficacy】 Tonifying kidney and strengthening spleen, warming yin and dispelling coldness to stop pain.

【适应证】 脾肾阳虚引起的腹痛泄泻。

【Indication】 Diarrhea with abdominal pain due to yang deficiency of spleen and kidney.

莱菔鸡金粥
Laifu JijinZhou
Radish Seedand Chicken's Gizzard-Membrane Porridge

【药物组成】 莱菔子 9 g,鸡内金 6 g,怀山药粉 50 g。莱菔子与鸡内金先加水煎煮 20 min,去渣,再加入怀山药粉煮沸成粥,白糖调味即可。每日 1 剂,趁热服食。

【Composition】 9 g Laifuzi(Radish seed) ,6 g Jineijin(Chicken's gizzard-membrane) , 50 g Huai Shanyao(Common yam rhizome)powder. Decoct radish seed and chicken's gizzard-membrane with water for 20 minutes,remove the dregs and add common yam rhizome powder, boil it for porridge,and flavor it with some sugar. Take one dose a day and take warm.

【功效】 顺气消食,健脾止泻。

【Efficacy】 Guiding qi downward and promoting digestion,strengthening spleen to check diarrhea.

【适应证】 腹痛肠鸣,泻下粪便臭如败卵,泻后痛减,脘腹胀满,嗳腐酸臭者。

【Indication】 Abdominal pain with rugitus,odor of stools like rotten eggs,pain relieved after diarrhea,distention and fullness of abdomen and gastric cavity,fetid and sour eructation.

食管癌 Esophagus Cancer

阿胶炖肉
E'JiaoDun Rou
Donkey–Hide Glue Stew Pork

【药物组成】 阿胶 6 g,瘦猪肉 100 g。将猪肉洗净切块,加水适量,慢火炖至肉熟烂,加入阿胶烊化,低盐调味。食肉喝汤,1 日 1 剂,连服 10 剂。

【Composition】 6 g E'jiao(Donkey–hide glue),100 g lean pork. Wash and cut the pork into pieces,add proper amount of water and decoct until the meat is tender,add donkey–hide glue and melt it by heat,flavor it with a little salt. Take the meat and soup one dose a day. Take 10 doses repeatedly.

【功效】 补血活血、滋阴润肺。

【Efficacy】 Nourishing blood to activate blood circulation,nourishing yin and moisturizing lung.

【适应证】 主治食道癌咳血日久,贫血以及全身虚弱等症的食管癌病人。

【Indication】 Esophageal cancer with excessive expectoration of blood,anemia and weakness.

清煮鱼翅
Qingzhu Yuchi
PlainBoiled Fin

【药物组成】 鱼翅 50 g,鸡汤 500 g,用清水将鱼翅洗净,放入鸡汤内煮熟,低盐调味,忌加酱油。喝汤吃鱼翅,日服 1 剂,连服 3~5 剂。

【Composition】 50 g Shark fin,500 g chicken soup,wash the shark fin and decoct it in chicken soup,add a little salt and no soy sauce. Take the soup and fin,one dose a day. Take for 3~5 doses repeatedly.

【功效】 益气补虚,开膈托毒。

【Efficacy】 Benefiting qi and improving asthenia,strengthening diaphragm to expel internal toxin

【适应证】 此方除治疗食道癌外,还可用于胃贲门癌者。

【Indication】 Esophageal cancer and gastric cardia cancer.

白萝卜蜂蜜饮
Bai Luobo Fengmi Yin
WhiteRadish Honey Decoction

【药物组成】 白萝卜 500 g,蜂蜜 30 g。将白萝卜放入清水中,刷洗干净,用温开水冲洗 3 次,切碎,压榨后用洁净纱布过滤,取其滤汁与蜂蜜拌和均匀,即成。早晚 2 次分服,空腹食尤佳。

【Composition】 500 g white radish, 30 g honey. Wash and scrub the white radish and rinse it 3 times with warm water, cut it up, squeeze it and filtered with clean gauze. Take its juice and mix with honey. Take twice daily in the morning and at night; better to take with empty stomach.

【功效】 抗癌利湿,化痰顺气。

【Efficacy】 Reducing dampness through diuresis for anti-cancer, dissipating phlegm and guiding qi downward.

【适应证】 通治各型食道癌以及消化道肿瘤等。

【Indication】 Treating various esophageal cancers and digestive tract cancers.

冬凌草蜂蜜饮
DonglingCao Fengmi Yin
RabdosiaRubescens Honey Decoction

【药物组成】 冬凌草 50 g,蜂蜜 30 g。将冬凌草洗净,晾干后切成小段,放入砂锅,加水适量,煎煮 2 次,每次 15 min,合并 2 次滤汁,放入容器,趁温热时兑入蜂蜜,调拌均匀即成。早晚 2 次分服。

【Composition】 50 g Donglingcao (Rabdosia rubescens), 30 g honey. Wash rabdosia rubescens and dry it in sunlight, cut into small pieces and put into earthen pot, add proper amount of water. Decoct it for 15 minutes twice and mix the juice together, put into a vessel and mix some honey in the warm juice and stir it. Take twice a day in the morning and at night.

【功效】 抗癌清热解毒。

【Efficacy】 Clearing away the heat-evil and expelling superficial evils for anti-cancer.

【适应证】 通治各型食管癌、胃癌等多种癌症。

【Indication】 Treating various esophageal cancers and stomach cancers.

枸杞乌骨鸡
Gouqi Wugu Ji
ChineseWolfberry and Black-Bone Chicken

【药物组成】 枸杞 30 g,乌骨鸡 100 g,调料适量。将枸杞乌骨鸡加调料后煮烂,然后打成匀浆或加适量淀粉或米汤,成薄糊状,煮沸即成,每日多次服用。

【Composition】 30 g Gouqi(Chinese wolfberry), 100 g black-bone chicken and proper amount of spice. Decoct fructus Lycii, black-bone chicken with spice until the meat is tender, then stir it into starch or add proper amount of starch or rice soup, make it into thin paste and get boiled. Take several times a day.

【功效】 补虚强身,滋阴退热

【Efficacy】 Improving asthenia for fitness, nourishing yin to relieve fever.

【适应证】 适用于食管癌体质虚弱者。

【Indication】 Esophageal cancer with weak body.

蒜鲫鱼
Suan Jiyu
Garlic Crucian

【药物组成】 活鲫鱼1条(约300 g),大蒜适量。鱼去肠杂留鳞,大蒜切成细块,填入鱼腹,纸包泥封,晒干。炭火烧干,研成细末即成。每日3克,每次3克,用米汤送服。

【Composition】 One live crucian(about 300 g), proper amount of garlic. Remove the internal organs and keep the scales of the fish, cut garlic into small pieces and put them in the fish stomach, wrap it with paper and sealed with mud, dried in sunlight. Bake it dry with charcoal and grind it into fine powder. Take 3 times daily, 3 g once; take with rice soup.

【功效】 解毒、消肿、补虚。

【Efficacy】 Detoxication, subsiding swelling and improving asthenia.

【适应证】 适宜于食道癌初期。

【Indication】 Early esophageal cancer.

紫苏醋散
ZisuCu San
Purple Perilla Vinegar Powder

【药物组成】 紫苏30 g,醋适量。将紫苏研成细末加水1500 mL,水煮过滤取汁。加等量醋后再煮干。每日3次,每次1.5 g。

【Composition】 30 g Zisu(Purple perilla) and proper amount of vinegar. Grind purple perilla into fine powder and decoct with water 1500 mL, filter and take the juice. Add the same amount of vinegar in it and boil again. Take 3 times a day, 1.5 g once.

【功效】 利咽、宽中。

【Efficacy】 Relieving sore-throat, and loosening the middle energizer.

【适应证】 适于食管癌吞咽困难者。

【Indication】 Esophageal cancer with difficult swallow.

鸡蛋菊花汤
Jidan Juhua Tang
Egg and Chrysanthemum Soup

【药物组成】 鸡蛋1个,菊花5 g,藕汁适量,陈醋少许。鸡蛋液与菊花、藕汁、陈醋调匀后,隔水蒸炖熟后即成,每日1次。

【Composition】 One egg, 5 g chrysanthemum, proper amount of lotus juice and a little mature vinegar. Mix egg with chrysanthemum, lotus juice and mature vinegar throughly, steam it with water seperately. Take once a day.

【功效】 止血活血,消肿止痛。

【Efficacy】 Stopping bleeding and activating blood circulation, subsiding swelling to relieve pain.

【适应证】 适用于食管癌咳嗽加重、呕吐明显者。

【Indication】 Esophageal cancer with serious cough and vomiting.

瓜蒌饼
Gualou Bing
Snakegourd Fruit Cake

【药物组成】 去籽枯蒌瓤 250 g,白糖 100 g,面粉 800 g。以小火煨熬蒌瓤,拌匀压成馅备用。面粉做成面团,包馅后制成面饼,烙熟或蒸熟食用,经常服食。

【Composition】 250 g Dried Gualou (snakegourd) pulp without seed, 100 g sugar, 800 g flour. Stew snakegourd pulp with gentle fire, stir and press it as stuffing. Make dough with flour, wrap the stuffing and make cakes, then bake or steam them. Take constantly.

【功效】 清热止咳。

【Efficacy】 Clearing the heat evil to stop cough.

【适应证】 适用于食管癌咳喘不止者。

【Indication】 Esophageal cancer with excessive cough.

循环系统疾病
Circulation System Disease

高血压 Hypertension

芹菜翠衣炒鳝片
Qincai Cuiyi Chao Shanpian
Celery Watermelon Peel Fry Eel

【药物组成】 黄鳝 120 g,西瓜翠衣 150 g,芹菜 150 g,姜、葱、蒜各少许。将黄鳝活剖,去内脏、脊骨及头,用少许盐腌去黏液,并放入开水中汆去血腥,切片;西瓜翠衣切条;芹菜去根叶,切段,均下热水中焯一下捞起备用。炒锅内加麻油,下姜、蒜茸及葱爆香,放入鳝片稍炒,再入西瓜翠衣、芹菜翻炒至熟,调味勾芡即可。

【Composition】 120 g Eel, 150 g watermelon peel, 150 g celery, a little ginger, green onion and garlic. Proccess live eel and take the internal organ, spine and the head off, preserve with some salt to remove the grume, get boiled in water to get rid of the bloody water and slice it. Cut watermelon peel into strips; take off the root and leaves of celery and cut it into pieces, boil them in the water. Add some sesame oil in the stir pot, fry ginger, garlic mince and green onion, then put in eel slices and fry it a while, add watermelon peel and celery and fry until all the ingredients are well-done. Spice and starch it.

【功效】 清热平肝,利尿降压。

【Efficacy】 Clearing away heat evil to pacify liver, diuresis and lowering blood pressure.

【适应证】 头晕胀痛,烦躁易怒,目眩耳鸣,面赤升火,口苦口干,夜眠不安者。

【Indication】 Dizziness with distention and pain in head, restlessness and being easy to anger, eye dizziness and tinnitus, reddish complexion due to upward fire, bitter and dry mouth, unpeaceful sleeping.

菊槐茶
Ju Huai Cha
Chryanthemum Flower and Sophora Flower Tea

【药物组成】 菊花、槐花、绿茶各 3 g。将上三味放入瓷杯中,以沸水冲泡,密盖浸泡 5 min 即可。每日 1 剂,不拘时频频饮服。

【Composition】 3 g Chryanthemum flower, 3 g sophora flower, 3 g green tea each. Put them in the porcelain cup and brew with boiling water, close the cover tightly for 5 minutes. Take one dose a day and take constantly at any time.

【功效】 平肝祛风,化痰降压。

【Efficacy】 Pacifying liver and dispelling wind evil, dissipating phlegm to lowering blood pressure.

【适应证】 痰浊内阻型高血压患者。

【Indication】 Phlegm-turbid high blood pressure.

首乌巴戟兔肉汤
Shouwu Baji Turou Tang
Fleece-Flower Root and Morinda Root Rabbit Meat

【药物组成】 兔肉500 g,制首乌30 g,巴戟天30 g,花生30 g,生姜4 片。兔肉洗净,切块,用开水汆去血水。把上物全部放入锅内,加清水适量,武火煮沸后,文火煮2~3 h,调味即可。随量饮汤食肉。

【Composition】 500 g Rabbit meat, 30 g prepared Shouwu (Fleece-flower root), 30 g Bajitian (Morinda root), 30 g peanut, 4 pieces of fresh ginger. Wash and cut the rabbit meat into pieces, get it boiled and remove the bloody water. Put all the ingredients in the pot, add proper amount of water and get boiled with high heat, then decoct with gentle fire for 2 ~ 3 hours, then spice it. Eat the meat and drink the soup as one wish.

【功效】 温补肝肾,养血益精。

【Efficacy】 Pacifying liver and dispelling wind evil, dissipating phlegm to lowering blood pressure.

【适应证】 阴阳两虚型高血压病。

【Indication】 Phlegm-turbid high blood pressure.

红萝卜海蜇粥
Hongluobo Haizhe Zhou
Carrot Jellyfish Porridge

【药物组成】 红萝卜120 g,海蜇皮60 g,粳米60 g。红萝卜削皮切片;海蜇皮漂净,切细条;粳米洗净。三物一起放入锅内,加清水适量,文火煮成粥,粥成后加调味品调味。作早晚餐或作点心食用。

【Composition】 120 g Take carrot, 60 g jellyfish and 60 g Jingmi (Non-glutinous rice). Peel and slice the carrot; rinse the jellyfish and slice it; wash non-glutinous rice. Put them in the pot and add proper amount of water, decoct porridge with gentle fire and spice it. Take as breakfast or supper, or take as dessert.

【功效】 化痰消滞,开胃健脾。

【Efficacy】 Dissipating phlegm and eliminating food stagnation, promoting appetite and strengthening spleen.

【适应证】 眩晕头痛,头目昏蒙,胸脘满闷,纳呆恶心,肢体困重,体倦嗜睡,口多痰涎者。

【Indication】 Dizziness and headache, head dizziness and blur eyesight, distention and fullness in breast and gastric cavity, anorexia and sickness, weakness in limbs and hypersomnia, excessive sputum in mouth.

丝瓜豆腐瘦肉粥
Sigua Doufu Shourou Zhou
Towel gourd Tofu Lean Pork Porridge

【药物组成】 猪瘦肉 60 g,丝瓜 250 g,嫩豆腐 2 块,葱花适量。将丝瓜去皮,切成厚片;豆腐切块;猪瘦肉切成薄片,加精盐、糖、芡粉拌匀。在锅内加清水适量,武火煮沸,先下豆腐煮沸后,再放入丝瓜、肉片,稍煮,至丝瓜、肉片刚熟,加葱花等调味即可。

【Composition】 60 g Lean port, 250 g towel gourd, 2 pieces of soft tofu and proper amount of green onion slices. Peel the towel gourd and cut it into thick slices; cut tofu into pieces and lean pork into thin slices; mix them with salt, sugar and starch. Add proper amount of water in the pot and get boiled with hiht heat, put tofu in it and get boiled, then add towel gourd, pork slices and boil until they are done, add some green onion slices to spice it.

【功效】 益气血,清虚热。

【Efficacy】 Benefiting qi and blood, clearing deficiency heat.

【适应证】 肝肾阴虚型高血压。

【Indication】 High blood pressure due to yin deficiency of liver and kidney.

泽泻粥
Zexie Zhou
Alismatis Porridge

【药物组成】 泽泻 10 g,南粳米 50 g,南粳米加水煮粥,待米花开后,调入泽泻粉,文火稍煮数沸。

【Composition】 10 g Zexie(Alismatis), 50 g Nan Jingmi(south non-glutinous rice). Decoct porridge with south non-glutinous rice and water, when the Jingmi is tender, add rhizome alismatis powder and boil for a while with slow fire.

【功效】 利水渗湿,消肿。

【Efficacy】 Removing dampness and promoting diuresis, subsiding swelling.

【适应证】 高血压。

【Indication】 High blood pressure.

橘皮饮
Jupi Yin
Orange Peel Drink

【药物组成】 橘皮、杏仁、老丝瓜各 10 g,白糖少许。将老丝瓜、橘皮洗净,杏仁去皮一同入锅,加水适量,置武火上烧沸,再用文火煮 20~30 min 去渣,用白糖调味。

【Composition】   10 g Orange peel, 10 g almond seed, 10 g old towel gourd, a little sugar. Wash the old towelgourd and orange peel, peel the almond seed and put these in the pot, add proper amount of water and get boiled with high heat. Then turn down the fire and cook for 20 ~ 30 minutes, remove the dregs.

【功效】   理气化痰,祛风通络。

【Efficacy】   Regulating qi to dissipating phlegm, dispelling wind evil to remove obstruction in the meridians.

【适应证】   高血压。

【Indication】   High blood pressure.

归芪蒸鸡饮
Guiqi Zheng Ji Yin
Chinese Angelica and Milkvetch Root Steam Chicken Decoction

【药物组成】   炙黄芪100 g,当归20 g,嫩母鸡1只。将黄芪、当归装入纱布袋,口扎紧。将鸡放入沸水锅内汆透、捞出,用凉水冲洗干净。将药袋装入鸡腹,鸡置于蒸盆内,加入葱、姜、盐、黄酒、陈皮、胡椒粉及适量清水,上笼隔水蒸约1 h,食时弃去药袋,调味即成。佐餐食用,分3次食完。

【Composition】   100 g honey-prepared Huangqi(Milkvetch root), 20 g Danggui(Chinese angelica), one young hen. Put milkvetch root and Chinese angelica in gauze bag and tie up the bag. Get the hen boiled in pot thoroughly and fish it out, washed with cold water. Put the drug bag in the stomach of the hen and steam it in the steamer, add green onion, ginger, salt, yellow wine, dried tangerine peel, pepper powder and proper amount of water, steam for an hour. Remove the drug bag and flavor it. Take with staple food and finish it in 3 times.

【功效】   温中补气,益血填精。

【Efficacy】   Warming the middle energizer to invigorating qi, benefiting blood and replenishing essence.

【适应证】   头昏眼花,面白少华,心悸气短,腰膝无力,夜尿频多,面部或下肢浮肿者。

【Indication】   Dizzy head and blur eyesight, dark facial complexion, palpitation and short breath, weakness in waist and knees, excessive night urination, edema in face or lower limbs.

菊花粥
Juhua Zhou
Chryanthemum Porridge

【药物组成】   菊花末15 g,粳米100 g。菊花去蒂,研成细末备用。粳米加水适量,用武火烧沸,改用文火慢熬,粥将成时调入菊花末,稍煮片刻即可。可作早晚餐食用。

【Composition】   15 g Chrysanthemum flower, 100 g Jingmi(Non-glutinous rice). Remove the stalks of chrysanthemum and grind it into fine powder. Add non-glutinous rice in proper amount of water and get boiled with high heat, then turn down the fire and decoct slowly, add chrysanthemum powder when the porridge is ready and boil for a short while. Take as breakfast or supper.

【功效】 清热疏风,清肝明目。

【Efficacy】 Clearing heat evil and expelling wind, clearing liver to brighten eyes.

【适应证】 ·肝阳上亢型高血压。

【Indication】 High blood pressure due to liver yang hyperactivity.

心悸 Palpitation

灵芝三七方
Lingzhi Sanqi Fang
Glossy Ganoderma and Sanchi Prescription

【药物组成】 灵芝 8 g,三七粉 3 g(水冲服)。

【Composition】 8 g Lingzhi(Glossy Ganoderma), 3 g Sanqi(Sanchi)powder(take with water).

【功效】 益气养心,活血通脉。

【Efficacy】 Benefiting qi and nourishing heart, activating and promoting blood circulation.

【适应证】 心气虚导致的心悸,形寒肢冷。

【Indication】 Palpitation due to deficiency of heart qi with coldness.

莲子百合猪心汤
Lianzi Baihe Zhuxin Zhou
Lotus Seed, Lily Bulb And Pig Heart Soup

【药物组成】 取莲子、百合各 30 g,与猪心切片 200 g 加水共煨汤,肉熟后调味即成。

【Composition】 30 g lotus seed, 30 g lily bulb, decoct with 200 g sliced pig heart and water. Spice it when the meat is tender.

【功效】 宁心安神。

【Efficacy】 Tranquilizing heart and calming nerves.

【适应证】 心悸、失眠、头昏等。

【Indication】 Palpitation, insomnia, dizziness.

莲心汤
Lianxin Tang
LotusPlumule Soup

【药物组成】 取莲子心 30 枚,酸枣 50 g,炙甘草 20 g,水煎。每晚睡前服,连服

10 天。

【Composition】　Take 30 pieces of lotus plumule,50 g wild jujube,20 g honey-prepared Gancao(liquorice root) and decoct with water. Take before sleep and take repeatedly for 10 days.

【功效】　宁心安神。

【Efficacy】　Tranquilizing heart and calming nerves.

【适应证】　肝火上延,心肾不交型患者。

【Indication】　Liver fire going upward,failure of the heart and kidney to integrate.

参芪丹参炖猪心
Shenqi Danshen Dun Zhuxin
Ginseng,Milkvetch Root and Red Sage Root Stew Pork Heart

【药物组成】　人参 10 g,黄芪 15 g,丹参 12 g,猪心 1 个,水适量,隔水炖 1 h,吃肉喝汤。

【Composition】　Take 10 g Renshen(Ginseng),15 g Huangqi(Milkvetch root),12 g Danshen(Red sage root),one pig heart and proper amount of water,stew them seperately with water. Eat the meat and drink the soup.

【功效】　补益气血、养心安神。

【Efficacy】　Tonifying and benefiting qi and blood,tranquilizing by nourishing the heart.

【适应证】　心血不足所致的心悸。

【Indication】　Palpation due to deficiency of heart blood.

菊花散
Juhua San
Chryanthemum flower powder

【药物组成】　菊花、石膏、川芎各 9 g,研磨为散,茶水调服。

【Composition】　9 g chryanthemum flower,9 g gypsum·and 9 g Chuanxiong(Sichuan lovage rhizome),grind them into powder and brew it with water.

【功效】　疏风清热。

【Efficacy】　Expelling wind evil to clearing heat.

【适应证】　风热感冒引起的头痛。

【Indication】　Headache due to wind-heat type common cold.

抗心梗合剂
Kang Xingeng Heji
Anti-myocardial Infarction Mixture

【药物组成】　黄芪、丹参各 30 g,党参、黄精、郁金、赤芍各 15 g。以上为 1 日量,水煎 2 次,去渣,浓缩为 100 mL,分 2 次服。

【Composition】 30 g Huangqi(Milkvetch root),30 g Danshen(red sage root)each,15 g Dangshen(Tangshen),15 g Huangjing(rhizome of king solomonseal),15 g Yujin(Turmeric root tuber),15 g Chishao(Red peony root)each. Take these as a daily amount. Decoct the drugs with water twice,remove the dregs and concentrate into 100 mL;take it twice.

【功效】 益气养阴,活血通络。

【Efficacy】 Supplementing qi and nourishing yin,promoting blood circulation to remove meridian obstruction.

【适应证】 急性心肌梗死。

【Indication】 Acute myocardial infarction.

阵发性心动过速方
Zhenfaxing Xindong Guosu Fang
Paroxysmal TachycardiaPrescription

【药物组成】 葛根 50 g,苦参、淫羊藿、麦冬各 30 g,生地黄、赤芍各 15 g,丹参 20 g。

【Composition】 Take 50 g Gegen(Kudzuvine root),30 g Kushen(Lavescent sophora root)(Kuh-seng),30 g Yin Yanghuo(Epimedium),30 g Maidong(Dwarf lilyturf tuber),20 g Sheng Dihuang(Dried rehamnnia root)and Chishao(Red peony root)15 g each,Danshen(red sage root).

【功效】 活血化瘀,补养气阴,调和阴阳。

【Efficacy】 Activating blood circulation to dissipate blood stasis,nourishing and replenishing qi yin,harmonizing yin and yang.

【适应证】 阵发性心动过速。

【Indication】 Paroxysmal tachycardia.

健身糖浆
Jianshen Tangjiang
Salubrity Sirop

【药物组成】 党参、赤芍各 30 g,黄精 24 g,红花、山楂 12 g,水煎服,或制成糖浆,以上为 1 日量。

【Composition】 30 g Dangshen(Tangshen)and 30 g Chishao(Red peony root),24 g Huangjing(Rhizome of king solomonseal),12 g Honghua(Safflower),12 g Shanzha(hawthorn fruit),decoct to take the juice or make it into sirop. Take it as a daily amont.

【功效】 益气活血,补虚止痛。

【Efficacy】 Benefiting qi and activating blood circulation,improving asthenia to stop pain.

【适应证】 冠心病心绞痛头晕、乏力者。

【Indication】 Coronary heart disease and angina pectoris with dizziness and powerless.

四味鹌鹑蛋羹
SiweiAnchundan Geng
Four Ingredients Quail Eggs Soup

【药物组成】　鹌鹑蛋10只,红参5 g,当归5 g,肉桂5 g,丹参5 g。将红参、当归、肉桂、丹参煎成药汁,取鹌鹑蛋打入瓷碗内,入药汁搅匀,加海米2~5 g,食盐、麻油少许,上蒸笼蒸熟。每日1次,7~10 d为1个疗程。

【Composition】　Take 10 quail eggs,5 g Hongshen(Red ginseng),5 g Danggui(Chinese angelica),5 g Rougui(Cassia bark) and 5 g Danshen(Red sage root). Decoct Red ginseng, Chinese angelica,Cassia bark,Red sage root and take the juice. Scatter quail eggs in a china bowl,add the drug juice and 2~5 g dried shrimps,a little salt and sesame and steam until it's done. Take once a day;take for 7~10 days for a period of treatment.

【功效】　温阳祛寒,化瘀止痛。

【Efficacy】　Warming the middle energizer to expelling coldness,dissolving stasis to stop pain.

【适应证】　心胸疼痛,受寒后加重,胸痛彻背,背痛彻心者。

【Indication】　Pain in chest and heart,especially after catching cold,pain in heart radiating to the back,or backache radiating to the heart.

灵芝三七山楂饮
Lingzhi Sanqi Shanzha Yin
Glossy Ganoderma,Sanchi and Hawthorn Fruit Decoction

【药物组成】　灵芝30 g,三七粉4 g,山楂汁200 mL。先将灵芝放入砂锅中,加适量清水,微火煎熬1 h,取汁,兑入三七粉和山楂汁即成。每日1剂,早晚各1次,服前摇匀。

【Composition】　30 g Lingzhi(Glossy ganoderma),4 g Sanqi(Sanchi) powder,200 mL Shanzha(Hawthorn fruit). Put glossy ganoderma in the earthen pot,add proper amount of water and dococt with gentle fire for an hour,take the juice and mix Sanchi powder and hawthorn fruit juice in it. Take one dose daily,in the morning and and at night,shake it befor taking.

【功效】　益气活血,通脉止痛。

【Efficacy】　Benefiting qi and activating blood circulation,promoting blood circulation to stop pain.

【适应证】　胸闷,心前区隐痛,心悸气短,体倦自汗,少气懒言,动则尤甚,面色少华,纳食不香者。

【Indication】　Dyspnea,pain in the precordial region,palpitation and short breath, tiredness and spontaneous perspiration,deficient breath and reluctant to speak,dark facial complexion,poor appetite.

人参富贵香酥雀
Renshen Fugui Xiangsu Que
Riches and Honour Ginseng Crispy Sparrow

【药物组成】 麻雀 10 只,红人参 5 g,制附片 5 g,肉桂 3 g,胡椒 1 g。上药捣成粗末,将药分装于洗净的麻雀腹内,装盘,加盐、葱、姜、蒜及五香粉适量,蒸 30 min 取出,弃药,入油锅内炸酥即成。每日 2～3 次,每次 1 只,可连服半个月。

【Composition】 Take 10 sparrows, 5 g Hong Renshen (Red ginseng), 5 g Zhi Fupian (Prepared monkshood), 3 g Rougui (Cassia bark), 1 g pepper, grind these drugs into coarse powder, divide into 10 parts and put into clean sparrow stomaches. Dish up and add proper amount of salt, green onion, ginger, garlic and five spice powder, steam for 30 minutes and remove the drugs, fry the sparrows in hot oil. Take 2～3 time a day, one sparrow once; take repeatedly for half a month.

【功效】 益气温阳,活血通络。

【Efficacy】 Benefiting qi and warming yang, promoting blood circulation to remove meridian obstruction.

【适应证】 心胸疼痛受寒后诱发,气短,胸闷,畏寒面青,手足不温者。

【Indication】 Pain in chest and heart induced after catching cold, short breath, dyspnea, chills and bluish complexion, coldness in hands and feet.

黄精玉竹牛肉汤
Huangjing Yuzhu Niurou Tang
Soupof King Solomonseal Rhizome, Fragrant Solomonseal Rhizome and Beef

【药物组成】 牛腿精肉 500 g,黄精 30 g,玉竹 15 g,龙眼肉 15 g,生姜 4 片。将黄精、玉竹、龙眼肉洗净;牛腿精肉洗净,切块,并用开水汆去膻味。把全部用料一齐放入锅内,加清水适量,武火煮沸后,文火煮 2～3 h,调味即可。饮汤食肉。

【Composition】 Take 500 g lean meat of cow legs, 30 g Huangjing (King solomonseal rhizome), 15 g Yuzhu (Fragrant solomonseal rhizome), 15 g Longyan Rou (Longan Aril), 4 pieces of fresh ginger. Wash king solomonseal rhizome, fragrant solomonseal rhizome and longan pulp, wash and cut up the lean meat of cow legs and get boiled to remove the smell. Put all the ingredients in the pot and add proper amount of water, boiled with high heat and decoct for 2～3 hours with gentle fire and flavor it. Eat the meat and drink the soup.

【功效】 益气养阴,养心安神。

【Efficacy】 Benefiting qi and nourishing yin, nourishing heart and calming nerves.

【适应证】 心悸心痛,气短自汗,头晕头痛,心烦不寐,口干少津者。

【Indication】 Palpitation and pain in heart, short breath and spontaneous perspiration, restlessness and insomnia, dry mouth with less saliva.

薤白粥
Xiebai Zhou
Longstamen Onion Bulb Soup

【药物组成】 薤白10 g,葱白2根,香菜适量,粳米100 g。将薤白、葱白切成3~4厘米的小段,与粳米同放锅内,加清水适量,文火煮粥,粥成后加入切碎的香菜稍煮即成。趁热服用。可作早晚餐服食。

【Composition】 Take 10 g Jiubai(Bulb of longstamen onion),2 green onion sticks, proper amount of caraway and 100 g Jingmi(Non-glutinous rice). Cut bulb of longstamen onion and onion sticks into pieces of 3 ~ 4 cm, put into the pot with non-glutinous rice and add proper amount of water, decoct these with slow fire. Add some sliced caraway when the porridge is well-done. Take warm and take as breakfast or supper.

【功效】 通阳散寒,行气导滞。

【Efficacy】 Activating yang and expelling coldness, promoting qi and guiding stagnation.

【适应证】 寒凝气滞型冠心病者。

【Indication】 Coronary heart disease due to cold obstruction causing qi stagnation.

瓜葛红花酒
Guage Honghua Jiu
Snakegourd Fruit and Safflower Wine

【药物组成】 瓜蒌皮25 g,葛根25 g,红花15 g,玄胡20 g,桃仁20 g,丹参30 g,檀香15 g。将上药拣净装一大瓶内,加入高粱酒800~1000 mL,泡1个月后取酒内服。每日晚服用,每次10 mL,同时用此酒擦膻中穴1次,连用7~10 d。

【Composition】 Take 25 g Gualou(Snakegourd Fruit) peel, 25 g Gegen(Kudzuvine root),15 g Honghua(Safflower),20 g Xuanhu(Corydalis tuber),20 g Taoren(peach kernel), 30 g Danshen(Red sage root),15 g Tanxiang(Sandalwood). Pick the clean drugs and put them in a big bottle, add 800 ~ 1000 mL sorghum wine in it and soak for a month. Take in the morning and at night,10 mL once, rub Tanzhong point with the wine once a day as well. Take 7 ~ 10 days repeatedly.

【功效】 化痰驱瘀,通络定痛。

【Efficacy】 Dissipating phlegm and expelling stasis, dredging collaterals and relieving pain.

【适应证】 胸闷窒痛,或轻或重,如刺如绞,痛有定处者。

【Indication】 Dyspnea with suffocated pain in certain place, mild or severe.

丹参茶
Danshen Cha
Red Sage Root Tea

【药物组成】 丹参9 g,绿茶3 g。将丹参制成粗末,与茶叶以沸水冲泡10 min,即可饮用。每日1剂,代茶饮。

【Composition】 Take 9 g Danshen(Red sage root)and 3 g green tea,grind red sage root into coarse powder and soak in boiling water with tea for 10 minutes. Take one dose a day as tea.

【功效】 活血祛瘀,止痛除烦。

【Efficacy】 Activating blood removing stasis,relieving pain and expelling annoyance.

【适应证】 气滞血瘀型冠心病患者。

【Indication】 Coronary heart disease due to qi-stagnancy and blood stasis.

人参银耳汤
Renshen Yin'er Tang
Ginseng andWhite Fungus Soup

【药物组成】 人参5 g,银耳10～15 g。银耳用温水浸泡12 h,洗净。人参去头,切成薄片,入砂锅中,用文火煮熬2 h,再加入银耳熬1 h即可。每日1剂,饮汤食银耳,分2次食完,连用10～15 d。

【Composition】 Take 5 g Renshen(Ginseng),10～15 g White fungus. Soak the white fungus in warm water for 12 hours and wash it,cut off the head of ginseng and slice it,put it in earthen pot and decoct with gentle fire for 2 hours,then add white fungus and decoct for an hour. Take one dose,twice a day;take the soup and white fungus. Take 10～15 days repeatedly.

【功效】 益气补血,生津宁神。

【Efficacy】 Benefiting qi and replenishing blood,generating bold fluid and calming nerves.

【适应证】 气血不足证型冠心病。

【Indication】 Coronary heart disease due to insufficiency of qi and blood.

神经系统疾病
NerveSystem Disease

头痛 Headache

桑菊薄竹饮
Sangju Bozhu Yin
Decoctionof Mulberry Leaf, Chryanthemum Flower, Mint and Bamboo Leaf

【药物组成】　桑叶 10 g,竹叶 15～30 g,菊花 10 g,白茅根 10 g,薄荷 6 g。将以上 5 味洗净,放入茶壶内,用沸水浸泡 10 min,即可。每日 1 剂,代茶饮连服 3～5 d。

【Composition】　Take 10 g Sangye (Mulberry leaf), 15～30 g bamboo leaf, 10 g chryanthemum flower, 10 g Baimao Gen (Cogongrass rhizome) and 6 g mint. Wash these drugs and put them in teapot, soak for 10 minutes. Take one dose a day as tea and take for 3～5 days repeatedly.

【功效】　疏风散热。

【Efficacy】　Expelling wind to dissipate heat.

【适应证】　头痛而胀,甚则痛如裂,发热,恶风,面红目赤,口渴喜饮,大便不畅或便秘者。

【Indication】　Headache with distention even worse like to be broken, having fever, and aversing to wind, reddish facial complexion and red eyes, thirst with excessive drinking, difficulty in stools or constipation.

川芎白芷炖鱼头
Chuanxiong Baizhi Dun Yutou
Sichuan Lovage Rhizome and Angelica Root Stew Carp Head

【药物组成】　鳙鱼(花鲢鱼)头 1 个,川芎 3～9 g,白芷 6～9 g。将川芎、白芷用纱布包,与鱼头共煮汤,文火炖至鱼头熟透,调味即可。饮汤食鱼头。

【Composition】　Take the head of a bighead carp (Silver carp), Chuanxiong (Sichuan lovage rhizome) 3～9 g, Baizhi (Angelica root) 6～9 g. Wrap Sichuan lovage rhizome and angelica root with gauze and decoct with the fish. Dencoct with gentle fire until the fish head is well-done and slice it. Eat the meat and drink the soup.

【功效】　疏风散寒。

【Efficacy】　Expelling wind to dissipate coldness.

【适应证】　头痛连及项背,恶风畏寒,遇风痛增,常喜裹头者。

【Indication】 Headache radiating to the neck and back, aversing to wind and coldness, being worse when meeting wind.

天麻鲤鱼头
Tianma Liyu Tou
Gastrodia Tuber and Carp Head

【药物组成】 天麻 25 g,川芎 10 g,茯苓 10 g,鲜鲤鱼 1 尾(约 1000 g)。将川芎、茯苓切片,与天麻一同放入二次米泔水中,浸泡 4~6 h,捞出天麻,置米饭上蒸透,切片,再将天麻片与川芎、茯苓一起放入洗净的鱼腹中,置盆内,加姜、葱蒸 30 min,按常规制作调味羹汤,浇于鱼上即成。佐餐食用。

【Composition】 Take 25 g Tianma(Gastrodia tuber), 10 g Chuanxiong(Sichuan lovage rhizome), 10 g Fuling(Tuckahoe) and a fresh carp(about 1000 g). Cut Sichuan lovage rhizome and Tuckahoe into pieces, soak in rice-washed-twice water with Gastrodia tuber for 4 ~ 6 hours, fish out Gastrodia tuber and steam it with rice and slice it. Then put gastrodia tuber slices with Sichuan lovage rhizome and tuckahoe into fish stomach, installed in a basin, add some ginger and green onion, steam for 30 minutes. Cook spice soup and pour it on the fish. Take with rice or bread.

【功效】 平肝宁神,活血止痛。

【Efficacy】 Soothing liver and tranquilizing nerves, promoting blood circulation to arrest pain.

【适应证】 头痛而眩,时作抽掣,两侧为重;常偏于一侧,心烦易怒,失眠或梦多不宁者。

【Indication】 Headache and dizziness, being worse on both sides; being often partial to one side, restlessness and being easy to anger, insomnia or unpeaceful sleeping with many dreams.

神经衰弱 Neurasthenia

清肝宁心汤
Qinggan Ningxin Tang
Clearing Liver and Tranquilizing Heart Soup

【药物组成】 钩藤 15 g,丹参 30 g,合欢皮 12 g,生珍珠母 20 g,夏枯草、酸枣仁各 15 g,炙甘草 3 g。水煎服,每日 1 剂,日 2 次。

【Composition】 Take 15 g Gouteng(Gambir Plant), 30 g Danshen(Red sage root), 12 g Hehuan Pi(silktree albizia bark), 20 g fresh Zhenzhumu(Mother-of-pearl) 15 g Xiakucao (Self heal), 15 g wild jujube seed, 3 g honey-prepared Gancao(Liquorice root). Decoct them with water; take one dose twice a day.

【功效】 清肝解郁,养心安神。

【Efficacy】 Clearing liver and relieving qi depression, tranquilizing by nourishing the heart.

【适应证】 肝郁气滞,热扰心神患者。

【Indication】 Stagnation of qi due to depression of the liver, tranquilizing by nourishing the heart.

百麦安神饮
BaimaiAnshen Yin
LilyBulb and Huai Wheat Mind Easing Decoction

【药物组成】 百合、淮小麦各 30 g,莲肉、夜交藤各 15 g,大枣 10 g,甘草 6 g。水煎服,每日 1 剂,日 2 次。

【Composition】 30 g lily bulb, 30 g Huai wheat, 15 g lotus seed 15 g Yejiaoteng(Tuber fleeceflower stem), 10 g Jujube, 6 g Gancao(Liquorice root). Decoct them and take one dose twice a day.

【功效】 益气养阴,清热安神。

【Efficacy】 Supplementing qi and nourishing yin, clearing heat and tranquilizing nerves.

【适应证】 气阴两虚,虚热内扰,心神失养的患者。

【Indication】 Qi-yin deficiency, disturbance of deficiency-heat inside the body, lack of nourishing of heart and spirit.

远志莲粉粥
Yuanzhi Lianfen Zhou
Milkwort Root and Lotus Seed Powder Porridge

【药物组成】 远志 30 g,莲子 15 g,粳米 50 g。将远志浸泡去心皮,与莲子研为细粉。粳米加适量水煮至粥将成时,放入远志和莲子粉,稍煮片刻即成。可作点心或随意食之。

【Composition】 30 g Yuanzhi(Milkwort root), 15 g lotus seed and 50 g Jingmi(Non-glutinous rice). Soak and remove the peel and core of Yuanzhi, grind into fine powder with lotus seed. Boil Jingmi(Non-glutinous rice) with water, add milkwort root and lotus seed powder when the porridge is done and boil a short while. Take as dessert or as one wishes.

【功效】 补中益心。

【Efficacy】 Strengthening the middle energizer and benefiting heart.

【适应证】 心脾亏虚型神经衰弱患者。

【Indication】 Neurastheria due to the deficiency of heart and spleen.

佛香梨

Foxiang Li

Fingered Citron and Nutgrass Galingale Rhizome Pear

【药物组成】 佛手 5 g,制香附 5 g,梨 2 个。将佛手、香附研末备用;梨去皮,切开剜空,各放入一半药末,合住放碗内,上锅蒸 10 min,即可食用。可作点心食用。

【Composition】 5 g Foshou(Fingered citron),5 g honey-prepared Xiangfu(Nutgrass falingale rhizome)and 2 pears. Grind fingered citron and nutgrass falingale rhizome into powder,peel core the pears,put the drugs in the pears seperately and cover the core,put them in the bowl and steam for 10 minutes. Take as dessert.

【功效】 疏肝和胃。

【Efficacy】 Soothing liver and regulating stomach.

【适应证】 肝气郁结型神经衰弱患者。

【Indication】 Neurastheria due to depression of liver-qi,stagnation of liver-qi.

怀山百合炖白鳝汤

Huaishan Baihe Dun Baishan Tang

Common Yam Rhizome and Lily Bulb Stew Eel Soup

【药物组成】 白鳝 1~2 条(约 250 g),怀山药、百合各 30 g。先将白鳝去内脏洗净,与怀山药、百合一起放瓦盅内,加清水适量,隔水炖熟,调味即可。佐餐食用。

【Composition】 1~2 eels(about 250 g),30 g Huai Shanyao(Common yam rhizome)and lily bulb each. Wash and remove the internal organs of eel,put in to the tile pot with common yam rhizome and lily bulb,add proper amount of water and stew seperately with water and spice it. Take with rice or bread.

【功效】 补虚健脾,养心安神。

【Efficacy】 Improving asthenia and strengthening spleen,tranquilizing by nourishing the heart.

【适应证】 精神疲劳,神经过敏,失眠,焦虑和忧郁伴有口淡无味,食欲不振,胁痛腹胀,恶心嗳气者。

【Indication】 Mental fatigue, being excessively sensitive, insomnia, anxiety and depression companied with tasteless of mouth and poor appetite,pain in flank and distention in abdomen,sickness and belching.

泌尿系统疾病
Urinary System Disease

前列腺炎及增生 Prostatitis and Prostatic Hyperplasia

黄芪甘草汤
Huangqi Gancao Tang
MilkvetchRoot and Liquorice Root Soup

【药物组成】 黄芪 120 g,甘草 30 g。

【Composition】 120 g Huangqi(Milkvetch root),30 g Gancao(Liquorice root).

【功效】 益气养阳,固本补元。

【Efficacy】 Benefiting qi and improving yang, strengthening the body essential and improving primordial qi.

【适应证】 老年人排尿时茎痛如刀割者,不论年深月久。

【Indication】 Acute pain in penis during urination.

田螺通淋汤
Tianluo Tonglin Tang
Fresh WatersnailStrangurtia Treating Soup

【药物组成】 田螺 250 g,鲜益母草 125 g,车前子 125 g。将田螺去尾尖洗净,车前子布包,加水适量,共煮汤。代茶饮用。

【Composition】 250 g fresh watersnail, 125 g fresh Yimucao (Motherwort), 125 g Cheqian Zi(Asiatic plantain seed). Wash the watersnail and take off its nail and tip, wrap Asiatic plantain seed with cloth, add proper amount of water and decoct them together. Drink it as tea.

【功效】 清热利湿,化瘀通淋。

【Efficacy】 Clearing away heat evil to reduce dampness through diuresis, dissolving stasis and dredging stranguria.

【适应证】 前列腺增生以尿少黄赤,点滴不畅,或闭塞不通,少腹胀满,烦躁不安,大便溏而不爽为主者。

【Indication】 Prostatic hyperplasia with less yellowish–red dripping urine; or urinary canal being blocked, distention and fullness in abdomen, restlessness, un–smooth loose stool.

苁蓉羊肉粥
Congrong Yangrou Zhou
Cistancheand Mutton Porridge

【药物组成】 肉苁蓉 10 g,精羊肉 60 g,粳米 60 g,葱白 2 根,生姜 3 片。分别把羊肉、肉苁蓉洗净,切细。先煎肉苁蓉取汁,去渣,再用肉苁蓉汁与羊肉、粳米一同煎煮,粥成时调味即可。空腹服食。

【Composition】 10 g Roucongrong(Cistanche),60 g lean mutton,60 g Jingmi(Non-glutinous rice),2 green onion sticks,3 pieces of fresh ginger. Wash and slice mutton and cistanche seperately. Decoct cistanche,remove the dregs and take the juice,then boil the juice with mutton and non-glutinous rice,flavor it when the soup is well-done. Take with empty stomach.

【功效】 温补肾阳。

【Efficacy】 Warming and reinforcing kidney yang.

【适应证】 前列腺增生以小便排出无力,淋沥不畅,面色无华,神疲倦怠,手足不温,腰膝冷痛为主者。

【Indication】 Prostatic hyperplasia with powerless and dripping urination, dark complexion,insipidity and fatigue, coldness in hands and feet, and cold pain in waist and knees.

丝瓜牡蛎汤
Sigua Muli Tang
Towel gourd Oyster Meat Soup

【药物组成】 丝瓜 450 g,牡蛎肉 150 g,味精、五香粉、湿淀粉、植物油、料酒、清汤、葱花、姜末、香油、食盐各适量。炒锅上火,油烧到六成热,下牡蛎片煸炒,烹入料酒,清汤,中火煮开,下丝瓜片、葱花、姜末,煮沸,加食盐、味精、五香粉,用湿淀粉勾芡,淋上香油,拌匀即可。

【Composition】 450 g towel gourd,150 g oyster meat, proper amount of monosodium glutamate,five spice powder, wet starch, vegetable oil, cooking wine, light soup, green onion slices,ginger mince,sesame oil and salt. Heat the pot until the oil is warm;put oyster slice in and fry it, add cooking wine, light soup and boil with moderate heat, then put towel gourd slices,green onion slices,giner mince and get boiled, add salt,monosodium glutamate and spice powder,starch it with wet starch. Then sprinkle some sesame oil and mix all the ingredients thoroughly.

【功效】 清热解毒,凉血和血,止渴降糖。

【Efficacy】 Clearing away the heat-evil and expelling superficial evils,cooling blood and stopping blood,quenching thirst and lowering blood sugar.

【适应证】 可作为前列腺炎患者食疗之用。

【Indication】 Dietary therapy for prostatitis.

癃闭茶
Longbi Cha
Retentionof Urine Tea

【药物组成】 肉桂 40 g,穿山甲 60 g,蜂蜜适量。将肉桂和穿山甲分别研成细粉和匀,用蜂蜜水冲。每次 3~5 g,1 日 2 次,代茶饮。

【Composition】 40 g Rougui(Cassia bark),60 g pangolin and proper amount of honey. Grind cassia bark and pangolin into fine powder seperately and mix them,brew it with honey water. Take 3~5 g once,twice a day. Take as tea.

【功效】 行瘀散结,通利水道。

【Efficacy】 Removing blood stasis,facilitating urination.

【适应证】 前列腺增生以小便努挣方出,或点滴全无,小腹刺痛,可有血尿或血精为主。

【Indication】 Prostatic hyperplasia with little urination,prickle in lower abdomen,and blood urine or hemospermia.

冬瓜薏米汤
Donggua Yimi Tang
Chinese waxgourd andCoix Seed Soup

【药物组成】 冬瓜 350 g,薏米 50 g,白糖适量。将冬瓜切成块,与薏米煎汤,用糖调味。以汤代茶饮。

【Composition】 350 g Chinese waxgourd,50 g Yimi(Coix seed)and proper amount of sugar. Cut waxgourd into pieces and decoct soup with coix seed,flaver it with sugar. Take the soup as tea.

【功效】 清热利湿。

【Efficacy】 Clearing away the heat evil to reduce dampness through diuresis.

【适应证】 膀胱湿热型前列腺增生。

【Indication】 Prostatic hyperplasia with damp heat of bladder.

薏米药粥
Yimi Yaozhou
Coix Seed Medicated Porridge

【药物组成】 党参 10 g,薏米 120 g,黄芪 120 g,生姜 12 g,大枣 10 g。将党参、黄芪用布包,大枣以冷水泡透,与薏米一起,置锅内,加水适量,用武火煎沸,下拍破的生姜,改用文火煨熬,至薏米熟烂即成。去药包。趁热空腹食粥。

【Composition】 10 g Dangshen(Tangshen),120 g Yimi(Coix seed),120 g Huangqi (Milkvetch root),12 g fresh ginger,10 g jujube. Wrap tangshen and milkvetch root with cloth, soak the jujube with cold water and put them in the pot with coix seed. Add proper amount of water and get boiled with high heat, then put in the broken fresh finger, boil with gentle fire until the coix seed is tender enough. Remove the drug wrap, take warm with empty stomach.

【功效】 健脾益气升阳。

【Efficacy】 Strengthening spleen, benefiting qi and invigorating yang.

【适应证】 前列腺增生以小便欲解不爽，或气坠脱肛，精神不振，少气懒言为主者。

【Indication】 Prostatic hyperplasia with difficult urination or proctoptosis due to qi downward, spiritlessness and being reluctant to speak.

知地麻鸭
Zhidima Ya
Anemarrhena Rhizome and Dried/Fresh Rehmannia Root Sheldrake

【药物组成】 生地 30 g, 知母 20 g, 牛膝 20 g, 麻鸭 1 只 (约 1000 g)。鸭子去毛、内脏、头、足，药物用纱布包好放入鸭腹内，置砂锅内，加水适量，用文火炖熟，调味。吃鸭肉饮汤。

【Composition】 30 g Shengdi (Dried/fresh rehmannia root), 20 g Zhimu (Anemarrhena rhizome), 20 g Niuxi (Achyranthes root), one sheldrake (about 1000 g). Take off the feather, internal organ, head and foot of the sheldrake, drugs wraped with gauze and put in the stomach of the sheldrake. Put the sheldrake in the earthen, add proper amount of water and boil with gentle fire, flaver it. Take the meat and soup.

【功效】 滋阴清热。

【Efficacy】 Nourishing yin and clearing heat.

【适应证】 前列腺增生以尿少黄赤，赤涩疼痛，或闭塞不通，手足心热，大便干结为主者。

【Indication】 Prostatic hyperplasia with less yellowish-red urine, unsmooth and painful; or urinary canal being blocked, feverish sensation over the palm and sole, dry stools.

尿道炎 Urethritis

黄芪茅根饮
Huangqi Maogen Yin
MilkvetchRoot and Cogongras Rhizome Decoction

【药物组成】 生黄芪 30 g, 白茅根 30 g, 肉苁蓉 20 g, 西瓜皮 60 g。上四味洗净放在砂锅中，加水适量煎煮成浓汁，加适量白糖调味。每日 1 剂，分 2 次服用。

【Composition】 30 g fresh Huangqi (Milkvetch root), 30 g Baimaogen (Cogongras rhizome) root, 20 g Roucongrong (Cistanche), 60 g watermelon peel. Wash these drugs and put them in the earthen pot, add proper amount of water and decoct it into thick juice. Take one dose twice a day.

【功效】 益脾温肾,利尿通淋。

【Efficacy】 Benefiting spleen and warming kidney, inducing diuresis for treating strangurtia.

【适应证】 小便赤涩不甚,淋漓不已,劳累即作者。

【Indication】 Hot and dripping urination, especially after work.

益肾粥
Yishen Zhou
Kidney Tonifying Porridge

【药物组成】 猪肾1个,冬葵叶100 g,粳米50 g。将猪肾洗净细切,先煎冬葵叶取汁,后入猪肾及粳米,煮作粥。每日1剂,分2次温热服食。

【Composition】 100 g one pig kidney, Dongkuiye(Mallow leaf), 50 g Jingmi(non-glutinous rice). Wash and slice the pig kidney, decoct mallow leaf and take the juice, put the pig kidney and non-glutinous rice in the juice and cook porridge. Take one dose twice a day after it's warmed.

【功效】 补益脾肾,利尿通淋。

【Efficacy】 Tonifying spleen and kidney, inducing diuresis for treating strangurtia.

【适应证】 淋漓涩痛,脾肾两虚者。

【Indication】 Unsmooth urination with pain and asthenia of both the spleen and kidney.

茅根赤豆粥
Maogen Chidou Zhou
Couchgrass Rootand Red Bean Porridge

【药物组成】 鲜茅根200 g,赤豆200 g,粳米200 g。鲜茅根加水煎,去渣取汁,入赤豆、粳米一同煮粥食用。每日1剂,分3~4次服用。

【Composition】 200 g fresh Maogen(Couchgrass root), 200 g red bean, 200 g Jingmi(Non-glutinous rice). Decoct fresh couchgrass root with water, remove the dregs and take the juice. Boil the juice with red bean and non-glutinous rice for porridge. Take one dose 3~4 times a day.

【功效】 清热凉血,利尿通淋。

【Efficacy】 Removing heat to cool blood, inducing diuresis for treating strangurtia.

【适应证】 小便频急,热涩刺痛,尿色红赤混浊者。

【Indication】 Frequent and urgent urination with hot pain and reddish, turbid urine.

利尿黄瓜汤
Liniao Huanggua Tang
Diuresis Inducing Cucumber Soup

【药物组成】 黄瓜 30 g,萹蓄 15 g,瞿麦 10 g。萹蓄、瞿麦水煎,去渣留汁,将药汁重新煮沸,余入黄瓜片,加调料,置冷后即可食用。每日 1 剂,佐餐食用。

【Composition】 30 g cucumber, 15 g Bianxu(Polygonum aviculare), 10 g Huomai(Pink herb). Decoct polygonum aviculare and pink herb with water, remove the dregs and take the juice, boil the juice again, add cucumber slices and flavors. Take after it is cold. Take one dose a day with meal.

【功效】 清热利尿。

【Efficacy】 Reducing fever to induce urination.

【适应证】 小便频数,尿色黄赤,灼热刺痛者。

【Indication】 Frequent urination with hot pain and yellowish-red urine.

参芪冬瓜汤
ShenqiDonggua Tang
Tangshen, Milkvetch Root and Chinese Waxgourd Soup

【药物组成】 党参 15 g,黄芪 20 g,冬瓜 50 g。将党参、黄芪放砂锅内,加水煎煮 15 min,去渣取汁,入冬瓜片,继续煎煮至冬瓜熟,调味即成。佐餐食用。

【Composition】 15 g Dangshen (Tangshen), 20 g Huangqi (Milkvetch root), 50 g Chinese waxgourd. Put Tangshen and milkvetch root in the earthen pot, decoct with water for 15 minutes, remove the dregs and take the juice, put Chinese waxgourd in the juice and decoct until it is well-done and flavor it. Take with meal.

【功效】 健脾益气利尿。

【Efficacy】 Strengthening spleen, benefiting qi and diuresis.

【适应证】 小便淋涩,点滴而出,混浊不黄,少腹坠胀,少气懒言者。

【Indication】 Unsmooth and drenching urination with turbid, upward distention in lower abdomen and being reluctant to speak.

车前粳米汤
Chenqian Jingmi Tang
Asiatic Plantain Seed and Non-Glutinous Rice Soup

【药物组成】 车前子 20 g,粳米 100 g。将车前子用布包好后煎汁。再将粳米入车前子煎汁中同煮为粥。每日早晚温热食用。

【Composition】 20 g Cheqianzi(Asiatic plantain seed), 100 g Jingmi(non-glutinous rice). Wrap Asiatic plantain seed with cloth and dococt to take the juice, boil the juice with non-glutinous rice for porridge. Take warm in the morning and at night.

【功效】　清热利水。

【Efficacy】　Clearing heat to alleviate water retention.

【适应证】　尿道刺痛。

【Indication】　Prickle in urinary tract.

枸杞红茶饮
Gouqi Hongcha Yin
ChineseWolfberry and Red Tea Drink

【药物组成】　枸杞子 50 g,茯苓 100 g,红茶 100 g。将枸杞子与茯苓共研为粗末,每次取 5～10 g,加红茶 6 g,用开水冲泡 10 min 即可。每日 2 次,代茶饮用。

【Composition】　Take 50 g Gouqizi(Chinese wolfberry fruit), 100 g Fuling(Tuckahoe), 100 g red tea. Grind Chinese wolfberry fruit and tuckahoe into coarse powder, get 5 ~ 10 g once, add red tea and brew with boiling water for 10 minutes. Take twice a day as tea.

【功效】　健脾益肾、利尿通淋。

【Efficacy】　Strengthening spleen and benefiting kidney, inducing diuresis for treating strangurtia.

【适应证】　淋漓涩痛,小便短赤者。

【Indication】　Unsmooth urination with pain, less and reddish urine.

尿血及尿路结石
Hematuria and Lithangiuria

川军猪胆汤
Chuanjun Zhudan Tang
RhubarbRoot and Pig Gall Soup

【药物组成】 大黄9 g(研末),猪胆汁6 g。先将猪胆汁加少许水煎服沸后,加入川军末调匀,制成如绿豆大的药丸。每次2丸,每日3次,温开水送服,至症状减轻后每次1丸,治愈为止。

【Composition】 8 g Dahuang(Rhubarb root, grinded) ,6 g pig gall. Get pig gall boiled with a little water and mix with Chuanjun(Rhubarb root) power throughly, make pills as the shape of mung bean. Take 2 pills once, 3 times a day. Take with warm water. Take 1 pill when the symptom is eased, take until cured.

【功效】 滋阴清热。

【Efficacy】 Nourishing yin and clearing heat.

【适应证】 尿血。

【Indication】 Hemuresis.

荸荠三金粥
Biqi Sanjin Zhou
Water Chestnutand Three Drugs Porridges

【药物组成】 取荸荠150 g,鸡内金20 g,金钱草30 g,海金沙15 g,粳米100 g,先用水煎金钱草和海金沙,过滤取汁备用。将荸荠捣烂挤汁、将鸡内金烘干研细,再将此荸荠汁、鸡内金粉和粳米加适量水煮粥,待粥半熟时加入药汁,煮至米烂粥稠后代早餐食用。

【Composition】 150 g Biqi (Water chestnut), 20 g Ji'neijin (Chicken's gizzard - membrane) ,30 g Jinqiancao(Christina loosestrife) ,15 g Hai Jinsha(Japanese fern spore) ,100 g Jingmi(Non-glutinous rice). Decoct christina loosestrife and Japanese fern spore with water firstly, filter and take the juice. Mash the water chestnut and squeeze the juice, parch and grind chicken's gizzard - membrane into powder, add water chestnut juice, chicken's gizzard - membrane powder, non-glutinous rice and proper amount of water to cook porridge. Mix the drug juice in it when it's half done, decoct until the rice is tender and porridge is thick.

【功效】 利尿通淋,止痛。

【Efficacy】 Inducing diuresis for treating strangurtia, stopping pain.

【适应证】　尿道结石。

【Indication】　Urinary calculi.

核桃粥
Hetao Zhou
Walnut Meat Porridge

【药物组成】　核桃仁 100 g,大米 100 g,冰糖 30 g,将大米淘洗干净,核桃去壳留仁,放入米锅内,加水 500 mL,冰糖打碎,放入锅内。把锅置武火上烧沸,用文火煮 30 min 成粥即成。每日 3 次,当主食。

【Composition】　100 g walnut meat, 100 g rice, 30 g crystal sugar, wash the rice, walnut shell removed, put them in the pot, add water 500 mL, smash the crystal sugar and put in the pot. Boiled with high heat and then turn down the fire, decoct porridge with gentle fire for 30 minutes. Take 3 times a day as staple food.

【功效】　补肺肾,排结石。

【Efficacy】　Tonifying lung and kidney, removing calculus.

【适应证】　尿道结石。

【Indication】　Urinary calculi.

肾炎 Nephritis

鲫鱼汤
Jiyu Tang
Crucian Soup

【药物组成】　鲫鱼 1 条,独头蒜 1 个,将鱼去内脏,装入大蒜,外用纸裹,放入谷糠内烧熟即可食用。每日 1 条,连服 1 周。

【Composition】　A crucian, a one-clove garlic, remove the internal organs of the fish, put garlic in it and wrap the fish with paper. Cook in millet hust until it is tender. Take a fish a day; take for a week repeatedly.

【功效】　益气健脾、清热解毒、利水消肿。

【Efficacy】　Nourishing qi to invigorate spleen, clearing away the heat-evil and expelling superficial evils, inducing diuresis to alleviate edema.

【适应证】　肾炎水肿。

【Indication】　Nephritis and edema.

茅根赤豆粥
Maogen Chidou Zhou
Porridgeof Couchgrass Root and Red Bean

【药物组成】 鲜茅根 200 g,赤小豆 200 g,粳米 100 g。先将鲜茅根洗净后切碎放入砂锅内,加清水适量,煎汁去渣;粳米、赤小豆淘洗干净后下入锅内,先用武火烧开,再转而用文火熬煮成稀粥。

【Composition】 200 g fresh Maogen(Couchgrass root),200 g red bean,100 g Jingmi(non-glutinous rice). Wash and cut up the couchgrass root,put in the earthern pot,add proper amount of water,decoct it and remove the dregs. Put non-glutinous rice and red bean in pot after washed,boil with high heat and decoct with gentle fire for porridge.

【功效】 益气健脾、利水消肿。

【Efficacy】 Nourishing qi to invigorate spleen,inducing diuresis to alleviate edema.

【适应证】 急性肾炎小便不利、水肿。

【Indication】 Acute nephritis with difficult urination and edema.

淮山茯苓鹌鹑汤
Huaishan Fuling Anchun Tang
Common Yam Rhizome, Tuckahoe and Quail Soup

【药物组成】 鹌鹑 1 只,怀山药 3 g,茯苓 15 g,精盐少许。将怀山药、茯苓洗净;鹌鹑宰杀后洗净;一起放入锅内,加清水适量,用武火煮沸后改用文火煮至鹌鹑熟烂,放入精盐调味即可。

【Composition】 A quail,3 g Huai Shanyao(Common yam rhizome),15 g Fuling(Tuckahoe)and a little salt. Wash common yam rhizome and Fuling(Tuckahoe),kill the quail and wash it;put them in the pot and add proper amount of water. Decoct with high heat and turn down the fire after it is boiled,decoct until the quail is tender,add some salt.

【功效】 益气健脾、利水消肿。

【Efficacy】 Nourishing qi to invigorate spleen,inducing diuresis to alleviate edema.

【适应证】 肾炎小便不利、水肿。

【Indication】 Nephritis with difficult urination and edema.

翠衣粥
Cuiyi Zhou
Green Peel Porridge

【药物组成】 西瓜翠衣 200 g,粳米 100 g,冰糖 30 g。首先将西瓜皮洗净,切丝。用纱布绞出汁液;粳米淘洗干净后放入锅内,加水适量,置武火烧沸,再用文火煮 40 min,放入西瓜汁及冰糖溶化即成。

【Composition】 200 g watermelon green peel,100 g Jingmi(non-glutinous rice),30 g crystal sugar. Wash the watermelon peel and slice it. Wring the juice with gauze; wash non-glutinous rice and put in the pot, add proper amount of water, decoct with high heat until it is boiled, turn down the fire and boil for 40 minutes. Mix watermelon juice and cystal suger.

【功效】 利水消肿。

【Efficacy】 Inducing diuresis to alleviate edema.

【适应证】 肾炎小便不利、水肿。

【Indication】 Nephritis with difficult urination and edema.

消蛋白尿粥
Xiao Dan bainiaoZhou
Proteinuria Alleviating Porridge

【药物组成】 芡实,糯米各 30 g,白果 10 枚,煮粥。每日 1 次,10 日为 1 疗程。间歇服 24 个疗程(食量少者芡实、糯米可用 15～20 g)。

【Composition】 30 g Qiansh(Gordon euryale seed), 30 g sticky rice each, 10 pieces of Baiguo(Gingko), decoct them for porridge. Take one time a day, 10 days for a period of treatment. Take 24 periods of treatment intermittently(use 15～20 g Gordon euryale seed and sticky rice respectively for people with small appetite).

【功效】 利水消肿。

【Efficacy】 Inducing diuresis to alleviate edema.

【适应证】 肾炎小便不利。

【Indication】 Nephritis with difficult urination.

生殖系统疾病 Genital System Diseases

产后病 Puerperal diseases

马齿苋汤
Machixian Tang
Purslane Soup

【药物组成】 鲜马齿苋汁 1 杯,蜂蜜 30 g。马齿苋煎沸后入蜂蜜和匀调服。

【Composition】 A cup of fresh Machixian(Purslane)juice,30 g honey. Decoct purslane and mix with honey throughly after it's boiled.

【功效】 祛湿止泻。

【Efficacy】 Eliminating dampness to stop diarrhea.

【适应证】 产后痢疾者。

【Indication】 Dysentery after childbirth.

姜术汤
JiangshuTang
Ginger and Largehead Atractylodes Rhizome Soup

【药物组成】 生姜 30 g,白术 25 g。

【Composition】 30 g fresh ginger,25 g Baizhu(Largehead atractylodes rhizome).

【功效】 健脾止呕。

【Efficacy】 Strengthening spleen to stop vomiting.

【适应证】 产后伤食者。

【Indication】 Improper dietary disorders after childbirth.

葱苏汤
CongsuTang
GreenOnion and Perilla Leaf Soup

【药物组成】 葱白 100 g,紫苏叶 9 g,红糖 50 g。

【Composition】 100 g Green onion,9 g Zisuye(Perilla leaf),50 g brown sugar.

【功效】 温中散寒止痛。

【Efficacy】 Warming the middle energizer,dispelling coldness and stopping pain.

【适应证】 风寒型产后身痛者。

【Indication】 Pain in body after childbirth due to wind cold.

香附汤
Xiangfu Tang
NutgrassFalingale Rhizome Soup

【药物组成】 香附 10 g，粳米 100 g。香附加水煮，去渣取汁，用药汁与粳米同煮为粥。可早晚餐食用。

【Composition】 10 g Xiangfu(Nutgrass falingale rhizome),100 g Jingmi(Non-glutinous rice). Decoct Nutgrass falingale rhizome,remove the dregs and take the juice,cook the juice with non-glutinous rice for porridge. Take as breakfast of supper.

【功效】 舒肝解郁。

【Efficacy】 Soothing liver to relieve qi stagnation.

【适应证】 肝气郁滞型不孕患者调理用。

【Indication】 Regulation for the sterility due to liver-li stagnation.

当归生姜羊肉汤
Danggui Shengjiang Yangrou Tang
ChineseAngelica, Fresh Ginger and Mutton Soup

【药物组成】 当归 9 g，生姜 15 g，羊肉 100 g。

【Composition】 9 g Danggui(Chinese angelica),15 g fresh ginger,100 g mutton.

【功效】 温中补血，祛寒止痛。

【Efficacy】 Warming the middle energizer and tonifying blood, dispelling cold and stopping pain.

【适应证】 寒疝腹痛者。

【Indication】 Abdominal pain due to cold hernia.

陈皮茯苓粥
Chenpi Fuling Zhou
DriedOrange Peel and Tuckahoe Porridge

【药物组成】 陈皮、茯苓各 10 g，粳米 100 g。将陈皮、茯苓先加水煮，去渣取汁，与粳米同煮为粥。作早晚餐食用。

【Composition】 10 g Chengpi(Dried orange peel) and Fuling(Tuckahoe) each,100 g Jingmi(Non-glutinous rice). Decoct dried orange peel and tuckahoe with water;remove the dregs and take the juice. Take as breakfast or supper.

【功效】 健脾燥湿，化痰祛脂。

【Efficacy】 Strengthening spleen and eliminating dampness, dissipating phlegm and eliminating fat.

【适应证】 痰湿内阻型不孕患者调理用。

【Indication】 Regulation for the sterility due to internal stagnation of phlegmatic dampness.

当归羊肉汤
Danggui Yangrou Tang
ChineseAngelica and Mutton Soup

【药物组成】 当归 9 g,生姜 15 g,羊肉 100 g,人参 15 g,黄芪 20 g。

【Composition】 9 g Danggui(Chinese angelica),15 g fresh ginger,100 g mutton,15 g Renshen(Ginseng),20 g Huangqi(Milkvetch root).

【功效】 益气养血,甘温清热。

【Efficacy】 Benefiting qi and nourishing blood,warming and clearing heat.

【适应证】 产后蓐劳,发热自汗者。

【Indication】 General debility during puerperium,having fever and spontaneous perspiration.

壮阳狗肉汤
ZhuangyangGourou Tang
Tonifying Yang Dog Meat Soup

【药物组成】 狗肉 2000 g,菟丝子 30 g,制附片 13 g。将狗肉整块下锅,用沸水煮透,捞入凉水内,洗净血水,控干水分,切成长方条。将锅置火上,放入狗肉、姜片热炒,烹入绍酒炝锅,然后倒入大锅内,同时把菟丝子、附片用纱布包好,放入锅内,加清汤、盐、味精、葱白,置武火上烧沸,去浮沫,改用文火炖 2 h,待狗肉炖至熟烂,挑出姜、葱白,调味,分装 10 份即成。每日 1 次,每次 1 份,晨起空腹食用,冬令尤宜多吃。

【Composition】 2000 g dog meat,30 g Tusizi(Dodder),13 g Fupian(Prepared monkshood).Put the the dog meat in the pot,boiled thoroughly with water,fish it out and put in cold water,wash up the bloody water and drain off the water,cut it into rectangular pieces. Put the dog meat in the pot,fry ginger firstly and then fry quickly with Shao wine,then pour them into a bigger pot. Wrap dodder and prepared monkshood with gauze,put them in the pot, add light soup,salt,monosodium glutamate,green onion stalk and boiled with high heat;remove the float,decoct with slow fire for 2 hours until the dog meat is tender,fish out ginger,green onion stalk;flaver it and devide it into 10 doses. Take one time a day,one dose a time. Take in the morning with empty stomach;take more especially in winter.

【功效】 温肾助阳,益精补虚。

【Efficacy】 Warming kidney and activating yang,benefiting essence and improving asthenia.

【适应证】 肾气亏虚型不孕患者调理。

【Indication】 Regulation for the sterility due to kidney-qi deficiency and consumption.

紫薇花牡蛎火腿汤散
Ziweihua Muli Huotuitang San
Crape Myrtle Flower, Oysterand Ham Soup

【药物组成】 紫薇花4朵,牡蛎净肉500 g,火腿末5 g,水发冬菇10 g,玉兰片10 g,胡椒粉、食盐、料酒、酱油、味精、鸡汤、姜片各适量。紫薇花去萼及杂质,洗净,切成细丝;牡蛎肉拣洗干净,沥干水分,切碎。火腿肉、玉兰片、冬菇分别洗净,切成片;将牡蛎、冬菇、玉兰片各用开水焯一下。锅烧热,放入鸡汤、料酒、酱油、姜片、食盐,大火煮沸,下入火腿、冬菇、玉兰片、牡蛎,烧沸,加入味精、紫薇花细丝,调好口味,撒上胡椒粉即成。

【Composition】 4 Ziwei Hua(Crape myrtle flower),500 g oyster meat,5 g minced ham, 10 g soaked mushroom,10 g Yulan Pian(Water–soaked bamboo slice),proper amount of pepper powder,salt,cooking wine,soy sauce,monosodium glutamate,chicken soup and ginger slice. Remove the calyx and the dregs of crape myrtle flower,wash and slice it,select and wash oyster meat,drain off the water and cut it up. Wash the ham,water–soaked bamboo slices and mushroom seperatey and then slice them;blanch them in boiling water separately. Heat the pot, put chicken soup,cooking wine,soy sauce,ginger slices,salt in the pot and get boiled,add ham, mashroom, water – soaked bamboo slices, oyster and boiled again, flavor it with monosodium glutamate and crape myrtle flower slices,splash some pepper powder.

【功效】 滋阴养血止血,健脾开胃解毒。

【Efficacy】 Nourishing yin, nourishing blood and stopping bleeding, strengthening spleen,promoting appetite and detoxication.

【适应证】 适用于产后虚损、烦热、产后血崩等症。

【Indication】 Consumptive disease and feverish dysphoria after childbirth,puerperal metrorrhagia.

花生炖猪爪
Huasheng Dun Zhuzhua
Peanut Stew Pig Foot

【药物组成】 花生米200 g,猪脚爪2只。将猪脚爪洗净,用刀划白,放入锅内,加花生米、盐、葱、姜、黄酒、清水,用武火烧沸后,转用文火熬至熟烂。随量食用。

【Composition】 200 g peanut,2 pig feet. Wash the pig feet,cut white with knife,put in the pot and add peanut,salt,green onion,ginger,yellow wine and water,boil with high heat, turn down the fire when the pig feet is tender. Take as one wish.

【功效】 益气养血通乳。

【Efficacy】 Benefiting qi,nourishing blood and promoting lactation.

【适应证】 产后乳少,甚或全无,乳汁清稀,乳房柔软无胀感,面色无华,神疲食少者。

【Indication】 Lack of or no breast milk after childbirth,thin milk,soft breast without the feeling of distention, dark complexion, spiritlessness and poor appetite.

蟹酒汤
Xie Jiu Tang
Crab Wine Soup

【药物组成】 蟹爪 200 g,黄酒和米醋适量。

【Composition】 200 g crab claw, proper amount of yellow wine and rice wine.

【功效】 补气活血。

【Efficacy】 Invigorating qi to activate blood circulation.

【适应证】 产后胎盘迟迟不出者。

【Indication】 Difficulty in placenta coming out.

归芪鲤鱼汤
Guiqi Liyu Tang
ChineseAngelica, Milkvetch Root and Carp Soup

【药物组成】 鲤鱼 1 条(约 500 g),当归 15 g,黄芪 50 g。将当归、黄芪用纱布包后与洗净的鱼同煮。饮汤吃肉。

【Composition】 Take a carp(500 g), 15 g Danggui(Chinese angelica), 50 g Huangqi (Milkvetch root). Wrap Chinese angelica and milkvetch root with gauze and boil with washed fish. Drink the soup and eat the meat.

【功效】 补气养血通乳。

【Efficacy】 Invigorating qi, nourishing blood and promoting lactation.

【适应证】 气血虚弱产后缺乳者。

【Indication】 Being lack of breast milk after childbirth due to qi and blood deficiency.

橘叶青皮猪蹄汤
Juye Qingpi Zhuti Tang
Orange Leaf, Green Tangerine Peel and Pig Foot Soup

【药物组成】 橘叶、青皮笞 10 g,猪蹄 1 只。先把猪蹄洗净,再与橘叶、青皮加水适量同煮,炖至猪蹄烂熟。饮汤吃肉,每日数次。

【Composition】 Take 10 g orange leaf and Qingpi(Green tangerine peel), one pig foot. Wash the pig foot and boil with orange leaf, green tangerine peel and proper amount of water, decoct until the pig foot is tender. Drink the soup and eat the meat several times a day.

【功效】 行气通乳。

【Efficacy】 Activating qi and promoting lactation.

【适应证】 产后乳少或无乳,乳房胀痛,胸胁胀满,食欲减退者。

【Indication】 Less or no breast mild after childbirth, distention and pain in breast, distention and fullness in chest and hypochondrium.

痛经 Dysmenorrhea

姜枣花椒汤
Jiangzao Huajiao Tang
Ginge, Jujube and Wild Pepper Soup

【药物组成】　干姜、大枣各 30 g,花椒 9 g。干姜切片,大枣去核,加水适量,煮沸,再放入花椒,改用文火煎汤。每日 1 剂,分 2 次温服,5 日为 1 个疗程。行经前 3 日饮服。

【Composition】　30 g dried ginger, 30 g jujube, 9 g wild pepper. Slice dried ginger, stone the jujube, add proper amount of water and get boiled, then put in wild pepper, turn down the fire and cook for porridge. Take one dose a day, devide it into 2 parts and take warm twice; take 5 days for a period of treatment. Take 3 days before period.

【功效】　温阳散寒化湿。

【Efficacy】　Warming yang, dispelling coldness and dissolving dampness.

【适应证】　寒湿凝滞型痛经。

【Indication】　Dysmenorrhea due to coldness and dampness stagnation.

归芪酒
Guiqi Jiu
ChineseAngelica and Milkvetch Root Wine

【药物组成】　当归、黄芪各 150 g,红枣 100 g。将黄芪、当归切片,与红枣一起置纱布袋内,投入盛酒容器,加酒 500 mL,加盖密封 7 日。每次饮 10 mL,每日 2 次,7 日为 1 个疗程,行经前 5 日开始饮服。以上剂量可用 3 个疗程。

【Composition】　Take 150 g Danggui(Chinese angelica) and Huangqi(Milkvetch root) each, 100 g red jujube. Slice milkvetch root and Chinese angelica, put into gauze bag with red jujube, installing in wine vessel and add 500 mL wine, seal it up for 7 days. Take 10 mL one time, twice a day, 7 days a period of treatment. Take 5 days before period. This dosage can be taken for 3 periods of treatment.

【功效】　益气养血,活血调经。

【Efficacy】　Benefiting qi and nourishing blood, promoting blood circulation to restore menstrual flow.

【适应证】　经后小腹隐隐作痛,月经量少,经色淡,质稀薄,面色苍白,精神倦怠者。

【Indication】　Pain lower abdominal after menstruation, less menstrual blood volume, light menstrual colour, thin menstrual blood, pale complexion, spiritlessness.

黑豆红花饮
HeidouHonghua Yin
Black Beanand Safflower Decoction

【药物组成】 黑豆30 g,红花6 g,红糖30 g。将黑豆、红花加清水适量,用武火煮沸4 min后,再用文火煮至黑豆烂熟,去黑豆、红花,加红糖调味即成。每次服2杯,每日2次。

【Composition】 Take 30 g black bean,6 g Honghua(Safflower),30 g brown sugar. Put black bean and safflower in proper amount of water and boil with high heat for 4 minutes,then turn down the fire and boil it until the black bean is tender,remove the black bean and safflower,add some brown sugar to flavor it. Take 2 cups a time,twice a day.

【功效】 活血化瘀,缓急止痛。

【Efficacy】 Activating blood circulation to dissipate blood stasis,relaxing tension and relieving pain.

【适应证】 经前或行经时小腹胀痛拒按,经量少或行而不畅,经色紫黯有血块,伴有经前胸胁胀痛者。

【Indication】 Unpressable pain in the lower abdomen before and during menstruation, less menstrual blood volume or difficult in menstruation,dark purple menstrual colour with coagulated blood,distention and pain in the chest and hypochondrium before menstruation.

椒附炖猪肚
Jiaofu Dun Zhudu
Pepper,Aconite Stew Pork Tripe

【药物组成】 猪肚150 g,附子2 g,川椒2 g,粳米30 g。将附子、川椒研末。猪肚洗净,装入药末、粳米及适量的葱,扎口入锅中,加水适量,微火煮至猪肚烂熟。佐餐食用。

【Composition】 Take 150 g pork tripe,2 g Fuzi(Aconite),2 g Sichuan pepper,30 g Jingmi(Non-glutinous rice),grind aconite and Sichuan pepper into powder. Wash pork tripe and put the powder,non-glutinous rice and proper amount of green onion in it,tie it off and put in the pot,add proper amount of water,boil with slow fire until the pork tripe is tender. Take with rice or bread.

【功效】 温经散寒止痛。

【Efficacy】 Warming meridians,dispelling coldness and stopping pain.

【适应证】 经前或经行中小腹疼痛,疼痛较剧,经量初少逐渐增多,色暗红带有血块,畏寒喜暖,得热则舒,腰脊疼痛,便溏者。

【Indication】 Unbearable pain in the lower abdomen before and during menstruation,less menstrual blood volume and more afterwards,dark red menstrual colour with coagulated blood, chills and favoring warmness,pain in waist and back,loose stool.

韭菜炒羊肝
Jiucai Chao Yanggan
Chinese Leek Fry Sheep Liver

【药物组成】 韭菜 150 g,羊肝 200 g。将羊肝切成小片,与韭菜一起于铁锅内急火烹炒,加入食盐、味精调味。佐餐食用。每日 1 次,连食 1 周为 1 个疗程。经行前 5 日开始食用。

【Composition】 150 g Jiucai(Chinese leek),200 g sheep liver,cut sheep liver into small pieces and fry with Chinese leek in iron pan with strong fire, add salt and monosodium glutamate to flavor it. Take with rice or bread. Take once a day;take one week repeatedly as a period of treatment.

【功效】 温补肝肾。

【Efficacy】 Warming and tonifying liver and kidney.

【适应证】 肝肾不足型痛经。

【Indication】 Dysmenorrheal due to deficiency of kidney and liver.

桃仁墨鱼
Taoren Moyu
Peach Kernel Cuttlefish

【药物组成】 墨鱼 150 g,桃仁 6 g。将墨鱼水泡后,去骨、皮后洗净,与桃仁一起放入锅内,加葱、姜、盐、清水,用武火烧沸后,改用文火,煮至墨鱼烂熟。佐餐食用,每日 1 次,经前连用 3 日。

【Composition】 150 g cuttlefish,6 g Taoren(Peach kernel). Soak cuttlefish in water, remove its bone and skin,wash and put it into pot with peach kernel,add green onion,ginger, salt and water;get boiled with high heat and turn down the fire,decoct until the cuttle fish is tender. Take with rice or bread once a day. Take for 3 days before period.

【功效】 养血活血,调经。

【Efficacy】 Nourishing blood and promoting blood circulation,regulating menstruation.

【适应证】 气血虚弱型痛经。

【Indication】 Dysmenorrheal due to weakness and deficiency of qi and blood.

枸杞炖兔肉
GouqiDun Turou
ChineseWolfberry Stew Rabbit Meat

【药物组成】 枸杞子 15 g,兔肉 250 g。将枸杞子和兔肉入适量水中,文火炖熟,用盐调味。饮汤吃肉,每日 1 次。

【Composition】 15 g Gouqizi Gouqizi(Chinese wolfberry fruit),250 g rabbit meat. Put Chinese wolfberry and rabbit meat in proper amount of water and decoct with slow water,flavor it with salt. Drink the soup and eat the meat, once a day.

【功效】　滋补肝肾,补气养血。

【Efficacy】　Tonifying liver and kidney, replenishing qi and nourishing blood.

【适应证】　经后小腹隐隐作痛,月经初潮较迟,经量少色淡,兼有腰酸肢软,头晕耳鸣者。

【Indication】　Little pain in the lower abdomen after menstruation, late menarche, less menstrual volume with light color, being accompanied with sore waist and weak limbs, dizzy head and tinnitus.

带下病

白果黄芪乌鸡汤
Baiguo Huangqi Wuji Tang
Ginkgo, Milkvetch Root Black-Bone Chicken Soup

【药物组成】　白果 30 g,黄芪 50 g,乌鸡 1 只(约 500 g),米酒 50 mL。将乌鸡去内脏、头足,洗净,把白果放入鸡腹中,用线缝口,与黄芪一起放入砂锅内,加酒及水适量,用文火炖熟,调味即可。分次饮汤食肉。

【Composition】　30 g Baiguo(Ginkgo), 50 g Huangqi(Milkvetch root), a black-bone chicken(about 500 g), 50 mL rice wine. Tripe off, head and foot off, and wash the chicken, put ginkgo in its stomach, stitch closure with lines and put into the earthern pot with Milkvetch root, add proper amount of wine and water, decoct with slow fire until it's tender and flavor it. Drink the soup and eat the meat with several times.

【功效】　健脾益气,固肾止带。

【Efficacy】　Strengthening spleen and benefiting qi, consolidating kidney and stopping leucorrhea.

【适应证】　带下量多,色白或淡黄,质稠无味,绵绵不断,面色萎黄,四肢不温,神倦乏力者。

【Indication】　More and excessive morbid leucorrhea with white or light yellow color, thickness with no smell, yellowish complexion, coldness in limbs, spiritlessness and weakness.

芡实核桃粥
Qianshi Hetao Zhou
Gordon Euryale Seedand Walnut Meat Porridge

【药物组成】　芡实粉 30 g,核桃肉 15 g,红枣 7 枚。将核桃肉打碎,红枣去核,芡实粉用凉开水打成糊状,放入滚开水中搅拌,再入核桃肉、红枣,煮成粥,加糖食用。每日 1 次,可作点心,连用半个月。

【Composition】　30 g Qianshi(Gordon euryale seed) powder, 15 g walnut meat, 7 red jujubes. Smash walnut meat into pieces, stone the jujubes and beat gordon euryale seed powder with cold boilded water to paste; stir it in boiling water, add walnut meat, red jujubes and boil into porridge, add some sugar. Take once a day as dessert, take for half a month repeatedly.

【功效】 益气温肾,止带。

【Efficacy】 Benefiting qi and warming kidney, stopping leucorrhea.

【适应证】 带下清稀量多,色白,有腥味,腰酸腿软,少腹冷,夜尿多,大便溏者。

【Indication】 Thin morbid leucorrhea with more volume, white color, offensive smell of fish, sore waist and weakness legs, coldness in the lower abdomen and loose stool.

茯苓车前粥
Fuling Cheqian Zhou
Tuckahoeand Asiatic Plantain Seed Porridge

【药物组成】 茯苓粉、车前子各30 g,粳米60 g。车前子用纱布包好,水煎半小时,去渣取汁,加粳米煮粥,粥成时加茯苓粉、白糖适量稍煮即可。每日空腹服2次。

【Composition】 30 g Fuling(Tuckahoe)powder, 30 g Cheqianzi(Asiatic plantain seed), 60 g Jingmi(Non-glutinous rice). Wrap Asiatic plantain seed with gauze and decoct with water for half an hour, remove the dregs and take the juice, add tuckahoe powder and sugar when it's ready and boil for a short while. Take twice a day with empty stomach.

【功效】 利水渗湿,清热解毒。

【Efficacy】 Removing dampness and promoting diuresis, clearing away the heat-evil and expelling superficial evils.

【适应证】 带下量多,色黄绿如脓,气味臭秽者。

【Indication】 Leucorrhea with more volume, yellowish-green color like pus and bed smell.

三味薏米羹
Sanwei YimiGeng
Three Drugs Coix Seed Soup

【药物组成】 薏米、山药、莲子各30 g。以上三味洗净,加水适量,用文火熬成粥。早晚食用,连用7 d。

【Composition】 30 g Yimi(Coix seed), 30 g Shanyao(Common yam rhizome), 30 g lotus seed, get them washed and add proper amount of water, decoct with slow fire to cook thick soup. Take in the morning and at night; take for 7 days repeatedly.

【功效】 健脾益气,化湿止带。

【Efficacy】 Strengthening spleen and benefiting qi, dissolving dampness and stopping leucorrhea.

【适应证】 脾虚湿型带下病。

【Indication】 Morbid leucorrhea due to deficiency and dampness of spleen.

芡实糯米鸡
Qianshi Nuomi Ji
GordonEuryale Seed and Sticky Rice Chicken

【药物组成】 芡实 50 g,莲子 50 g,乌骨鸡 1 只(约 500 g),糯米 100 g。将乌骨鸡去内脏,洗净,将莲子、芡实、糯米放入鸡腹中,用线缝口,放在砂锅内,加水适量,用文火炖烂熟,调味即可。分次酌量食用。连服 2 周。

【Composition】 50 g Qianshi(Gordon euryale seed),50 g lotus seed, a black – bone chicken(about 500 g),100 g sticky rice. Wash and tripe off the chicken,put lutus seed,gordon euryale seed and sticky rice in its stomach and seam it with lines. Put the chicken in earthern pot and add proper amount of water,decoct with slow fire until gets tender and flavor it. Take appropriate amount for several times. Take for 2 weeks.

【功效】 健脾补肾,除湿止带。

【Efficacy】 Strengthening spleen and tonifying kidney,dissolving dampness and stopping leucorrhea.

【适应证】 肾气不足型带下病。

【Indication】 Morbid leucorrhea due to deficiency of kidney qi.

内分泌及代谢系统疾病
Endocrine and Metabolic System Diseases

高血脂 Hyperlipidemia

紫菜豆腐汤
Zicai Doufu Tang
LaverTofu Soup

【药物组成】　紫菜 20 g,猪瘦肉 50 g,嫩豆腐 100 g。紫菜撕成小片,豆腐切成条,猪肉切成薄片。锅中放鲜汤,用中火烧开,加入紫菜、豆腐,水沸再入猪肉片,肉片将熟入味精,淋入香油调味。佐餐食用。

【Composition】　20 g laver,50 g lean pork,100 g soft tofu. Tear laver into small pieces, cut tofu into strips and pork into thin slices. Cook delicious soup with moderate heat,add laver and tofu,get boiled and put in the pork slice,and put some SMG when it's done, add some sesame oil. Take with rice or bread.

【功效】　软坚化痰,清热降脂。

【Efficacy】　Softening hard mass and dissipating phlegm,clearing heat and reducing blood fat.

【适应证】　痰浊内盛的高血脂患者。

【Indication】　Hyperlipemia due to internally abundant turbid phlegm.

二花桑楂汁
Er'hua Sangzha Yin
TwoFlowers,Mulberry Leaf and Hawthorn Fruit Decoction

【药物组成】　金银花 6 g,菊花 6 g,桑叶 4 g,生山楂 6 g,冰糖 20 g。将金银花、菊花、桑叶、生山楂用清水洗去灰渣,用白洁纱布包扎好,放入锅内煎 10 min,加入冰糖溶化即成。每日 1 剂,代茶频饮。10~30 日为 1 个疗程。

【Composition】　6 g Jinyinhua(Honeysuckle),6 g chrysanthemum flower,4 g Sangye (Mulberry leaf),6 g fresh Shanzha(Hawthorn fruit),20 g crystal sugar,wash the first 4 drugs to remove the ashes,wrap them with gauze and decoct in the pot for 10 minutes,add crystal suger in it. Take one dose a day as tea and take constantly. Take 10~30 days for a period of treatment.

【功效】　清肝明目,降脂。

【Efficacy】　Clearing liver to brightening eyes,reducing fat.

【适应证】 阴亏阳亢且伴血脂水平较高的患者。

【Indication】 Patients with yang hypera ctivities and high blood fat.

决明子汁
Juemingzi Zhi
Cassia Seed Juice

【药物组成】 决明子50 g水煎取汁。

【Composition】 Take 50 g Juemingzi(Cassia seed), dococt and take the juice.

【功效】 清热明目降脂。

【Efficacy】 Clearing liver to brightening eyes, reducing fat.

【适应证】 高血脂患者。

【Indication】 Hyperlipemia.

田三七粥
Tiansanqi Zhou
Sanchi Porridge

【药物组成】 田三七粉3 g,粳米50 g,白糖适量。粳米加水适量,煮至粥成,入三七粉和白糖,稍煮即可。每日1剂,分2次热服。1个月为1个疗程。

【Composition】 3 g Sanqi(Sanchi)powder, 50 g Jingmi(Non-glutinous rice), proper amount of sugar. Decoct non-glutinous rice with proper amount of water to cook porridge, mix sanchi powder and sugar in it and boil for a short while. Devide one dose into two parts and take twice a day after it's warmed. Take one month for a period of treatment.

【功效】 活血散瘀。

【Efficacy】 Activating blood flow and removing blood stasis.

【适应证】 血瘀络痹者。

【Indication】 Patients with blood stasis and arthromyodynia in collaterals.

降脂减肥茶
Jiangzhi Jianfei Cha
Lipid Decreasing and Weight Reducing Tea

【药物组成】 干荷叶60 g,生山楂、生薏米各10 g,花生叶15 g,橘皮5 g,茶叶60 g。将上药共为细末,以沸水冲泡代茶饮。每日1剂,不拘时频饮。

【Composition】 60 g Dried lotus leaf, 10 g fresh Shanzha(Hawthorn fruit), 10 g fresh Yimi(Coix seed), 15 g peanut leaf, 5 g orange peel, 60 g tea, grind these into fine powder and brew with boiling water. Take as tea one dose a day; take constantly.

【功效】 清热消食,降脂化湿。

【Efficacy】 Clearing heat, promoting digestion, reducing blood fat and dissolving dampness.

【适应证】 形体肥胖,面有油光,头脑昏重,咯吐痰涎,恶心呕吐,胸闷脘痞,肢麻沉重者。

【Indication】 Patients with fat figure, greasy complexion, drowsiness in head, spitting phlegm and sputum, sickness and vomiting, depression in chest and gastric cavity, numb and heavy limbs.

冬青山楂茶
Dongqing Shanzha Cha
Holly Root Hawthorn Tea

【药物组成】 毛冬青 25 g,山楂 30 g。将二物洗净,水煎代茶饮。每日 1 剂,不拘时频饮。

【Composition】 25 g Mao Dongqing(Hairy holly root), 30 g Shanzha(Hawthorn fruit), washes them and decoct with water. Take one dose a day and take constantly as tea.

【功效】 活血化瘀,消积化痰。

【Efficacy】 Activating blood circulation to dissipate blood stasis, removing food retention and dissipating phlegm.

【适应证】 胸闷刺痛,头痛,肢体麻木或有蚁行感的患者。

【Indication】 Depression in chest with stabbing pain, headache, numb limbs or like ants moving in them.

健脾饮
Jianpi Yin
Spleen Invigorating Decoction

【药物组成】 橘皮 10 g,荷叶 15 g,炒山楂 3 g,生麦芽 15 g,白糖适量。橘皮、荷叶切丝,和山楂、麦芽一起,加水 500 ml 煎煮 30 min,去渣留汁,加入白糖即可。每日 1 剂,代茶饮。

【Composition】 Take 10 g orange peel, 15 g lotus leaf, 3 g fried Shanzha (Hawthorn fruit), 15 g fresh malt and proper amount of sugar. Slice orange peel and lotus leaf and decoct with hawthorn fruit, malt and 500 ml water for 30 minutes. Take the juice and remove the dregs, add some sugar. Take one dose a day as tea.

【功效】 健脾导滞,升清降浊。

【Efficacy】 Strengthening spleen and guiding stagnation, ascending the clear and descending the turbid.

【适应证】 脾气虚弱且血脂水平较高的患者。

【Indication】 Patients with deficiency of spleen qi and high blood fat.

昆布海藻汤
Kunbu Haizao Tang
Tangle and Kelp Soup

【药物组成】 昆布、海藻各 30 g,黄豆 150 g。

【Composition】 30 g tangle,30 g kelp,150 g soybean.

【功效】 消痰利水,健脾宽中。

【Efficacy】 Dissolving phlegm to alleviate water retention, strengthening spleen to relaxing the middle energizer.

【适应证】 血脂较高的患者。

【Indication】 Patients with high blood fat.

糖尿病 Diabetes

二丹汤
Er'dan Tang
Two Dan Soup

【药物组成】 牡丹、丹参、玄参各 20 g,茯苓、柏子仁各 9 g。

【Composition】 20 g Peony,20 g Danshen(Red sage root),20 g Xuanshen(Figwort root),9 g Fuling(Tuckahoe),9 g Baiziren(Arborvitate seed)

【功效】 滋阴清热,生津止渴。

【Efficacy】 Nourishing yin and clearing away heat,promoting the production of body fluid to quench thirst.

【适应证】 消渴欲饮水者。

【Indication】 People with wasting thirst and excessive drinking.

止消渴速溶饮
Zhixiaoke Surong Yin
Thirst Quenching Instant Powder Decoction

【药物组成】 鲜冬瓜皮、西瓜皮各 1000 g,瓜蒌根 250 g,白糖 500 g。鲜冬瓜皮、西瓜皮削去外层硬皮,切成薄片,瓜蒌根捣碎,先以冷水泡透以后同放入锅内,加水适量,煮 1 h,去渣,再以小火继续煎煮浓缩,至较稠黏将要干锅时停火,待温,加入干燥的白糖粉,把煎液吸净,拌匀,晒干,压碎,装瓶备用。每日数次,每次 10 g,以沸水冲化,频频代茶饮服。

【Composition】 1000 g fresh Chinese waxgourd peel,1000 g watermelon peel,250 g Gualou Gen(Snakegourd root),500 g sugar. Chip off the tough layer of Chinese waxgourd peel and Watermelon peel,cut them into fine pieces,and mash the snakegourd root into pieces. Soak them with cold water and put in the pot, decoct with proper amount of water for an hour, remove the dregs and decoct with small fire until it concentrates. Turn off the fire until it's thick and sticky. Add some dried sugar powder when it's lukewarm. Take all the juice, mix thoroughly, dry in the sun, grind into pieces and install in the bottle. Take several times a day, 10 g one time, brew with boiling water and take as tea constantly.

【功效】　清热生津止渴。

【Efficacy】　Removing heat to promote salivation and quench thirst.

【适应证】　口渴引饮,随饮随渴,尿频量多者。

【Indication】　Excessive thirst, frequency of urination with large volume.

乌梅五参汤
Wumei Wushen Tang
DarkPlum and Five Ginsheng Soup

【药物组成】　党参15 g,丹参30 g,元参、沙参各10 g,玉竹参12 g,乌梅30 枚。

【Composition】　15 g Dangshen (Tangshen), 30 g Danshen (Red sage root), 10 g Yuanshen(Scrophularia), 10 g Shashen(Root of straight ladybell), 12 g Yuzhu Shen(Fragrant solomonseal rhizome), 30 pieces of Wumei(Dark plum fruit).

【功效】　降糖。

【Efficacy】　Lowering blood sugar.

【适应证】　糖尿病引起的各种不适。

【Indication】　Various uncomforts due to diabetes.

菠菜银耳汤
Bocai Yin'er Tang
Spinach and White fungus Soup

【药物组成】　菠菜根100 g,银耳10 g。菠菜根洗净,银耳发泡,共煎汤服食。每日1～2 次,佐餐食用。可连服3～4 周。

【Composition】　100 g Spinach root, 10 g White fungus, wash the spinach root and soak white fungus in the water, cook soup with them. Take 1～2 times one day with meal. Take 3～4 weeks repeatedly.

【功效】　滋阴润燥,生津止渴。

【Efficacy】　Nourishing yin and moisturizing dryness – syndrome, promoting fluid production to quench thirst.

【适应证】　燥火伤肺型糖尿病者。

【Indication】　Diabetes due to lung damage caused by dryness-fire.

银耳玉竹汤
Yin'er Yuzhu Tang
White Fungusand Fragrant Solomonseal Rhizome Soup

【药物组成】 银耳 15 g,玉竹 25 g,冰糖适量。银耳用清水浸泡至软,洗净,与玉竹、冰糖同入砂锅内加适量清水煮汤。温服,日服 2 次。

【Composition】 Get 15 g white fungus, 25 g Yuzhu (Fragrant solomonseal rhizome), proper amount of crystal sugar. Soak white fungus in water till its tender and wash it, decoct with fragrant solomonseal rhizome and crystal sugar in the earthern pot with proper amount of water to cook soup. Take warm twice a day.

【功效】 滋阴消热。

【Efficacy】 Nourishing yin and relieving fever.

【适应证】 适合胃阴不足而口干、口渴者服用。

【Indication】 Deficiency of stomach yin, dry mouth and excessive drinking.

百合枇杷藕羹
Baihe Pipa Ou Geng
Lily Bulb, Loquatand Lotus Root Soup

【药物组成】 鲜百合 30 g,枇杷 30 g,鲜藕 10 g,桂花 2 g。藕切成片,枇杷去核,与鲜百合加水同煮,熟时用淀粉勾芡成羹。食用时调入桂花。可作早晚餐或作点心食用。

【Composition】 30 g Fresh lily bulb, 30 g loquat, 10 g fresh lotus root, 2 g sweet osmanthus flower. Slice lotus into pieces, stone the loquat and decoct with fresh lily bulb, dressing with starchy sauce when it's well – done. Add some sweet osmanthus flower before eating. Take in the morning and at night or take as dessert.

【功效】 清热润肺,生津止渴。

【Efficacy】 Clearing heat and moisturizing lung, promoting fluid production to quench thirst.

【适应证】 多食易饥,形体消瘦,烦热汗出,大便干燥,喜饮尿频者。

【Indication】 Eating much but being easy to hunger, emaciated figure, feverish dysphoria to sweat, dry stools, excessive drinking and frequent urination.

参冬鸡蛋清
Shendong Jidanqing
Ginseng Egg White

【药物组成】 人参 6 g,天门冬 30 g,鸡蛋 1 个,将人参和天门冬研末,与鸡蛋清调匀。

【Composition】 6 g Renshen (Ginseng), 30 g Tianmendong (Cochinchinese Asparagus Root), one egg. Grind Ginseng and cochinchinese asparagus root into powder, mix with egg white thoroughly.

【功效】 益气养心。

【Efficacy】 Benefiting qi and nourishing heart.

【适应证】 糖尿病伴心气不足者。

【Indication】 Diabetes with deficiency of heart qi.

<h2 style="text-align:center">葛根粉粥</h2>
<h3 style="text-align:center">Gegenfen Zhou</h3>
<h3 style="text-align:center">Kudzuvine Root Powder Porridge</h3>

【药物组成】 葛根粉30 g,粳米100 g。粳米加水适量武火煮沸,改文火再煮半小时加葛根粉拌匀,至米烂成粥即可。每日早晚服用,可连服3~4周。

【Composition】 30 g Gegen powder (Kudzuvine root), 100 g Jingmi (non – glutinous rice). Decoct non-glutinous rice with water until it get boiled, turn down the fire and decoct for half an hour, mix kudzuvine root powder thoroughly and decoct until the rice is tender enough. Take in the moring and at night, take for 3~4 weeks repeatedly.

【功效】 清热生津,除烦止渴。

【Efficacy】 Removing heat to promote salivation, eliminating restlessness and quenching thirst.

【适应证】 胃燥津伤型糖尿病。

【Indication】 Diabetes caused by damage of body fluid due to dryness in stomach.

<h2 style="text-align:center">鳖鱼滋肾汤</h2>
<h3 style="text-align:center">Bieyu Zishen Tang</h3>
<h3 style="text-align:center">TurtleKidney Nourishing Soup</h3>

【药物组成】 鳖鱼1只(500 g左右),枸杞子30 g,熟地黄15 g。将鳖鱼切块,加枸杞、地黄、料酒和清水适量,先用武火烧开后改用文火煨炖至肉熟透即可。可佐餐食用或单食。

【Composition】 One turtle (500 g), 30 g Gou Qizi, 15 g Shu Dihuang (prepared rehmannia root). Cut the turtle into pieces, add Chinese wolfberry fruit, prepared rehmannia root, cooking wine and proper amount of water; cook with high heat before its boiled and turn down the fire and decoct until the meat is tender. Take with rice or bread or take seperately.

【功效】 滋补肝肾,滋阴养血。

【Efficacy】 Nourishing and tonifying liver and kidney, nourishing yin and blood.

【适应证】 尿频量多,尿如脂膏,口干唇燥不多饮,形体虚弱,腰膝无力者。

【Indication】 Frequent urination with large volume, mobilgrease urine, dry mouth but drinking less, emaciated body, weakness of waist and knees.

苦瓜片
Kugua Pian
Bitter Gourd Pill

【药物组成】 苦瓜若干,将苦瓜干碾粉制成片,每片含干粉 0.5 g,每次口服 15~25 片,日服 3 次,餐前 1 h 服用,2 个月为一疗程。

【Composition】 Some bitter gourd. Grind dried bitter gourd into powder and make pills with the powder. Each pill contain 0.5 g dried powder, take 15~25 pills once, take 3 times a day before meal, take 2 month for a period of treatment.

【功效】 清热解毒,降血糖。

【Efficacy】 Clearing away the heat-evil and expelling superficial evils, lowering blood sugar.

【适应证】 糖尿病。

【Indication】 Diabetes.

山药玉竹鸽肉汤
Shanyao YuzhuGerou Tang
CommonYam Rhizome,Fragrant Solomonseal Rhizome and Pigeon Meat Soup

【药物组成】 白鸽 1 只,怀山药 30 g,玉竹 20 g。白鸽洗净入锅,加山药、玉竹、清水适量,煮至鸽肉烂熟后,放入食盐、味精调味即可。每日 1 次,食肉喝汤,可常服。

【Composition】 One pigeon,30 g Huai Shanyao(Common yam rhizome),20 g Yuzhu (Fragrant solomonseal rhizome). Wash the pigeon, add common yam rhizome, fragrant solomonseal rhizome and proper amount of water, decoct until the pigeon is tender; add some salt and monosodium glutamate. Take once a day, eat the meat and drink the soup, take constantly.

【功效】 养阴益气,滋补肝肾。

【Efficacy】 Nourishing yin and benefiting qi, nourishing and tonifying liver and kidney.

【适应证】 肝肾阴虚型糖尿病。

【Indication】 Diabetes due to yin deficiency of liver and kidney.

鲜奶玉露
Xiannai Yulu
Fresh Milk Jade Dew

【药物组成】 牛奶 1000 g,炸胡桃仁 40 g,生胡桃仁 20 g,粳米 50 g。粳米淘净,用水浸泡 1 h,捞起沥干水分,将四物放在一起搅拌均匀,用小石磨磨细,再用细筛滤出细茸待用。锅内加水煮沸,将牛奶胡桃茸慢慢倒入锅内,边倒边搅拌,稍沸即成。早晚服食,连服 3~4 周。

【Composition】 1000 g Milk,40 g fried walnut kernel,20 g fresh walnut kernel,50 g

Jingmi(Non-glutinous rice). Wash and soak non-glutinous rice in water for an hour, fish out and drain off the water. Mix these drugs thoroughly and grind them with stone mill, filter out the minced drugs with fine screen. Boil some water in the pot, put in the milk and minced drugs while stirring; turn off the fire when it's boiled. Take in the moring and at night for 3 ~ 4 weeks repeatedly.

【功效】 补脾益肾,温阳滋阴。

【Efficacy】 Tonifying spleen and benefiting kidney, warming yang and nourishing yin.

【适应证】 小溲频数,混浊如膏者。

【Indication】 Frequent urination with turbid urine like paste.

脂肪肝病 Fatty Liver Disease

何首乌粥
Heshouwu Zhou
Fleece-Flower Root Porridge

【药物组成】 何首乌 20 g,粳米 50 g,大枣 2 枚。将何首乌洗净晒干,打碎备用,再将粳米、红枣加清水 600 mL,放入锅内煮成稀粥,兑入何首乌末搅匀,文火煮数沸,早晨空腹温热服食。

【Composition】 20 g Heshouwu(Fleece-flower root), 50 g Jingmi(Non-glutinous rice), 2 jujubes. Get fleece-flower root washed and dried in the sun, grind into pieces. Decoct non-glutinous rice and jujube with 600 mL water in the pot to make porridge, add fleece-flower root powder, boiled with slow fire. Take warmed in the morning with empty stomach.

【功效】 益气健脾,活血化瘀。

【Efficacy】 Nourishing qi to invigorate spleen, activating blood circulation to dissipate blood stasis.

【适应证】 脂肪肝患者伴脾胃虚弱者。

【Indication】 Fatty liver with deficiency and weakness in spleen and stomach.

赤小豆鲤鱼汤
Chixiaodou Liyu Tang
Soup of Red Bean and Carp

【药物组成】 赤小豆 150 g,鲤鱼 1 条(约 500 g),玫瑰花 6 g。将鲤鱼活杀去肠杂,与余两味加水适量,共煮至烂熟。去花调味,分 2 ~ 3 次服食。

【Composition】 150 g red bean, a carp(about 500 g), 6 g rose flower. Kill the live fish and remove the internal organs, add some water and boil it with the other two drugs until they become tender. Remove the rose flower and take it for 2 ~ 3 times.

【功效】 清热利湿。

【Efficacy】　Clearing away the heat to reduce dampness through diuresis.

【适应证】　脂肪肝患者伴腹胀明显者。

【Indication】　Fatty liver with obvious abdominal distention.

灵芝河蚌
Lingzhi Hebang
Glossy Ganodermaand Freshwater Mussel

【药物组成】　煮冰糖取灵芝 20 g,蚌肉 250 g,冰糖 60 g。将河蚌去壳取肉,用清水洗净待用。灵芝入砂锅加水煎煮约 1 h,取浓汁加入蚌肉再煮,放入冰糖,待溶化即成,饮汤吃肉。

【Composition】　Take 20 g Lingzhi(Glossy ganoderma),250 g freshwater mussel,60 g crystal sugar. Take the meat and remove the shell of freshwater mussel,washed with water. Decoct glossy ganoderma with water in earthern pot for an hour,take the juice and put mussel meat in the pot to boil again,put in crystal sugar and turn off the fire after it is melt. Drink the soup and eat the meat.

【功效】　补气清肝,化瘀除湿。

【Efficacy】　Invigorating qi and clearing liver, dissolving stasis and eliminating dampness.

【适应证】　脂肪肝患者伴气虚者。

【Indication】　Fatty liver with qi deficiency.

兔肉煨山药
Turou Wei Shanyao
Rabbit Meat Stew Common Yam Rhizome

【药物组成】　取兔肉 500 g,怀山药 50 g,盐少许。将兔肉洗净切块,与怀山药共煮,沸后改用文火煨,直至烂熟,饮汤吃肉。

【Composition】　Take 500 g rabbit meat,50 g Huai Shanyao(Common yam rhizome),a little salt. Wash and cut up the rabbit meat into pieces,decoct with common yam rhizome,use slow fire after it is boiled,decoct until it is well-done,drink the juice and eat the meat.

【功效】　健脾益气,开胃。

【Efficacy】　Strengthening spleen and benefiting qi,promoting appetite.

【适应证】　脂肪肝伴食欲不振明显者。

【Indication】　Fatty liver with obvious poor appetite.

肥胖病 Obesity

菊楂决明饮汤
JuZha Jueming Yin Tang
Chrysanthemum, Hawthorn Fruit and Cassia Seed Decoction

【药物组成】 菊花 10 g,生山楂片 15 g,草决明子 15 g。将草决明子打碎,与菊花、生山楂片共放锅中,水煎代茶饮。每日 1 剂,代茶频饮。

【Composition】 10 g chrysanthemum, 15 g fresh Shanzha(Hawthorn fruit)slice, 15 g Caojuemingzi (Cassia seed). Grind cassia seed and decoct with chrysanthemum and fresh hawthorn fruit in the pot, take the juice as tea. Take one dose a day and take constantly.

【功效】 活血化瘀,降脂减肥。

【Efficacy】 Activating blood circulation to dissipate blood stasis, reducing fat to lose weight.

【适应证】 气滞血瘀型肥胖症。

【Indication】 Obesity with qi-stagnancy and blood stasis.

降脂饮
Jiangzhi Yin
Lipid-Decreasing Decoction

【药物组成】 枸杞子 10 g,首乌 15 g,草决明 15 g,山楂 15 g,丹参 20 g。上药共放砂锅中,加水适量以文火煎煮,取汁约 1500 mL,储于保温瓶中。

【Composition】 10 g Gouqizi (Chinese wolfberry fruit), 15 g Shouwu (fleece-flower root), 15 g Caojueming(Cassia seed), 15 g Shanzha(Howkthon fruit), 20 g Danshen(Red sage root). Decoct these drugs in earthen pot with proper amount of water and slow fire, get about 1500 mL juice, installed in thermos.

【功效】 活血化瘀,轻身减肥。

【Efficacy】 Activating blood circulation to dissipate blood stasis, losing weight.

【适应证】 形体肥胖,头晕头痛,胸痛胸闷,两胁胀痛,走窜疼痛者。

【Indication】 Obesity with dizziness and pain in head, pain and oppression in chest, and moving pain in both flanks.

减肥茶
Jianfei Cha
Weight-loss Tea

【药物组成】 干荷叶 60 g,生山楂 10 g,生薏米 10 g,橘皮 5 g。上药共制细末,混合,放入热水瓶中,用沸水冲泡即可。每日 1 剂,不拘时代茶饮。

【Composition】 60 g dried lotus leaf, 10 g fresh Shanzha (Howkthon fruit), 10 g fresh Yimi (Coix seed), 5 g orange peel. Grind these drugs into fine powder, installed in thermos. Brew with boiling water. Take one dose a day as tea at any time.

【功效】 理气行水,降脂化浊。

【Efficacy】 Regulating qi and moving water, reducing fat and eliminating the turbid.

【适应证】 体形肥胖,气短,神疲,痰多而黏稠,胸脘痞闷者。

【Indication】 Obesity, short breath, spiritlessness, excessive thick phlegm, distention and oppression in chest and gastric cavity.

三花减肥茶
Sanhua Jianfei Cha
Three Flowers Weight-loss Tea

【药物组成】 玫瑰花、玳玳花、茉莉花、川芎、荷叶各等份。将上药切碎,共研粗末,用滤泡纸袋分装,每袋 3～5 g。每日 1 小袋,放置茶杯中,用沸水冲泡 10 min 后,代茶饮服。

【Composition】 Take rose flower, Daidai Hua (Sour orange flower), jasmine flower, Chuanxiong (Sichuan lovage rhizome) and lotus leaf for the same amount. Chop them into pieces and grind into coarse powder. Devide and wrap them up with follicular bags, 3～5 g each bag. Take one bag a day, install it in a cup and brew with boiling water for 10 minute, take as tea.

【功效】 宽胸理气,利湿化痰,降脂减肥。

【Efficacy】 Relaxing chest and regulating qi, reducing dampness through diuresis and dissolving phlegm, reducing fat to lose weight.

【适应证】 形体肥胖,面赤或见粉刺痤疮,烦渴引饮不止,食纳超常者。

【Indication】 Obesity, reddish complexion with acnes, excessive thirst and drinking, over eating.

什锦乌龙粥
Shijin Wulong Zhou
Porridgeof Mixed Drugs and Oolong Tea

【药物组成】 生薏米 30 g,冬瓜仁 100 g,红小豆 20 g。干荷叶、乌龙茶适量。干荷叶、乌龙茶用粗纱布包好备用。将生薏米、冬瓜仁、红小豆洗净一起放锅内加水煮熬至熟,再放入用粗纱布包好的干荷叶及乌龙茶再煎 7～8 min,取出纱布包即可食用。每日早晚食用。

【Composition】 30 g Fresh Yimi (Coix seed), 100 g Chinese waxgourd seed, 20 g red bean, proper amount of dried lotus and oolong tea. Wrap dried lotus and oolong tea with coarse gauze. Wash fresh coix seed, Chinese waxgourd seed and red bean and put them in pot, decoct them with water until it's well-done, then put lotus leaf and oolong tea in it and decoct for 7～8 minutes. Fish out the mesh gauze parcel. Take in the morning and at night.

【功效】 健脾利湿。

【Efficacy】 Strengthening spleen to reduce dampness through diuresis.

【适应证】 痰湿困脾型肥胖症者。

【Indication】 Obesity due to phlegmatic dampness in spleen.

乌龙茶
Wulong Cha
Oolong Tea

【药物组成】 乌龙茶 3 g;槐角 18 g,首乌 30 g,冬瓜皮 18 g,山楂肉 15 g。先将槐角、首乌、冬瓜皮、山楂肉四味加适量清水煎沸 20 min,取药汁冲泡乌龙茶即成。每日 1 剂,不拘时饮服。

【Composition】 3 g oolong tea, 18 g Huaijiao (Sophora fruit), 30 g Shouwu (Fleece-flower root), 18 g Chinese waxgourd peel, Shanzha Rou (Hawkthorn pulp) 15 g. Decoct sophora fruit, fleece-flower root, Chinese waxgourd peel and hawkthon pulp with proper amount of water for 20 minutes, take the juice to brew oolong tea. Take one dose a day at any time.

【功效】 消脂减肥,健身益寿。

【Efficacy】 Reducing fat to lose weight, keeping fitness to lengthen lives.

【适应证】 体形肥胖,痰多而黏稠,胸脘痞闷,身重嗜睡者。

【Indication】 Obesity, excessive thick phlegm, distention and oppression in chest and gastric cavity, drowsiness.

雪羹萝卜汤
Xuegeng Luobo Tang
White Radish Soup

【药物组成】 荸荠 30 g,白萝卜 30 g,海蜇 30 g。三者切碎块,文火煮 1 h 至三者均烂即可。可随意食之。

【Composition】 30 g Biqi (Water chestnut), 30 g white radish, 30 g jellyfish, chop these into pieces, decoct for an hour until it's tender. Take as one prefers.

【功效】 清热化痰,利湿通便。

【Efficacy】 Clear away heat to dissolve phlegm, reducing dampness through diuresis.

【适应证】 脾胃热盛型肥胖症者。

【Indication】 Obesity due to excessive heat in spleen and stomach.

甲状腺功能亢进病 Thyroid function hyperfunction sickness

佛手粥
Foshou Zhou
Finger Citron Porridge

【药物组成】 佛手 9 g,海藻 15 g,粳米 60 g,红糖适量。将佛手、海藻用适量水煎汁去渣后,再加入粳米、红糖煮成粥即成。每日 1 剂,连服 10 ~ 15 d。

【Composition】 9 g Foshou(Finger citron),15 g kelp,60 g Jingmi(non-glutinous rice) and proper amount of brown sugar. Decoct finger citron and varech with proper amount of water and remove the dregs,add non-glutinous rice and brown sugar to cook porridge. Take one dose a day and take for 10 ~ 15 days repeatedly.

【功效】 疏肝清热,理气解郁。

【Efficacy】 Soothing liver and clearing heat,regulating qi to reduce stagnation.

【适应证】 甲状腺功能亢进者。

【Indication】 Hyperthyroidism.

昆布海藻饮
Kunbu Haizao Yin
Tangle and Kelp Decoction

【药物组成】 昆布、海藻、牡蛎用水煎汁。每日 1 次,连服数日。

【Composition】 Boil tangle,kelp and oyster with water to get the juice. Take once a day and take repeatedly for several days.

【功效】 疏肝清热,理气解郁。

【Efficacy】 Soothing liver and clearing heat,regulating qi to reduce stagnation.

【适应证】 甲状腺功能亢进者。

【Indication】 Hyperthyroidism.

青柿子羹
Qing Shizi Geng
Green Persimmon Soup

【药物组成】 青柿子 1000 g,蜂蜜适量。青柿子去柄洗净,捣烂并绞成汁,放锅中煎煮浓缩至黏稠,再加入蜂蜜 1 倍,继续煎至黏稠时,离火冷却、装瓶备。

每日 2 次,每次 1 汤匙,以沸水冲服,连服 10 ~ 15 d。

【Composition】 1000 g green persimmon,proper amount of honey. Wash the persimmon and remove its petiole,grind and mince it into juice,decoct it in the pot until it's thick,add honey with the same amount;decoct it until it's thick again. Turn off the fire and cool it down. Put it in bottle and take twice a day with one spoon once. Take with boiled water. Take for 10 ~ 15 days repeatedly.

【功效】 清热泻火。

【Efficacy】 Clearing heat to reduce fire.

【适应证】 甲状腺功能亢进伴烦躁不安、性急易怒、面部烘热者。

【Indication】 Hyperthyroidism with restlessness,hastiness and irritability,baking heat in face.

川贝海带粥
Chuanbei Haidai Zhou
PorridgeCirrhosae and Kelp

【药物组成】 川贝、海带、丹参各 15 g,薏米 30 g,冬瓜 60 g,红糖适量。川贝、丹参先煎汤后去渣,入其他味煮粥吃。每日晨起空腹温服,连服 15～20 d。

【Composition】 15 g Chuanbei(Cirrhosae),15 g kelp,15 g Danshen(Red sage root),30 g Yimi(Coix seed),60 g Chinese waxgourd,proper amount of brown sugar. Decoct cirrhosae and red sage root,remove the dregs and add the rest drugs,cook the porridge. Take warmed in the morning with empty stomach. Take for 15～20 days repeatedly.

【功效】 消痰软坚,健脾利湿。

【Efficacy】 Dispelling phlegm to soften abdominal mass,strengthening spleen to reduce dampness through diuresis.

【适应证】 甲状腺功能亢伴颈部肿大、恶心、便溏者。

【Indication】 Hyperthyroidism with deroncus,sickness and loose stool.

其他杂病
Other miscellaneous disease

疲劳 Fatigue

生脉补气汤
Shengmai Buqi Tang
Pulse-promoting and Qi-Invigorating Soup

【药物组成】 党参10 g,桂圆3 g。

【Composition】 10 g Dangshen(Tangshen),3 g longan.

【功效】 益气健脾。

【Efficacy】 Nourishing qi to invigorate spleen.

【适应证】 亚健康患者。

【Indication】 Subhealth.

失眠 Isomnia

三味安眠汤
Sanwei Anmian Tang
Three-drugs Sleeping Soup

【药物组成】 酸枣仁15 g,麦门冬、远志各5 g。

【Composition】 15 g wild jujude seed,5 g Maimen Dong,5 g Yuanzhi(milkwort root).

【功效】 滋阴安神。

【Efficacy】 Nourishing yin and calming nerves.

【适应证】 入睡困难者。

【Indication】 Difficulty in falling asleep.

百合柏仁汤
Baihe Bairen Tang
Decoction of Lily bulb and Arborvitate Seed

【药物组成】 百合 20 g,夏枯草 15 g,柏子仁 10 g,蜂蜜适量。

【Composition】 20 g Lily bulb,15 g Xiakucao(Self heal),10 g Baiziren(Arborvitate seed),proper amount of honey.

【功效】 清泄肝火,养心安神。

【Efficacy】 Clearing and dispersing liver fire,tranquilizing by nourishing the heart.

【适应证】 肝火上攻引起的烦躁易怒失眠者。

【Indication】 Insomnia with restlessness and irritability due to liver fire going upward.

生地黄粥
Shengdihuang Zhou
Dried Rehamnnia Root Porridge

【药物组成】 生地黄汁 30 mL,酸枣仁 60 g,大米 150 g。

【Composition】 30 mL Sheng Dihuang juice(Dried rehamnnia root),60 g wild jujude seed,150 g rice.

【功效】 补养心血,滋阴宁神。

【Efficacy】 Tonifying or nourishing heart blood,nourishing yin and calming nerves.

【适应证】 四肢无力,心烦不得卧者。

【Indication】 Weakness in limbs and restlessness,being reluctant to take a rest.

莲肉龙眼饮
Lianrou Longyan Yin
Decoction of Lotus Seed Pulp and Longan Aril

【药物组成】 莲子肉 9 g,龙眼肉 15 g,百合 12 g,五味子 9 g。

【Composition】 9 g Lotus seed pulp,15 g Longan aril,12 g lily bulb,9 g Wuweizi(Chinese magnoliavine fruit).

【功效】 安神宁心。

【Efficacy】 Calming nerves and tranquilizing heart.

【适应证】 心阴虚所致的失眠。

【Indication】 Insomnia caused by heart yin deficiency.

百合枣仁饮
Baihe ZaorenYin
Decoction of Lily Bulb and Wild Jujube Seed

【药物组成】 百合 400 g,酸枣仁 20 g。

【功效】 养血安神。

【Efficacy】 Nourishing blood and calming nerves.

【适应证】 血虚引起的失眠。

【Indication】 Insomnia due to blood deficiency.

人参粥
Renshen Zhou
Ginseng Porridge

【药物组成】 人参 3 g,大米 100 g,冰糖适量。将人参研为细末备用。先取大米煮粥,待熟时调入人参末、冰糖,再煮一二沸即成。

【Composition】 3 g Renshen(Ginseng),100 g rice,proper amount of crystal sugar. Grind ginseng into fine powder for backup. Cook porridge with rice and add ginseng and crystal sugar when it's well-done,get boiled again for a short while.

【功效】 健脾益气。

【Efficacy】 Strengthening spleen and benefiting qi.

【适应证】 适用于脾胃亏虚所致的心悸、健忘等。

【Indication】 Palpitation and forgetfulness due to deficiency and consumption of spleen and stomach.

口腔溃疡 Mouth ulcer

乌梅生地绿豆糕
Wumei Shengdi Lùdou
Dark Plum,Dried/Fresh Rehmannia Rootand Mung Bean Candy

【药物组成】 乌梅 50 g,生地 30 g,绿豆 500 g,豆沙 250 g。将乌梅用沸水浸泡 3 min,取出切成小丁或片。生地切细,与乌梅拌匀。绿豆用沸水烫后,放在淘箩里擦去外皮,并用清水漂去。将绿豆放在钵内,加清水上蒸笼蒸 3 h,待酥透后取出,除去水分,在筛上擦成绿豆沙。将特制的木框放在案板上,衬以白纸一张,先放一半绿豆沙,铺均匀,撒上乌梅、生地,中间铺一层豆沙,再将其余的绿豆沙铺上,揿结实,最后把白糖撒在表面。把糕切成小方块。作点心吃。

【Composition】 50 g Wumei(Dark plum fruit),30 g Shengdi(Dried/fresh rehmannia root),500 g mung bean,250 g bean paste. Soak dark plum fruit in hot water for 3 minute,fish out and cut into pieces. Slice dried/fresh rehmannia root,mix with dark plum fruit thoroughly. Heat up mung bean in hot water,rub the peel in basket,rinse out the peel with water. Steam the mung bean in steamer for 3 hours,take out after it's well-done. Get rid of the water in the mung bean and grind it into paste. Put a piece of paper on the breadboard,get a special wooden-frame on the paper. Spread half of the mung bean paste thoroughly,then dark plum fruit and dried/fresh rehmannia root, then add the rest bean paste. Press it into solid, spread sugar on the suface. Cut the candy into pieces and take as dim sum.

【功效】 滋阴清热,解毒敛疮。

【Efficacy】 Nourishing yin and clearing heat, detoxication and astringing sores.

【适应证】 口腔溃疡周围黏膜淡红,疼痛轻微者。

【Indication】 Mouth ulcer with reddish mucous membrane and little pain.

耳鸣、耳聋 Tinnitus and Deaf

黄精聪耳粥
Huangjing Conger Zhou
Rhizome of king solomonseal Audition-improving Porridge

【药物组成】 黄精 15 g,茯苓 15 g,葛根 10 g,糯米 150 g。将上四味加水浸泡 30 min,用文火煮成粥。早晚分食。

【Composition】 15 g Huangjing (Rhizome of king solomonseal), 15 g Fuling (Tuckahoe), 10 g Gegen (Kudzuvine root), 150 g Sticky rice. Soak these drugs with water for 30 g, boil with slow fire into porridge. Take in the morning and at night.

【功效】 健脾益气,升阳聪耳。

【Efficacy】 Strengthening spleen and benefiting qi, ascending yang and making ears sensitive.

【适应证】 耳鸣、耳聋,劳而更甚,或在蹲下站起时较甚,耳内有空虚感觉,倦怠乏力,纳少,食后腹胀,大便时溏,面色萎黄者。

【Indication】 Tinnitus and deaf, being more serious while laboring or standing up, usually accompanied by powerlessness, poor eating, distention in abdomen after eating, loose stool and yellowish complexion.

胡桃芝麻糊
Hutao Zhima Hu
Paste of Walnut Kernel and Black Sesame

【药物组成】 胡桃仁 12 g,黑芝麻 30 g,面粉 30 g. 。先将胡桃仁、黑芝麻分别碾碎;另将面粉放在锅内炒熟,最后将胡桃仁、黑芝麻、面粉及白糖下起搅拌均匀即可。每日 1 次,用时以少量开水冲泡成糊状。

【Composition】 .12 g walnut kernel, 30 g black sesame, 30 g wheat flour. Grind walnut kernel and black sesame, fry wheat flour thoroughly, mix walnut kernel, black sesame and sugar. Brew the drug with a little hot water into paste. Take one dose a day.

【功效】 滋阴养血,补肾聪耳。

【Efficacy】 Nourishing yin and blood, tonifying kidney and making ears more sensitive.

【适应证】 肾虚亏损之耳鸣、耳聋者。

【Indication】 Tinnitus and deaf due to deficiency and consumption of kidney.

红枸杞红花酒
Honggouqi Honghua Jiu
Chinese Wolfberry Fruit and Safflower Wine

【药物组成】 枸杞子 50 g,红花 20 g,低度白酒 300 ml。将红花、枸杞子一同浸泡于白酒内,1 个月后即可。随量饮用。

【Composition】 50 g Gouqizi(Chinese wolfberry fruit),20 g Honghua(Safflower),300 ml Low-alcohol liquor. Soak safflower and Chinese wolfberry fruit in the liquor for a month. Take with proper amount.

【功效】 养血活血,通窍聪耳。

【Efficacy】 Nourishing blood and promoting blood circulation,getting through orifices to make ears more sensitive.

【适应证】 肾精亏损型耳鸣、耳聋者。

【Indication】 Tinnitus and deaf due to damage of kidney-essence.

枸杞蒸鸡
Gouqi Zhengji
Chicken Steamedwith Chinese wolfberry fruit

【药物组成】 枸杞子 30 g,山茱萸 15 g,嫩鸡半只(约 600 g),香肠 50 g。将香肠切片,鸡剁成 3 厘米见方的鸡块,加入酱油、蚝油、食油、料酒、白糖、生粉、食盐、麻油、胡椒粉拌匀,腌渍 15 min。把枸杞子、山茱萸、香肠片、姜片与鸡块拌匀,放在盆内,加盖进入微波炉,用高功率火转 8 min。取出,翻动一下鸡块,撒少许葱段,再转 1 min 即可。佐餐食用。

【Composition】 30 g Gouqizi(Chinese wolfberry fruit),15 g Shan Zhuyu(Dogwood),half young chicken(about 600 g),50 g sausage. Slice the sausage,and cut the chicken into pieces of 3 cm square,mix with some soy sauce,oyster juice,oil,cooking wine,sugar,starch,salt,peppermint oil;sesame oil and pepper powder for 15 minutes. Mix Chinese wolfberry fruit,Dogwood,sausage slice,ginger slices and chicken throughly and put them in a basin with a cover. Cook in the microwave oven with high power for 8 eights. Take out the basin, stir the chicken and sprinkle a few green onion pieces on it. Cook for one more minute in the oven. Take together with rice or bread.

【功效】 养阴补肾,通窍聪耳。

【Efficacy】 Nourishing yin to supplement kidney,getting through orifices to make ears more sensitive.

【适应证】 耳鸣、耳聋以耳内常闻蝉鸣之声,由微渐重,夜间较甚,以致虚烦失眠,听力渐减者。

【Indication】 Tinnitus, deaf or cicada sound in the ears, being worse at night, causing insomnia and decrease of hearing.

生地青梅饮
Shengdi Qingmei Yin
Decoction of Dried/Fresh Rehmannia Root and Green Plums

【药物组成】 生地15 g,石斛10 g,甘草2 g,青梅30 g。将生地、石斛、甘草、青梅加水适量,同煮20 min,去渣取汁。每日1剂,分2~3次饮服,可连用数日。

【Composition】 15 g Shengdi (Dried/fresh rehmannia root), 10 g Shihu (Dendrobium stem), 2 g Gancao (Liquorice root), 30 g green plums. Boil Shengdi (dried/fresh rehmannia root), Shihu (Dendrobium stem), Gancao (Liquorice root) and green plums with proper amount of water for 20 minutes, remove the dregs and take the juice. Take one dose a day for 2~3 times. Take for several days repeatedly.

【功效】 养阴清热,降火敛疮。

【Efficacy】 Eliminating heat by nourishing yin, reducing fire and astringing sores.

【适应证】 口腔溃疡属于阴虚火旺者。

【Indication】 Mouth ulcer due to excessive fire caused by deficiency yin.

竹茹陈皮粥
Zhuru Chenpi Zhou
Porridge of Bamboo Shavings and Dried Orange Peel

【药物组成】 竹茹10 g,陈皮10 g,粳米50 g。陈皮切细丝备用;竹茹加水煎煮,去渣取汁,用其汁与粳米一起煮粥,待粥将成时,倒入陈皮丝,稍煮即可。早晚分食。

【Composition】 10 g Zhuru (Bamboo shavings), 10 g Chenpi (Dried orange peel), 50 g Jingmi (Non-glutinous rice). Slice the dried orange peel, boil bamboo shavings with water and take the juice, mix the juice with non-glutinous rice and boil for porridge. Add dried orange peel slices before its done, boil a little bit. Divide it into two parts, take in the morning and at night.

【功效】 清热化痰,和胃除烦。

【Efficacy】 Eliminating phlegm by clearing heat, regulating stomach to eliminate restlessness.

【适应证】 痰火郁结型耳鸣、耳聋患者。

【Indication】 Tinnitus and deaf due to stagnation of phlegmatic fire.

芹菜粥
Qincai Zhou
Celery Porridge

【药物组成】 连根芹菜120 g,粳米250 g。芹菜洗净,切碎,与粳米一起加水适量煮粥。早晚分食,每日 1 剂,连用数剂。

【Composition】 120 g celery with root, 250 g Jingmi (Non–glutinous rice). Wash and cup up the celery, boil with non–glutinous rice for porridge. Divide one dose into two parts, take in the morning and at night. Take repeatedly for several days.

【功效】 清肝泻火。

【Efficacy】 Clearing liver to reduce fire.

【适应证】 耳鸣如闻潮声,或如风雷声,耳聋时轻时重,每于郁怒后耳鸣、耳聋突发性加重者。

【Indication】 Tinnitus, being like the sound of tides or the sounds of wind and thunder, being worse after anger.

栀子窝头
Zhizi Wuotou
CapeJasmine Fruit Bun

【药物组成】 细玉米面 500 g,黄豆粉 150 g,白糖 200 g,桂花酱 5 g,栀子粉 25 g。将以上五物倒在一起拌匀,加温水适量和成面团,揉匀后,搓成圆条,再揪成 50 g1 个的小面团,制成小窝头,上屉用旺火蒸熟。早晚作主食。

【Composition】 500 g Fine corn powder, 150 g soybean powder, 200 g sugar, 5 g Guihua (Sweet osmanthus flower) jam, 25 g Zhizi (Cape jasmine fruit) powder. Mix these drugs throughly and make dough with proper amount of warm water, knead the dough throughly and make it into strips, then small doughs 50 g each. Make buns by steaming with roaring fire. Take as main meal for breakfast or supper.

【功效】 清心泻肝,解毒。

【Efficacy】 Clearing heart and liver, detoxication.

【适应证】 肝火上扰型耳鸣、耳聋者。

【Indication】 Tinnitus and deaf due to disturbing upward of liver–fire.

皮肤病 Skin Disease

茅根绿豆饮
Maogen Lùdou Yin
Decoctionof Couchgrass Root and Mung Bean

【药物组成】 鲜茅根 30 g,绿豆 50 g,泽泻 15 g,冰糖 20 g。白茅根切段,与泽泻一起先煮 20 min,捞去药渣,再入绿豆、冰糖,煮至绿豆开花蜕皮后,过滤去渣取汁。每日 1 剂,温饮药汁。

【Composition】 30 g Fresh Maogen(Couchgrass root), 50 g mung bean, 15 g Zexie(Alismatis), 20 g crystal sugar. Cut Couchgrass root into pieces and boiled with alismatis for 20 minutes. Fish up the dregs and add mung bean, crystal sugar, boiled until the mungbean is well –done. Remove the dregs and take the juice. Take one dose a day with the juice warmed.

【功效】 清热除湿,凉血解毒。

【Efficacy】 Clearing heat and eliminating dampness, cooling blood for detoxication.

【适应证】 皮肤瘙痒,红斑迭起,粟疹攒聚,水疱丛生,湿烂,基底鲜红者。

【Indication】 Itching skin, excessive erythema, miliaria, blister everywhere, dampness and rottenness with bright red flesh.

绿豆海带汤
Lǜ dou Haidai Tang
Soup of Mung Bean and Kelp

【药物组成】 绿豆 30 g,海带 30 g,鱼腥草 15 g,薏米 30 g,冰糖适量。将海带切丝,鱼腥草布包,与绿豆、薏米同放锅中煎煮,至海带烂、绿豆开花时取出鱼腥草。食用前用白糖调味。每日 1 剂,连用 10 日。

【Composition】 30 g Mung bean, 30 g kelp, 15 g Yuxing Cao (Heartleaf Houttuynia), 30 g Yimi (Coix seed), proper amount of crystal sugar. Slice the kelp and wrap the Heartleaf Houttuynia with cloth, decocted with mung bean and Coix seed. Take out of Heartleaf Houttuynia when mung bean and Coix seed are thoroughly cooked. Mix with sugar before eating. Take one dose a day and take 10 days repeatedly.

【功效】 清热除湿止痒。

【Efficacy】 Clearing heat, eliminating dampness and relieving itching.

【适应证】 湿热蕴结型湿疹者。

【Indication】 Eczema due to accumulation or stagnation of damp heat.

未病先防 Preventive Treatment of Disease

菊黄银花汤
Juhuang Yinhua Tang
Decoctionof Kalimeris, Rhizome of King Solomonseal Leaf and Honeysuckle

【药物组成】 田边菊、黄荆叶、金银花藤各 9 g。

【Composition】 9 g Tianbian Ju (Kalimeris), 9 g Huangjingye (Rhizome of king solomonseal leaf), 9 g Jinyinhua (Honeysuckle).

【功效】 清热解毒。

【Efficacy】 clearing away the heat–evil and expelling superficial evils.

【适应证】 流行性感冒者。

【Indication】 Influenza.

犁头草合剂
Litoucao Heji
Viola bisseti Maxim Mixture

【药物组成】 犁头草、忍冬藤、车前草各 15 g。

【Composition】 15 g Litoucao (Viola bisseti maxim) , 15 g Rendongteng (Honeysuckle stem) , 15 g Cheqiancao (Plantain herb) .

【功效】 解毒透疹。

【Efficacy】 Detoxication and promoting eruptions.

【适应证】 预防麻疹。

【Indication】 Preventing measles.

大青连根汤
Daqing Liangen Tang
Decoctionof Dyers Wood Leaf , Weeping Forsythia Capsule and Isatis

【药物组成】 大青叶、连翘、板蓝根各 9 g。

【Composition】 9 g Daqingye (Dyers woad leaf) , 9 g Lianqiao (Weeping forsythia capsule) , 9 g Banlangen (Isatis) .

【功效】 解毒透疹。

【Efficacy】 Detoxication and promoting eruptions.

【适应证】 预防麻疹。

【Indication】 Preventing measles.

大青二花汤
Daqing Erhua Tang
Decoction of Dyers Wood Leaf and Two Flowers

【药物组成】 大青叶 15 g,金银花、野菊花各 9 g。

【Composition】 15 g Daqingye (Dyers woad leaf) , 9 g Jinyinhua (Honeysuckle) , 9 g wild chrysanthemum.

【功效】 清热解毒。

【Efficacy】 Clearing away the heat-evil and expelling superficial evils.

【适应证】 预防痄腮(流行性腮腺炎)。

【Indication】 Epidemic parotitis.

清凉饮汤
Qingliang Yintang
Cool and Refreshing Decoction

【药物组成】 荷叶、白茅根各 2500 g,桑叶、香薷、淡竹叶、夏枯草各 1260 g,青蒿、薄荷各 500 g。将各药切细混匀,按 1∶1 比例制成合剂,加红糖适量,并加防腐剂备用,每服 80 ml,日服 2～3 次。

【Composition】　2500 g Lotus leaf, 2500 g Baimaogen (Cogongras rhizome), 1260 g Sangye (Mulberry leaf), 1260 g Xiangru (Herba Moslae), 1260 g Danzhuye (Lophatherum herb), 1260 g Xiakucao (Self heal), 500 g Qinghao (Artemisia Selengensis0, 1260 g mint. Chop up these drugs and mix them with the same amount each, adding proper amount of brown sugar and preservative. Take 80 ml one dose, 2～3 times a day.

【功效】　清热,除烦,祛暑。

【Efficacy】　Clearing heat, eliminating restlessness, dispelling summer heat.

【适应证】　预防中暑。

【Indication】　Preventing heat stroke.

历代医方的养生方摘录
Excerpt of Medical Prescription of Past dynasties in Health Preserving

十精丸
Shijing Wan
Ten Essential Substances Pill

【方剂出处】　《普济方》,方名十精者,是言此十种药物乃天、地,人、日,月,山、石,水、草、药之精华。本方为唐,宋代以后的延年益寿的代表方。

【Source of Prescription】　"Universal Relief Prescription", the name ten essential substances refers this 10 drugs are the essence of the sky, earth, people, sun, moon, mountain, stone, water, grass and drug. This prescription is on behalf of the longevity prescription of the Tang and Song Dynasty.

【药物组成】　枸杞子,熟地黄、桂心木、菊花、山茱萸,菟丝子、肉苁蓉、汉椒,柏子仁、白茯苓各等分,共碾为极细末,酒糊为丸,如梧桐子大。每服 30 丸,空心温酒送下,盐汤亦可,妇人醋汤服。

【Composition】　Gouqizi (Chinese wolfberry fruit), Shu Dihuang (prepared rehmannia root), Guixinmu, chryanthemum flower, Shanzhuyu (Dogwood), Tushizi (Dodder), Roucongrong (Cistanche), Han pepper, Baiziren (Arborvitate seed), Bai Fuling (White tuckahoe) each with same amount, grinded into fine powder, mix some wine to make pill as the size of Wutong Zi (Phoenix tree seed). Take 30 pills once with warm wine and empty stomach, or with salt soup; woman with vinegar soup.

【功效】　温肾助阳,滋精填髓,养心益智,疏风明目。

【Efficacy】　Warming kidney and activating yang, nourishing essence and replenishing marrow, nourishing heart to develop intelligence or wisdom, dispelling wind and brightening eyes.

【适应证】 中老年人肾阳不足,精神衰减,须发早白,头昏目眩,健忘失眠者。久服可使头白返黑,面如童颜,四肢轻健。

【Indication】 Syndromes of the old such as insufficiency of kidney-yang, decrease of spirit, early-white beard and hair, lightheadedness or dizziness, forgetfulness and insomnia. Long-term dose can blacken hair, make complexion childlike and limbs brisk and vigorous.

八仙茶
Baxian Cha
The Eight Immortals Tea

【方剂出处】 《韩氏医通》

【Source of Prescription】 Hanshi Yitong; Han's Clear View of Medicine

【药物组成】 粳米,黄粟米,黄豆,赤小豆,绿豆各750 g,细茶500 g,净芝麻375 g,净花椒75 g,净小茴香150 g,泡干白姜,炒白盐各30 g。先将粳米等前5味炒香熟,然后共研为极细粉末,和合一处,外加麦面,炒黄熟,与前11味等分拌匀,瓷坛收贮。胡桃仁、南枣、松子仁、白砂糖之类,任意加入。每服50克,一日3次,白开水冲服。

【Composition】 750 g Jingmi(Non-glutinous rice), 750 g yellow millet, 750 g soybean, 750 g red bean, 750 g green been each, 500 g tea bust, 375 g clean sesame, 75 g clean wild pepper, 150 g clean fennel, 30 g soaked dry white ginger, 30 g fried white salt. Parch the previous 5 drugs thoroughly with fragrant and grinded into fine powder, mix all the drugs with wheat powder and fried thoroughly until turned yellow. Mix well with the previous 11 drugs of equal portions and installed in porcelain bottles. Add walnut meat, South jujube and white sugar freely. Take 50 g one dose, 3 times a day with boiled water.

【功效】 益精悦颜,保元固肾。

【Efficacy】 Benefiting essence and making complexion good, sustaining primordial qi and consolidating kidney.

【适应证】 四、五十岁中寿之人延缓衰老之用,药性平和,可以常服用。

【Indication】 Delaying senility for the middle-aged with its mild drug nature.

万氏延寿丹
Wanshi Yanshou Dan
Wan'S Life-Prolonging Pill

【方剂出处】 《万氏积善堂秘验滋补诸方》

【Source of Prescription】 Wanshi Jishantang Miyan Zibu Zhufang; Wan's Jishan Tang secret tonic prescription

【药物组成】 川乌、南木香各30 g,苍术、花椒、小茴香、白茯苓各60 g。取苍术用竹刀刮去外反,花椒炒一下,小茴香微炒。上药6味,共为细末,酒糊为丸,如梧桐子大,每服80丸,温酒盐汤下,空腹服。

【Composition】 30 g Chuanwu(Prepared Sichuan aconite root), 30 g Nan Muxiang (South aucklandia root),60 g Cangzhu(Atractylodes rhizome),60 g wild pepper,60 g fennel, 60 g Bai Fuling(Tuckahoe). Scrape the skin of atractylodes rhizome with bamboo knife; fry it with wild pepper and then gently fried with fennel. Grind these 6 drugs into fine powder, wine to make pill as the size of Wutong Zi(Phoenix tree seed). Take 80 g once with warm wine or salt soup, empty stomach.

【功效】 温肾助阳,暖脾和中,兼益心智。

【Efficacy】 Warming kidney and activating yang, warming spleen and harmonizing the middle energizer, benefiting the development of intelligence and wisdom.

【适应证】 中老年人脾肾阳虚,形寒喜暖,腰膝冷痛,小便频数,夜尿频多,须发早白,精神倦怠,纳少便溏者服用。

【Indication】 Symptoms of the middle – aged and the old such as yang deficiency of spleen and kidney, cold body favoring warmth, coldness and pain in waist and knees, excessive urination and nocturia, early white beard and hair, spiritlessness, poor eating and loose stool.

无价保真丸
Wujia Baozhen Wan
Priceless Fidelity Pill

【方剂出处】 《验方新编》

【Source of Prescription】 Yanfang Xinbian; New Compilationof Proved Recipes

【药物组成】 制熟地120 g,酒浸金石斛90 g,全当归75 g,酒浸炒川芎、姜汁炒杜仲、人乳拌蒸白茯苓各45 g,酒炒甘草,酒炒金樱子,仙灵脾各30 g。以上各药俱用顶好烧酒制。杜仲另研为末,同各药末加入生白蜜共捣一千杵,丸如梧桐子大。每服10 g,空腹好酒送下。

【Composition】 120 g Prepared Shudi(Chinese foxglove),90 g wine – soaked Jin Shihu (Dendrobium stem),75 g Quan Danggui(Chinese angelica),45 g wine – soaked Chuanxiong (Sichuan lovage rhizome),45 g ginger – fried Duzhong(Bark of eucommia),45 g human milk mixed and steemed Bai Fuling(Tuckahoe),30 g wine – fried Gancao(Liquorice root),30 g wine – fried Jinyyingzi(Cherokee rose fruit),30 g XianLingpi(Epimedium). All these prepared drugs processed with wine of top quality. Grind bark of eucommia into powder, mixed with the previous drugs and raw honey, pestled one thousand times and get pills as the size of Wutong Zi (Phoenix tree seed). Take 10 g one dose with top quality wine and empty stomach.

【功效】 益精补髓,兴阳益寿。

【Efficacy】 Benefiting essence and replenishing marrow, promoting yang and lengthening life.

【适应证】 药性平和,一般人均可服用。

【Indication】 Mild drug nature for everyone.

长生神芝膏
Changsheng Shenzhi Gao
Longevity GodMagical Paste

【方剂出处】 《药酒与膏滋》

【Source of Prescription】 Yaojiu Yu Gaozi;Medicated Wine and Soft Extract

【药物组成】 白术1000 g,苍术500 g,人参90 g。前2味药,共切碎,放入坛中,用水浸一天,次日放入砂锅煎汁,共煎3次,过滤去渣,合并药汁,用小火缓缓炼之熬成膏。人参用水煎汁,煎5次,浓缩煎汁,熬膏入前膏,和匀,煎透。人参也可磨成极细粉末,和入前2味药的膏汁中,拌匀即得。瓷瓶盛贮。每服10 g,一日2次,白开水冲服,或含化均可。

【Composition】 1000 g Baizhu(Largehead atractylodes rhizome),500 g Cangzhu(Atractylodes),90 g Renshen(Ginseng). Cut up the previous two drugs and soak with water in jar for a day. Decocted in earthen pot and get the juice for 3 times,filtered and merge the juice, decocted with slow fire to get ointmen. Decoct ginseng 5 times with water and concentrated the juice. Mix and decoct the previous ointment with it thoroughly. Or grind ginseng into fine powder,mixed with the previous 2 ointment and installed in porcelain bottles. Take 10 g one dose,twice a day. Take with boiled water or melted in the mouth.

【功效】 大补元气,延缓衰老。

【Efficacy】 Replenishing primordial qi,delaying senility.

【适应证】 男女一切体虚之调理补养,凡食少倦怠,虚咳气喘,失眠健忘,少气懒言,大便溏薄均可服用,久服延缓衰老。

【Indication】 Regulating and promoting body deficiency,being used by people with poor eating and tireness,deficiency cough and asthma,insomnia and forgetfulness,short breath and being reluctant to speak,and loose stool. Long-term dose can delay senility.

周公百岁酒
Zhougong Baisui Jiu
Zhou'S One Hundred Years'Old Wine

【方剂出处】 《药方杂录》

【Source of Prescription】 Yaofang Zalu;Prescription Miscellany

【药物组成】 蜜炙黄芪、茯神各60 g,当归、熟地、生地各36 g,党参、麦冬、茯苓、白术、枣皮、川芎,炙龟板、防风、枸杞子,广陈皮各30 g,肉桂18 g,五味子、羌活各24 g,红枣,冰糖各1kg。上药共研粗末,红枣去核,浸入高粱烧酒1万克中,浸半月后服。每服20 ml,一日2次。

【Composition】 60 g Honey-prepared Huangqi(milkvetch root),60 g Fushen(Poria with hostwood),36 g Danggui(Chinese angelica),36 g Shudi(Chinese foxglove),36 g Shengdi (Dried/fresh rehmannia root),30 g Dangshen(Tangshen),30 g Maidong(Dwarf lilyturf root),

30 g Fuling(Tuckahoe),30 g Baizhu(Largehead atractylodes rhizome),30 g jujube peel,30 g Chuanxiong(Sichuan lovage rhizome),30 g Zhiguiban(Stir-baked tortoise plastron),30 g Fangfeng(Ledebouriella root),30 g Gouqizi(Chinese wolfberry fruit),30 g Guang Chenpi (Dried orange peel).18 g Rougui(Cassia bark),24 g Wuweizi(Chinese magnoliavine fruit), 24 g Qianghuo(Notopterygium),1kg red jujube and crystal sugar. Grind these drugs into coarse powder and 10000 g jujube stoned,soaked in sorghum wine for half a month. Take 20 ml one dose,twice a day.

【功效】 补气活血。

【Efficacy】 Replenishing qi and activating blood circulation.

【适应证】 一般人均可服用。

【Indication】 For everyone.

虫草酒
Chongcao Jiu
CaterpillarFungus Wine

【方剂出处】 《药补和食补》

【Source of Prescription】 Yaobu He Shibu;Drug and Diet Tonification

【药物组成】 冬虫夏草10 g。将上药共研粗末,浸500 g白酒内,半月后服。每日服 30 ml。服完后可再加入白酒500 g浸服。

【Composition】 Take 10 g Dongchong Xiacao(Caterpillar fungus),grinded into coarse powder and soaked in 500 g white wine for half a month. Take 30 g one day. Add 500 g white wine after it's finished.

【功效】 补益肾阳,滋养肺阴。

【Efficacy】 Tonifying kidney-yang,nourishing lung-yin.

【适应证】 年老体弱,慢性咳嗽气喘,咯血盗汗,贫血虚弱,阳痿遗精,老人畏寒,涕 多泪出等症。

【Indication】 Physical weakness of the aged,chronic cough and asthma,hemoptysis and night sweat,weakness due to anemia,impotence and seminal emission,chills of the old, excessive nasal discharge and tearing.

红枣膏
Hongzao Gao
Red Jujube Ointment

【方剂出处】 《药用果品》

【Source of Prescription】 Yaoyong Guopin;Medicinal Fruit

【药物组成】 大红枣500 g。将大枣去核,加水煮烂,熬成膏状,加白糖500 g,拌匀 使溶即成。每服15 g,一日2次,白开水冲服。

【Composition】 500 g Big jujube. Stone the jujube and boiled to concentrate into ointment. Mix and melt with 500 g white sugar. Take 15 g one dose, twice a day, with boiled water.

【功效】 健脾和胃,补气养血。

【Efficacy】 Strengthening the spleen and harmonizing the stomach, replenishing qi and nourishing blood.

【适应证】 中老年人脾胃虚弱,气血不足,面色萎黄,倦怠乏力,心悸健忘,失眠多梦,饮食减少,腹胀便溏,皮肤紫癜,易于出血等。

【Indication】 Syndromes of the old such as deficiency and weakness of the spleen and stomach, deficiency of qi and blood, yellowish complexion, tireness and weakness, palpitation and forgetfulness, insomnia and excessive dreaming, poor eating, distention in the abdomen and loose stool, easy bleeding of skin with purpura.

红颜酒(不老汤)
Hongyan Jiu
Beauty Wine(Immortal Soup)

【方剂出处】 《万病回春》

【Source of Prescription】 Wanbing Huichun; Curative Measures for All Diseases

【药物组成】 胡桃仁、小红枣、白蜜各 60 g,光杏仁、酥油各 30 g,白酒 1500 g。先以白蜜、酥油溶化,入酒和匀,随将其余三药研碎,入酒内,密封,浸 21 天。每次服 15 ml,一日 2 次。

【Composition】 60 g walnut meat, 60 g small jujube, 60 g white honey, 30 g apricot kernel, 30 g butter, 1500 g white wine. Melt white honey, butter and mixed them with wine. Then grind those 3 drugs into powder and sealed and soaked in the wine for 21 days. Take 15 ml one dose, twice a day.

【功效】 益气补髓,强筋健骨。

【Efficacy】 Benefiting qi and replenishing marrow, strengthening bones and muscles.

【适应证】 一般可用来防治肾虚腰痛。久服令人面色红润,壮腰健步,青春常驻,为延缓衰老和摄生保健之佳品。

【Indication】 Generally being used to treat lumbago due to deficiency of the kidney.

青娥丸
Qing'e Wan
Qing'e Pill

【方剂出处】 《和剂局方》

【Source of Prescription】 Heji Jufang; Prescription of peaceful benevolent dispensary

【药物组成】 胡桃 20 个,酒浸炒补骨脂 250 g,蒜 120 g,杜仲 100 g。将胡桃去皮膜,杜仲刮去外层粗皮,用姜汁浸炒,大蒜熬膏。上药共磨为极细末,用蒜膏为丸,每服 6 g,空腹温酒送下,妇人淡醋汤送下。

【Composition】 20 pieces of walnut, 250 g wine-soaked fried Buguzhi(Psoralen), 120 g garlic, 100 g Duzhong(Bark of eucommia). Peeled walnut and bark of eucommia, soaked and fried with ginger, decoct garlic ointmen. Grind these drugs into fine powder and mix with garlic ointment to get pill. Take 6 g one dose with warm wine and empty stomach. Woman take with light vinegar soup.

【功效】 壮筋骨,活血脉,乌须发,益颜色。

【Efficacy】 Strengthening bone and musculature, activating blood circulation, blackening beard and hair, benefiting complexion.

【适应证】 老年肾阳亏虚,腰酸膝软,久服可以延缓衰老。

【Indication】 Deficiency of kidney yang, sore waist and weak knees of the old, delaying senility with long-term doses.

刺五加酒
CiwujiaJiu
Acanthopanax Wine

【方剂出处】 《药酒与膏滋》

【Source of Prescription】 Yaojiu Yu Gaozi; Medicated Wine and Soft Extract

【药物组成】 刺五加 30 g。研成粗末,加白酒 500 g,浸泡半月后服。每服 15 ml,一日 2 次。

【Composition】 50 g Ciwujia, grinded into coarse powder, soaked in 500 g liquor for half a month. Take 15 g once, twice a day.

【功效】 益气健脾,舒筋活络。

【Efficacy】 Nourishing qi to invigorate spleen, relaxing tendons and activating meridians.

【适应证】 患有多种慢性病者服本酒后能增强体力,减轻疲劳,促进睡眠,增加食欲,提高视力和听力,故长期小剂量服用,有益于健康。

【Indication】 Increasing physical strength for those with chronic disease, recovering fatigue, promoting sleep quality, promoting appetite, improving eyesight and hearing, benefiting health with long-term doses.

参杞膏
Shenqi Gao
Ointment of Tangshen and Chinese Wolfberry

【方剂出处】 《中成药研究》

【Source of Prescription】 Zhongchengyao Yanjiu; Chinese patent medicine research

【药物组成】 党参 500 g,枸杞子 250 g。上药共研粗末,加水煎熬,过滤,共 3 次,压榨残渣,合并药液,浓缩,加炼蜜;250 g 收膏。每服 15 g,一日 2 次,白开水冲服。

【Composition】 500 g Dangshen(Tangshen), 250 g Gouqizi(Chinese wolfberry). Grind these drugs into coarse powder, decocted with water and filtered 3 times and get dregs squeezed. Merge the juice and concentrate it to 250 g to get ointment. Take 15 g one dose, twice a day with boiled water.

【功效】 补肝明目,滋肾润肺。

【Efficacy】 Tonifying liver and improving eyesight, nourishing kidney and moisturizing lung.

【适应证】 肝肾阴亏,头晕目眩,腰背酸痛等症,久服可补虚益精,延缓衰老。

【Indication】 Yin deficiency of liver and kidney, dizziness, aching pain in waist and back; improving asthenia, benefiting essence and delaying senility with long-term doses.

药酒秘方
Yaojiu Mifang
Secret Recipeof Medicated Wine

【方剂出处】 《经验良方》

【Source of Prescription】 Jingyan Liangfang; Experienced and effctive recipe

【药物组成】 生羊肾1具,沙苑蒺藜,桂圆肉,仙灵脾、仙茅、薏苡仁各120克。用低度洋河大曲2000克浸半月。随员时时饮之,以不醉为度。

【Composition】 One raw sheep kidney, 120 g Shayuan Jili (Complanate astragalus seed), 120 g longan meet, 120 g Xianlingpi (Epimedium), 120 g Xianmao (Curculigo rhizome), 120 g Yiyiren(Coix seed). Steep the drugs in 2000 g Yanghe wine for half a month. Take constantly without drunk.

【功效】 延龄益肾,乌须黑发。

【Efficacy】 Delaying senility, blackening beard and hair.

【适应证】 足痹,老年下肢酸软,腰膝酸痛,男子不育等症。

【Indication】 Pedal numbness, weakness of lower limbs, aching pain of waist and knees, intertility.

保健抗老简化方
BaojianKanglao Jianhua Fang
Health-Protectingand Anti-Ageing Simplified Priscription

【方剂出处】 《云南中医杂志》

【Source of Prescription】 Yunna Zhongyi Zazhi; Yunnan Journal of Traditional Chinese Medicine

【药物组成】 茯神、黄芪、芡实、党参、五味子、黄精、首乌、枸杞、玉竹,黑豆、紫河车,葡萄干,白术,丹参、熟地、菟丝子、莲子,山萸肉,炙草,山药、柏子仁,龙眼肉,生地、乌梅。共生药25味。均采用临床常规剂量。制药系参照近代加工方法,极尽古方制炙之能事,使药力疗效较平常丸散可大至五六倍之多。

【Composition】 Fushen (Poria with hostwood), Huangqi (Milkvetch root), Qianshi (Gordon euryale seed), Dangshen (Tangshen), Wuweizi (Chinese magnoliavine fruit),

Huangjing(Rhizome of king solomonseal), Shouwu(Fleece – flower root), Gouqi(Chinese wolfberry), Yuzhu (Fragrant solomonseal rhizome), black bean, Ziheche (Dried human placemta), raisin, Baizhu(Largehead atractylodes rhizome), Danshen(Red sage root), Shudi (Chinese foxglove), Tusizi(Dodder), lotus seed, Shanyu Rou(Pulp of dogwood fruit), Zhicao (Honey-fried licorice root), Shanyao(Common yam rhizome), Baiziren(Arborvitate seed), longan meet, Shengdi(Dried/fresh rehmannia root), Wumei(Dark plum fruit), all together 25 drugs. Take clinical usual dose. Process the drugs according to modern methods and use as much ancient processing ideas as possible, to promote its effect 5 ~ 6 times as effective as the common drugs.

【功效】　疏通经络,补益脏腑。

【Efficacy】　Dredging meridians,tonifying viscera.

【适应证】　一般人均可服用。药方虽简化,功效甚宏,贵在久服,则可愈身远之病。

【Indication】　Being available for everyone. Simple formula with good effects can keep healthy.

神仙不老丸
Shenxian Bulao Wan
Immortal Gods Pill

【方剂出处】　《寿亲养老新书》

【Source of Prescription】　Shouqin Yanglao Xin Shu The New Book for Prolonging Parent'S Life and Nourishing the Eldly.

【药物组成】　人参须,酒炒菟丝子、全当归各60 g,枸杞子、柏子仁、石菖蒲、地骨皮、熟地黄、生地、巴戟天各30 g,川牛膝、杜仲各45 g。上药用慢火焙干,共研极细末,炼蜜为丸,如梧桐子大。每日空腹服10 g,温酒盐汤任下。

【Composition】　60 g Renshen Xu(Ginseng), 60 g wine – fried Tusizi(Dodder), 60 g Quan Danggui(Chinese angelica), 30 g Gouqizi(Chinese wolfberry fruit), 30 g Baiziren (Arborvitate seed), 30 g Shi Changpu(Grassleaf sweelflag rhizome), 30 g Digupi(Wofberry bark), 30 g Shu Dihuang(Prepared rehmannia root), 30 g Shengdi(Dried/fresh rehmannia root), 30 g Bajitian(Morinda root), 45 g Chuan Niuxi(Achyranthes root), 45 g Duzhong(Bark of eucommia). Bake these drugs to dry with slow fire, grinded into fine powder, mixed with honey to get pills as the size of Wutong Zi(Phoenix tree seed). Take 10 g with warm wine or salt water. Take with empty stomach.

【功效】　益气养阴,乌须黑发。

【Efficacy】　Supplementing qi and nourishing yin,blackening beard and hair.

【适应证】　本方药性平和,一般人均可服用。

【Indication】　Mild nature for everyone.

神仙五子丸
Shenxian WuziWan
The Gods Five Sons Pill

【方剂出处】 《烟霞圣效方》

【Source of Prescription】 Yanxia Shengxiao Fang; Magic Prescriptions On The Earth

【药物组成】 覆盆子,五味子,醋炒蛇床子、酒炒菟丝子、巴戟天、白茯苓,川断、酒炒肉苁蓉,酒炒牛膝、枸杞子、山药,熟地,肉桂、槟榔、熟附片,麸炒枳实、炮姜各 30 g。上药共为极细末。炼蜜为丸,如桐子大。每服 30 丸,一日 2 次,空腹温酒送服。

【Composition】 30 g Fupenzi(Korean raspberry),30 g Wuweizi(Chinese magnoliavine fruit),30 g vinegar-fried Shengchuang Zi(Cnidium seed),30 g wine-fried Tusizi(Dodder), 30 g Bajitian(Morinda root),30 g Bai Fuling(Tuckahoe),Chuanduan(Dipsacus root),30 g wine-fried Roucongrong(Cistanche),30 g wine-fried Nuixi(Achyranthes root),30 g Gouqizi (Chinese wolfberry),30 g Shanyao(Common yam rhizome),30 g Shudi(Chinese foxglove),30 g Rougui(Cassia bark),30 g Areca seeds,30 g Shu Fupian(Prepared monkshood),30 g bran-fried Zhishi(Immature orange fruit);30 g baked ginger. Grind these drugs into fine power, mixed with honey to make pill,as the shape of Wutong Zi(Phoenix tree seed). Take 30 pills a dose,twice a day. Take with warm wine with empty stomach.

【功效】 温肾助阳,生精益髓。

【Efficacy】 Warming kidney and activating yang,generating essence and benefiting marrow.

【适应证】 老年肾阳不足,气阴两亏,腰膝冷痛,下肢无力,食少纳呆,须发早白者。

【Indication】 Symptoms of the aged such as deficiency of kidney yang, qi and yin deficiency,cold pain of waist and knees,weakness of lower limbs,poor appetite and anorexia, and early-white of beard and hair.

益气聪明丸
Yiqi Congming Wan
Qi-benefiting and Smart Pill

【方剂出处】 《证治准绳》

【Source of Prescription】 Zhengzhi Zhunsheng; Standards for Diagnosis and Treatment

【药物组成】 党参、黄芪各 100 克,升麻 550 克,葛根 225 克,蔓荆子 11.2 克,白芍药,酒炒川柏各 75 克,炙甘草 12 克。上药共研极细末,炼蜜为丸,如梧桐子大。每服 10 克,一日 2 次,白开水送下。

【Composition】 100 g Dangshen(Tangshen),100 g Huangqi(Milkvetch root),550 g Shengma(Cimicifuga rhizome),225 g Gegen(Kudzuvine root),11.2 g Manjing Zi(Chastetree fruit), 75 g Baisao jiu (White paeony root wine), 75 g parched Chuanbai (Sichuan phellodendron),12 g honey-fried Gancao(Liquorice root). Grind these drugs into fine powder, mix with honey to make pill as the shape of Wutong Zi(Phoenix tree seed). Take 10 one dose, twice a day with boiled water.

【功效】 补中益气,明目健脑。

【Efficacy】 Tonifying the middle energizer and benefiting qi,improving eyesight and intelligence or wisdom.

【适应证】 脑动脉硬化症患者出现的中气不足,如眩晕,耳鸣,头痛、头重等症。本丸久服,其效尤著。

【Indication】 Insufficiency of middle-energizer qi of those with cerebral arteriosclerosis such as dizziness,tinnitus,headache,heaviness of head etc.

容颜不老丹
Rongyan Bulao Dan
Agerasia Pill

【方剂出处】 《奇效良方》

【Source of Prescription】 Qixiao Liangfang;Miraculous and Effective Prescription

【药物组成】 生姜50 g,大枣25 g,白盐6 g,甘草9 g,丁香、沉香各5 g,茴香12 g。上药共切碎,加水煎取药汁。每日两剂,早上空腹时服用。

【Composition】 50 g Ginger,25 g Jujube,6 g salt,9 g Gancao(Liquorice root),5 g clove,5 g Chenxiang(Agalloch eaglewood),12 g fennel. Cut up these drugs and dedoct with water to take the juice. Take 5 doses a day,take with empty stomach in the morning.

【功效】 温补脾肾,扶正固本。

【Efficacy】 Pryetic tonification of spleen and kidney,support healthy qi.

【适应证】 中老年人脾肾阳虚,形寒喜暖,腰膝酸痛,精力衰减,食少便溏者。

【Indication】 Symptoms of the middle-aged and the old such as spleen-kidney yang deficiency,cold body favoring warmth,aching pain in waist and knees,decrease of spirit and power,poor eating and loose stool.

决明子茶
Jueming ZiCha
Cassia Seed Tea

【方剂出处】 《全国中草药汇编》

【Source of Prescription】 Quanguo Zhongcaoyao Huibian;National Chinese Medical Herb Collection

【药物组成】 决明子15 g,夏枯草9 g。将决明子炒至稍鼓起,微有香气,放凉,打碎,或研成粗末。夏枯草切碎。每日1剂,冲白开水当茶饮。

【Composition】 15 g Juemingzi(Cassia seed),9 g Xiakucao(Self heal). Stir-fry cassia seed until bulge slightly and emit a slight aroma,let cool,shatter or grind into coarse powder. Shredding self heal. One dose a day. Take with boiled water as tea.

【功效】 清肝明目,润肠通便。

【Efficacy】 Clearing liver and improving eyesight, loosening bowel to relieve constipation.

【适应证】 适用于高脂血症,高血压患者,可作为保健药茶长期服用。

【Indication】 Hyperlipemia, high blood pressure, being as health-protective drink.

还童茶
Huantong Cha
Rejuvenation Tea

【方剂出处】 《药茶与药露》

【Source of Prescription】 Yaocha Yu Yaolu; Herb Tea and Distilled Herb water

【药物组成】 槐角1000 g。每年秋季,采摘果实,除去枝梗,果柄,挑选饱满壮实之荚果作为原料。然后用热水迅速淘洗去土,常温晾干,以表面无水为宜。再将槐果均匀地铺于铁丝筛上,烘烤至深黄色,然后再上蒸笼,以水蒸气蒸至发黑亮时出锅,再烘干至棕红色,除尽水分。最后将槐果豆荚轧破,将其内黑色种子脱去。取干燥之果皮轧碎,过筛,分装,每袋10克。每次3 g,一日2次,白开水冲茶,时时饮服。本品可连泡2次,颜色以棕红色至浅黄色为宜。

【Composition】 1000 g Huaijiao (Sophora fruit). Every fall, Pick fresh and fat fruit, remove the branches and stems, washed with hot water to remove the soil, dried at room temperature until no water on the surface. Then spread sophora fruit evenly on wire sieve, baking into deep yellow color, and then put in the steamer. Steam until the steam water turn to black, and then parched to reddish brown, wipe out the water. Break their pod and get rid of the black seed. Take the dry peel, get crushed, screened and packed in bags of 10 grams. Take 3 g a dose, 2 times a day. Take after mixed with boiled water and take constantly. It can be mixed twice with water until the color turns brown-red to light yellow.

【功效】 益肾明目荣发。

【Efficacy】 Benefiting kidney, improving eyesight and improving luster of hair.

【适应证】 适用于老年性血管硬化,冠心病,高血压,痔漏出血等。

【Indication】 Symptoms of the old as sclerosis of blood vessels, coronary heart disease, high blood pressure and anus fistula with bleeding.

铁笛膏
Tiedi gao
Iron FluteOintment

【方剂出处】 《古今医方集成》

【Source of Prescription】 Gujin Yifang Jicheng

【药物组成】 苏薄荷120 g,甘草、百药煎、桔梗各60 g,川芎,连翘各75 g,诃子肉、砂仁、大黄各30 g。上药共研粗末,加水共煎3次,分次过滤,去渣,合并滤液,用小火煎熬，浓缩至膏状，加炼蜜 240 g 收膏，瓷瓶收贮。每服 9 g，含化，或白开水送下，一日 3 次。

【Composition】　120 g Su mint,60 g Gancao(Liquorice root),60 g Baiyao Jian(Chinese gall leaven),60 g Jiegeng(Platycodon root),75 g Chuanxiong(Sichuan lovage rhizome),75 g Lianqiao(Weeping forsythia capsule),30 g Hezirou(Myrobalan fruit),30 g Sharen(Amomum fruit),30 g Dahuang(Rhubarb root). Grind these drugs into coarse powder. boil three times with water,filter and remove the dregs,then combined the filtrate,decoct with slow fire to get ointment,add 240 g refining honey to extract the ointment,Install in porcelain bottles. Take 9 g once,or with warm water,three times a day.

【功效】　清肺利咽。

【Efficacy】　Clearing lung and relieving sore-throat.

【适应证】　年老体弱，肺虚内热，喉痛声哑，口燥咽干，或语言过多，呼叫耗伤所致失音声哑，也可作为慢性歌喉疾患的保健佳品。

【Indication】　Physical weakness of the old,lung deficiency with internal heat,laryngalgia and hoarseness,dry mouth and pharynx,or aphonia and hoarseness due to pyperphasia and shouting,being good choice of singers with chronic throat diseases.

蒲公英丸
Pugong Ying Wan
Dandelion Pill

【方剂出处】　《延龄纂要》

【Source of Prescription】　Yangling Zuanyao;Age-delaying Prescriptions Compilation

【药物组成】　蒲公英 500 克，香附 15 克，青盐 10 克。取蒲公英连根带叶，洗净，加香附，共研极细末，加青盐和匀为丸。每服 15 克，一日 3；次，白开水送下。

【Composition】　500 g of Pugongying(Dandelion),15 g Xiangfu(Nutgrass falingale rhizome),10 g halite. Take dandelion roots,leaves and get washed. Grind with nutgrass falingale rhizome into fine powder,mix with halite for the pills. Take 15 g per dose,3 times a day with warm water

【功效】　乌须黑发，健骨强筋。

【Efficacy】　Blackening beard and hair,strengthening bones and tendons.

【适应证】　适用于免疫力低下者。

【Indication】　Hypoimmunity.

神仙服百花方
Shenxian Fu Baihua Fang
Flowers Prescription for Gods

【方剂出处】　《太平圣惠方》

【Source of Prescription】　Taiping Shenghui Fang;Taiping Holy Prescriptions for Universal Relief

【药物组成】　桃花、蒺藜花、甘菊花、枸杞叶、枸杞花、枸杞子、枸杞根各等分。上药共阴干,研极细粉末。每服 10 g,一日 3 次,用白开水调服。

【Composition】　Peach flower,Baijili Hua(Tribulus flower),Ganju hua(Chrysanthemum flower),Gouqi Ye(Chinese wolfberry leaf),Gouqi Hua(Chinese wolfberry flower),Gouqi Zi(Chinese wolfberry fruit),Gouqi Gen(Chinese wolfberry root)with the same amount. Get the drugs dried in the shade and grind into fine powder. Take 10 g Per dose,3 times a day. Mix with warm water.

【功效】　养血活血,润肤耐老。

【Efficacy】　Nourishing blood and promoting blood circulation,moistening skin and resisting aging.

【适应证】　一般人可服用,尤适用于免疫力低下者。

【Indication】　Being available for everyone,especially for those with hypoimmunity.

逡巡酒
Qunxun Jiu
Instant Wine

【方剂出处】　《本草纲目》

【Source of Prescription】　Bencao Gangmu;Compendium of Materia Medica

【药物组成】　桃花50 g,马兰花82 g,芝麻花100 g,黄菊花工50 g,光桃仁6 g,米酒5 kg。将上药共研粗末,置瓷坛中,加酒浸泡,浸 10 天后服。每服 30 mL,一日 2 次。

【Composition】　50 g Peach flower,82 g Malan Hua(Flagger flower),100 g sesame flower,50 g yellow chrysanthemums flower,6 g walnuts,5kg rice wine. Grind these drugs into coarse powder, installed in porcelain altar, soaked in wine, take 10 days later. Take 30 mL once,2 times a day.

【功效】　补虚益气,活血祛风。

【Efficacy】　Improving asthenia and benefiting qi, activating blood circulation and dispelling wind.

【适应证】　适用于年老体弱,头昏目眩,肢节酸痛,关节屈伸不利,大便干结等症。久服益寿耐老,青春常驻。

【Indication】　Being available for the the old with weak body, dizziness, arthralgia of limbs,inflexibility of joints,dry stool,resisting aging with long-term doses.

九节菖蒲茶
Jiujie Changpu Cha
Rhizoma Anemones Altaicae Tea

【方剂出处】　《药茶与药露》

【Source of Prescription】　Yaocha Yu Yaolu;Herb Tea and Distilled Herb water

【药物组成】　九节菖蒲 1.5 g,酸梅肉 2 个,大枣肉 2 个,赤砂糖适量。先将菖蒲切片,放茶杯内,再把大枣、酸梅肉、赤砂糖一齐放入水内煮沸,再倒入茶杯内,盖紧,15 min 后服,每日 1 剂。

【Composition】 1.5 g Jiujie Changpu(Rhizoma anemones altaicae),2 pieces of plum meat,2 pieces of jujube meat,proper amount of brown sugar. Slice the rhizoma anemones altaicae,then put jujube,plum meat,brown sugar together into the water to boil,then pour in the cup and fasten the lid. Take after 15 minutes. Take one dose a day.

【功效】 健脾化痰。

【Efficacy】 Strengthening spleen and dissolving phlegm.

【适应证】 适用于年老体弱,脾虚食少,身倦肢乏,纳谷不香,夜寐不安者。

【Indication】 Being available for the old with weak body,poor eating due to deficiency of spleen,weakness of body and limbs,poor appetite and restless sleep.

三山丸
San Shan Wan
San Shan Pill

【方剂出处】 《奇效良方》

【Source of Prescription】 Qixiao Liangfang;Miraculous and Effective Prescription

【药物组成】 苍术、香附各 60 g,何首乌、小茴香,炒川椒、川楝子、煅牡蛎,炮姜各 30 g。先将苍术用米泔水浸一宿,再用清水洗净,晒干。上药共为细末,酒煮面糊为丸,如梧桐子大。每服 30 丸,一日 2 次,空腹用淡盐汤送下。

【Composition】 60 g Cangzhu(Atractylodes rhizome),60 g Xiangfu(Nutgrass falingale rhizome),30 g Heshouwu(Fleece-flower root),30 g fennel,30 g fried Sichuan pepper,30 g Chuanlianzi(Sichuan toosendan fruit), 30 g calcined oyster, 30 g baked ginger. Soak atractylodes rhizome with rice-washed water for a night,get washed and dried in sunlight. Grind these drugs into fine powder,boil with wine to form pills as the size of Wutong Zi(Phoenix tree seed). Take 30 pills one dose twice a day. Take with light salt water with empty stomach.

【功效】 健脾化痰,温肾壮阳。

【Efficacy】 Invigorating spleen to remove phlegm,warming kidney to invigorate yang.

【适应证】 痰湿体质者。

【Indication】 Being available for those with phlegmatic dampness.

三花减肥茶
Sanhua Jianfei Cha
Three Flowers dietic tea

【方剂出处】 《中成药研究》

【Source of Prescription】 Zhongchengyao Yanjiu;Chinese Patent Drugs Research

【药物组成】 玫瑰花,茉莉花,玫瑰花、川芎、荷叶各 30 克。共研细末。每次 6 克,每天 1 次,放置茶杯内,用白开水冲泡,不要放在保温杯内,时时饮服。

【Composition】 30 g Roses, jasmine, 30 g Daidai Hua (Sour orange flower), 30 g Chuanxiong(Sichuan lovage rhizome), 30 g lotus leaf. Mix them together and grind into fine powder. Take 6 g a day. Brewed with hot water in the cup and take constantly, do not put in vacuum cup.

【功效】 宽胸利气,祛痰逐饮,利水消肿,活血养胃,降脂提神。理想的减肥保健饮料。

【Efficacy】 Loosening chest and making qi moving downward, expelling phlegm stagnation, inducing diuresis to alleviate edema, activating blood circulation and nourishing stomach, reducing fat for refreshment, being ideal drink to lose weight.

【适应证】 肥人多痰湿者。

【Indication】 Being available for the fat with phlegmatic dampness.

长生丹
Changsheng Dan
Life–Prolonging Pill

【方剂出处】 《老年病》

【Source of Prescription】 Laonian Bing, Disease of Old People

【药物组成】 大附子15克,清半夏30克。取大附子用清水漂洗,每日换水2～3次,浸3～5天,去皮尖,用铜刀切,日晒干。再取生半夏以水泡浸至无麻辣味为度,搅拌搓去外皮,晾干,切片。上二味药,在石臼中共捣为细末,用生面粉60克、生姜自然汁适量,和匀,制丸如芡实大,阴干,日日转动。每服6丸,一日2次,空腹服,白开水或黄酒送下。

【Composition】 15 g Da Fuzi (Aconite), 30 g Qing Banxia (Pinellia tuber). Rinse aconite with water, renew the water 2～3 times, soak 3～5 days, remove the peel and tips with copper knife, get dried in sunlight. Steep pinellia tuber in water until no spicy and hot taste in it. Stir and remove the covering. Dry in sunlight and sliced. Grind the 2 drugs into superfine powder. Mix 60 g flour with proper amount of ginger juice evenly. Make pills as the size of Qianshi(Gordon euryale seed), dry in the shade and roll them day by day. Take 6 pills once, twice a day with empty stomach. Swallow with boiled water or yellow wine.

【功效】 温补脾气。

【Efficacy】 Warming and tonifying spleen qi.

【适应证】 中老年人阴寒内盛,四肢冰凉,身体衰弱,胸腹冷痛者。

【Indication】 Being available for the middle aged and the old with internally vigorous cold pathogen, cold limbs, weak body and cold pain in chest and abdomen.

长生神鼎玉液膏
Changsheng Shending Yuye Gao
Longevity Sacred Vessal and Precious Beverages Ointment

【方剂出处】　《遵生八笺》

【Source of Prescription】　Zunsheng Bajian;Eight Commentaries on Regimen

【药物组成】　白术 1kg,苍术 500 g。二药同用土炒令色黄,然后用木石臼捣碎入缸中,用清水浸 24 h,次入砂锅煎汁,过滤取汁,药淹加水再煎,绢滤取汁,药汁合并,用桑柴火缓缓熬炼成膏,瓷瓶收贮。每服 10 g,一日 2 次,白开水冲服。

【Composition】　1kg Baizhu (Largehead atractylodes rhizome), 500 g Cangzhu (Atractylodes rhizome). Stir-bake these drugs with earth until get yellow. Grind them in wood/stone mortar, soak in water for 24 hours, boil in earthen pot and get the juice. Water down the drugs and reboil, filter to get juice with cloth. Mix these juice together, decoct with mulberry firewood to get ointment. Gather in chinaware. Take 10 g once, twice a day. Swallow with boiled water.

【功效】　健脾化湿,开胃进食。

【Efficacy】　Invigorating spleen to eliminate dampness, promoting appetite.

【适应证】　年高体弱,饮食减少,易于感冒,咳嗽痰白,身倦肢乏,下肢水肿等症,久服可延缓衰老。

【Indication】　Symptoms of the old such as weak body, poor eating, being easy to catch cold, cough with white phlegm, fatigue and weakness of body and oedema legs; delaying aging with long-term doses.

长寿粉
Changshou Fen
Life-prolonging Powder

【方剂出处】　《串雅外编》

【Source of Prescription】　Chuanya Wai Bian;External Therapies of Folk Medicine

【药物组成】　芡实、苡仁,莲子各 250 g,山药 500 g,糯米 500 g,人参、茯苓各 90 g,白糖适量。上药共研极细末,每日调服 30 g。如不欲调服,以水打成丸如元宵服。一日 2 次。

【Composition】　250 g Qianshi(Gordon euryale seed),250 g Yiren(Coix seed),250 g lotus seed,500 g Shanyao(Common yam rhizome),500 g sticky rice,90 g ginseng,90 g Fuling (Tuckahoe),white sugar proper amount. Grind these drugs into superfine powder. Take 30 g once. Swallow after mix with water or make pills with water as the size of yuanxiao. Take twice a day.

【功效】　补脾益气,固肾涩精。

【Efficacy】　Invigorating the spleen and benefiting qi, strengthening kidney.

【适应证】 适用于老年人脾肾不足,身倦肢乏,自汗气短,腰酸齿落,妇女带多,食少便溏者。

【Indication】 Being available for the old with deficiency of spleen and kidney, fatigue and weakness of body, spontaneous perspiration, aching waist and falling of teeth, leukorrhagia, poor eating and loose stool.

玉芝徐老丸
Yuzhi Xulao Wan
Yuzhi Xu Lao Pill

【方剂出处】 《御药院方》

【Source of Prescription】 Yuyao Yuan Fang; The Imperial Medicine and Prescription

【药物组成】 天南星、干姜各 15 g,姜半夏、白矾、大黄各 30 g,细蛤粉 60 g,牵牛 18 g,黄柏 45 g。先取天南星以生姜片和匀煮透,至中心无白色星点为度,切片阴干。牵牛子研碎去皮不用。然后 1∶8 味药共研为极细粉末,水丸如绿豆大。每服土 2 丸,一日 2 次,温开水送下,饭后服。

【Composition】 15 g Tiannanxing (Jackinthepulpit tuber), dried ginger each, 30 g Jiang Banxia (Pinellia tuber), white alum, Dahuang (Rhubarb root) each, 60 g Xihafen (Fine clamshell powder) each, 18 g Qianniu (Morning glory seed) each, 45 g Huangbai (Amur corktree bark) each. Mix jackinthepulpit tuber with ginger splices and boil them until no white spots on jackinthepulpit tuber. Slice and dry it in the shade. Peel and grind morning glory seed. Then put these two drugs as 1∶8 and grind them into superfine powder. Make pills as the size of mung bean. Take 2 pills once, twice a day. Swallow with warm water after meals.

【功效】 化痰消食,顺气调血。

【Efficacy】 Dissipating phlegm and promoting digestion, guiding qi downward and regulating blood.

【适应证】 脾虚湿盛者。

【Indication】 Damp abundance due to splenic dampness.

交感丹
Jiaogan Dan
Jiaogan Pill

【方剂出处】 《寿亲养老新书》

【Source of Prescription】 Shouqin yanglao xin shu; The New Book for Prolonging Parent'S Life and Nourishing the Eldly

【药物组成】 茯神土 20 g,香附 500 g。茯神取肉厚实,松根小者为佳,香附取个大、色棕褐、质坚实、香气浓者为佳,用石碾碾去毛皮,置锅内用火炒至表面黄色即可。共为细末,炼蜜为丸,如梧桐子大。每服 5 g,一日 2 次,白开水送下。

【Composition】 20 g Fushen Tu (Poria with hostwood), 500 g Xiangfu (Nutgrass falingale rhizome). Choose poria with hostwood with thick meet and small pine stump, nutgrass falingale rhizome with big size, dark brown color, solid quality and intense fragrant. Remove their skin with stone roller; stir-fry them until their surface turns yellow. Grind these drugs into fine powder and mix refined honey to make pillers, as the size of Wutong Zi(Phoenix tree seed). Take with boiled water, 5 g once, twice a day.

【功效】 健脾化湿,舒郁安神。

【Efficacy】 Invigorating spleen to eliminate dampness, dispelling qi stagnation to calm nerves.

【适应证】 脾虚失眠者。

【Indication】 Insomnia due to spleen deficiency.

延年茯苓饮
Yannian Fuling Yin
Life-Prolonging Tuckahoe Decoction

【方剂出处】 《外台秘要》

【Source of Prescription】 Waitai Miyao;(Waitai Secret Prescriptions)

【药物组成】 茯苓、白术各90 g,党参、炒枳实各60 g,生姜120 g,陈皮45 g。上药共切碎,加水煎熬3次,合并煎液,浓缩。分3次服,每天1次。

【Composition】 90 g Fuling(Tuckahoe), Baizhu(Largehead atractylodes rhizome) each, 60 g Dangshen(Tangshen), fried Zhishi(Immature orange fruit) each, 120 g ginger, 45 g Chenpi(Dried tangerine peel). Cut up these drugs and get them boiled 3 times in water. Merge the juice and concentrate it. Take one third each time, one time a day.

【功效】 健脾化痰。

【Efficacy】 Invigorating spleen to remove phlegm.

【适应证】 适用于年高体虚,痰温素盛,胸闷咳嗽,痰浊粘腻,身倦肢乏,饮食减少,大便溏薄者调服。久服本方以化痰延年。

【Indication】 Weak body of the old, abundant phlegm, dyspnea and cough, turbid and sticking phlegm, fatigue and powerless body, poor eating, thin and loose stool, lengthening life span with long-term doses.

米莲散
Milian San
Sticky Rice and Lotus Seed Powder

【方剂出处】 《杂病源流犀烛》

【Source of Prescription】 Zabing Yuanliu Xi Zhu; Miscellaneous Diseases Origin Rhinoceros Candle

【药物组成】 糯米15 g,莲子肉10个。共为极细末,用米酒适量送服,每日1次。或以墨汁作丸服。

【Composition】 15 g sticky rice, 10 lotus seeds. Grind them into superfine powder. Take with rice wine, once a day; or mix with ink to make pills.

【功效】 益气安神。

【Efficacy】 Benefiting qi an calming nerves.

【适应证】 适用于年老体弱,脾气虚弱,湿阻中焦,纳少便溏,失眠等症。

【Indication】 Being available for weak body of the old, deficiency of spleen qi, damp blockage of middle energizer, poor eating and loose stool, and insomnia.

苍术膏
Cangzhu Gao
Atractylodes rhizome Ointment

【方剂出处】 《卫生杂兴方》

【Source of Prescription】 Weisheng Zaxing Fang; Health varied effective Prescriptions

【药物组成】 苍术 2000 g。取上药浸去粗皮,洗净晒干,碾成粗末,用米泔水浸一宿,洗净,以慢火煎熬,滤去渣,浓缩,加入适量炼蜜,同煎成膏。每服 15 g,一日 2 次,用白开水调服。

【Composition】 2000 g Cangzhu(Atractylodes rhizome) to remove the raw bark, wash and dry it in sunlight, grind it into coarse powder. Soak in rice-washed water for one night, wash and decoct with slow fire, strain its dregs and concentrate it. Mix with proper amount of refined honey and boil it into cream. Take 15 g once, twice a day. Take after mixed with boiled water.

【功效】 健脾化湿。

【Efficacy】 Invigorating spleen to eliminate dampness.

【适应证】 适用于中老年人食少纳呆,四肢无力,湿气身痛,口角流涎,脚趾湿气搔痒,每有良效。

【Indication】 Being available for the old with poor eating and anorexia, powerless limbs, painful body due to dampness, angular salivation, itching toes due to dampness.

扶老强中丸
Fulao Qiangzhong Wan
Eldly-helping and Stomach-strengthening Pill

【方剂出处】 《老年病》

【Source of Prescription】 Laonian Bingc; Disease of Old People

【药物组成】 吴茱萸、干姜各 120 g,麦芽 300 g,六神曲 600 g。上药共研极细末,炼蜜为丸,如梧桐子大,每服 40 丸,一日 2 次,白开水送下。

【Composition】 120 g Wu Zhuyu(Evodia fruit), 120 g dried ginger each, 300 g malt, 600 g Liu Shenqu(Medicated leaven). Grind all these drugs into superfine powder, mix refine honey with the power to make pills, as the size of Wutong Zi(Phoenix tree seed). Take 40 pills once, twice a day, swallow down with boiled water.

【功效】　温中助运。

【Efficacy】　Warming the middle energizer and promoting digestion.

【适应证】　适用于脾胃虚寒,食积停滞,胸脘痞满,腹胀时痛,嗳腐吞酸,饮食不化,身倦肢乏,大便溏薄者。

【Indication】　Spleen-stomach insufficiency-cold, food stagnation, fullness in chest and gastric cavity, distention and pain in abdomen, fetid eructation and acid regurgitation, poor digestion, fatigue body and weak limbs, and loose stool.

沉香永寿丸
Chenxiang Yongshou Wan
Agalloch Eaglewood Life-prolonging Pill

【方剂出处】　《奇效良方》

【Source of Prescription】　Qixiao Liangfang;　Miraculous and Effective Prescription

【药物组成】　莲肉、苍术各 500 g,白茯苓 20 g,沉香、熟地黄、木香各 30 g,五味子、小茴香、川楝子、枸杞子、山药、柏子仁、破故纸各 60 g,青盐 15 g。取莲肉先用酒浸一日,后装入雄猪肚内,缝合,却将莲肉添水煮熟,取出晒干,肚子不用。苍术分作四份,1 份酒浸,1 份泔水浸,1 份盐水浸,1 份醋浸,浸 5～10 d,焙干。然后,上药共研极细末,用酒煮糊和丸,如梧桐子大。每服 50 丸,加至 70 丸,一日 2 次,空腹用温酒或盐汤送下。

【Composition】　500 g lotus, 500 g Cangzhu (Atractylodes), 120 g Bai Fuling (Tuckahoe), 30 g Chenxiang (Agalloch eaglewood), 30 g Shu Dihuang (prepared rehmannia root) 30 g Muxiang (Common aucklandia root), 60 g Wuweizi (Chinese magnoliavine fruit), 60 g fennel, 60 g Chuan Dongzi (Fructus meliae toosendan), 60 g Gouqizi (Chinese wolfberry fruit), 60 g Shanyao (Common yam rhizome), 60 g Baiziren (Arborvitate seed), 60 g Poguzhi (Psoralea), 15 g Qingyan (Halite). Steep the lotus in wine for a day; put and stitch it into male pig tripe. Boil the lotus and take it out and get dried in sunlight, abandon the tripe. Divide the atractylodes into four parts, steep one part in wine, one in slop, one in salt water, and one in vinegar for 5～10 days, and then bake them to dry. Grind all these drugs into superfine powder, boil them with wine into brei, and make them into pills as the size of Wutong Zi (Phoenix tree seed). Take 50～70 pills once, twice a day on an empty stomach with warm wine or salt soup.

【功效】　补脾化痰,滋养气血,补肾理气,填补精髓。

【Efficacy】　Invigorating the spleen and dissolving phlegm, nourishing qi and blood, tonifying kidney and regulating qi, replenishing essence and marrow.

【适应证】　中老年脾肾虚弱者。

【Indication】　Deficiency of the spleen and kidney of the old.

茯苓面
Fuling Mian
Tuckahoe Flour

【方剂出处】 《老年病》

【Source of Prescription】 Laonian Bingc；Disease of Old People

【药物组成】 茯苓、蜂蜜各 300 g。茯苓研为极细末，加蜂蜜合为面。每服 15 g，一日 2 次，温开水送服。

【Composition】 300 g Fuling（Tuckahoe），300 g honey. Grind tuchahoe into superfine powder；mix it with honey to make flour. Take twice a day with warm water，15 g once.

【功效】 健脾补中，利水渗湿。

【Efficacy】 Strengthening spleen and tonifying the middle energizer，removing dampness and promoting diuresis.

【适应证】 免疫力低下者。

【Indication】 Hypoimmunity.

三仁粥
Sanren Zhou
Three Kernels Porridge

【方剂出处】 《杂病源流犀烛》

【Source of Prescription】 Za Bing Yuan Liu Xi Zhu；Miscellaneous Diseases Origin Rhinoceros Candle

【药物组成】 桃仁、海松子仁各 4 g，郁李仁 3 g。先把桃仁置沸水锅中煮至外皮微皱，捞出，浸入凉水中，去皮。取郁李仁去杂质，淘净，然后研碎。以上 3 味药加水共研取汁，加粳米 100 g，煮粥。每日 1 剂。

【Composition】 4 g Taoren（Peach kernel），4 g Korean pine seed，3 g brush-cherry seed. Put peach kernels into boiling water，fish out and put into cool water until their husk start to winkle，peel them. Remove the impurity in brush-cherry seed，wash and grind them. Grind these 3 drugs together with water and take out their juice. Boil them with 100 g nonglutinous rice. Take 1 dose a day.

【功效】 润肠通便。

【Efficacy】 Loosening bowel to relieve constipation.

【适应证】 适用于年老体弱，津亏血少，肠燥便秘者。

【Indication】 Being available for the old with weak body，deficiency of body fluid and blood，constipation due to dryness of the intestine.

山楂酒
Shanzha Jiu
Hawthorn Wine

【方剂出处】 《药酒与膏滋》

【Source of Prescription】 Yaojiu Yu Gaozi; Medicated Wine and Soft Extract

【药物组成】 山楂、桂圆肉各 250 g,红枣、红糖各 30 g。前 3 味;去核,研成泥,加米酒 1000 g,浸 10 d 后服用。每服 50 mL,一日 2 次。

【Composition】 250 g Hawthorn, 250 g longan pulp, 30 g red jujube, 30 g brown sugar. Stone and grind the first 3 drugs into mud, soaked in rice wine 1000 g for 10 days. Take twice a day, 50 mL once.

【功效】 消食散瘀,补益气血。

【Efficacy】 Promoting digestion and eliminating stasis to activate blood circulation, tonifying qi and blood.

【适应证】 适用于年老体弱,头晕目眩,颈部转动不利,腰背酸痛,脘腹胀闷,肉食积滞,血脂偏高者长期服用。

【Indication】 Being available for the old with weak body, dizziness, inflexible neck, aching pain of waist and back, distention and depression of gastric cavity and abdomen, meat stagnation, and high blood fat.

杏仁煎
Xingren Jian
Apricot Kernel Decoction

【方剂出处】 《杨氏家藏方》

【Source of Prescription】 Yang's Jia Cang Fang; Yang's Prescription Collection

【药物组成】 甜杏仁 100 克,胡桃肉 200 克。将杏仁去皮尖,微炒,胡桃肉去皮。上 2 味药加入生蜜少许,同研细,制成小丸,每丸重 3 克。每晚临卧前服 1 丸,细嚼和津液顿咽,久服效佳。

【Composition】 100 g sweet apricot kernel, 200 g walnut meet. Peel the apricot kernel, get rid of the bud and parch with a slow fire, peel the walnut meet. Grind these 2 drugs with a little raw honey and make them into pills, 3 g each pill. Take 1 pill every night before bedtime by nibbling and swallowing it down with saliva. Long term usage is recommended.

【功效】 消食行滞,令人聪明。

【Efficacy】 Promoting digestion and removing food stagnation, promoting intelligence or wisdom.

【适应证】 适用于老年津液亏虚,纳少便秘,咳嗽气喘者服用。

【Indication】 Being available for the old with deficiency and consumption of bold fluid, poor eating and constipation, cough and asthma.

活血通络方保健汤
Health-care Soup of Blood Circulation
Promoting and Meridian Obstruction Removing

【方剂出处】 《浙江中医杂志》

【Source of Prescription】 Zhejiang Zhongyi Zazhi; Zhejiang Journal of Traditional Chinese Medicine

【药物组成】 紫丹参,制首乌,北沙参各 15 g。加水煎成 800 ml,作为一天饮料,分次饮用。

【Composition】15 g Zi Danshen (Red sage root), 15 g prepared Shouwu (Fleece-flower root), 15 g Bei Shashen (Coastal glehnia root), decoct these drugs with water into 300 ml. Take several times a day as a daily doze.

【功效】 活血安神。

【Efficacy】 Activating blood circulation and calming nerves.

【适应证】 心血管系统失常、脂质代谢紊乱者。

【Indication】 Abnormal cardiovascular system, metabolic disorder of lipide.